AF904102

Encyclopedia of Veterinary Science

Volume I

Encyclopedia of Veterinary Science
Volume I

Edited by **Mel Roth**

hayle medical

New York

Published by Hayle Medical,
30 West, 37th Street, Suite 612,
New York, NY 10018, USA
www.haylemedical.com

Encyclopedia of Veterinary Science: Volume I
Edited by Mel Roth

© 2015 Hayle Medical

International Standard Book Number: 978-1-63241-210-2 (Hardback)

This book contains information obtained from authentic and highly regarded sources. Copyright for all individual chapters remain with the respective authors as indicated. A wide variety of references are listed. Permission and sources are indicated; for detailed attributions, please refer to the permissions page. Reasonable efforts have been made to publish reliable data and information, but the authors, editors and publisher cannot assume any responsibility for the validity of all materials or the consequences of their use.

The publisher's policy is to use permanent paper from mills that operate a sustainable forestry policy. Furthermore, the publisher ensures that the text paper and cover boards used have met acceptable environmental accreditation standards.

Trademark Notice: Registered trademark of products or corporate names are used only for explanation and identification without intent to infringe.

Printed in the United States of America.

Contents

Preface

Veterinary science is a discipline of medical science which studies about the prevention, diagnosis, and treatments of diseases, disorders, and different types of injuries in animals. This field has a wide scope, as all the animals including land animals, birds, aquatic animals, and sometimes insects as well are included in the list, irrespective of whether they are wild or domestic. Veterinary science is practiced all over the globe. However, from professionals to humans with very basic knowledge, all are involved in the treatment and healthcare of animals. Veterinary science is also very helpful in human healthcare as many diseases, especially zoonotic diseases - which are infectious diseases, that are transmitted to humans by animals. Sometimes veterinary sciences are combined with epidemiology to find better solutions for both human healthcare and animal healthcare.

If we turn the pages of history all over the world, the first written records of veterinary medicine can be traced to Vedic literature in ancient India and the Egyptian Papyrus of Kahun. In earlier days, veterinary sciences were mainly focused on the care and treatment of horses due to their extreme economic significance. It was finally in the year 1762 in France, that Veterinary Science established itself as an academic discipline, by laying the foundation of the first veterinary college by Claude Bourgelat.

The topics discussed in this book cover various aspects of animal healthcare. I especially wish to acknowledge the contributing authors, without whom a work of this magnitude would clearly not have been realizable. I thank all the authors for allocating their scarce time to this project. I hope that this book proves to be a resourceful guide for both basic and advanced concepts in veterinary science. I do believe that the contents in this book will be helpful to many researchers in this field around the world.

Editor

1

Colistin Resistance in *Escherichia coli* and *Salmonella enterica* Strains Isolated from Swine in Brazil

Adriano Savoia Morales,[1] Juliana Fragoso de Araújo,[1] Vasco Túlio de Moura Gomes,[1] Adrienny Trindade Reis Costa,[2] Dália dos Prazeres Rodrigues,[3] Thais Sebastiana Porfida Ferreira,[1] Pedro Henrique Nogueira de Lima Filsner,[1] Maria Roberta Felizardo,[1] and Andrea Micke Moreno[1]

[1] *Laboratório de Sanidade Suína e Virologia, Faculdade de Medicina Veterinária e Zootecnia (FMVZ), Universidade de São Paulo (USP), 05508 270 São Paulo, SP, Brazil*
[2] *Instituto de Pesquisas Veterinárias Especializadas-IPEVE, Rua Esmeralda, 786, 304111-191 Belo Horizonte, MG, Brazil*
[3] *Laboratório de Enterobactérias, FIOCRUZ, Avenida Brasil, 4365, Pavilhão Rocha Lima, 3° andar, Manguinhos, 21040-360 Rio de Janeiro, RJ, Brazil*

Correspondence should be addressed to Andrea Micke Moreno, morenoam@usp.br

Academic Editors: L. L. Barton and G. C. Ulett

Reports about acquired resistance to colistin in different bacteria species are increasing, including *E. coli* of animal origin, but reports of resistance in wild *S. enterica* of different serotypes from swine are not found in the literature. Results obtained with one hundred and twenty-six *E. coli* strains from diseased swine and one hundred and twenty-four *S. enterica* strains from diseased and carrier swine showed a frequency of 6.3% and 21% of colistin-resistant strains, respectively. When comparing the disk diffusion test with the agar dilution test to evaluate the strains, it was confirmed that the disk diffusion test is not recommended to evaluate colistin resistance as described previously. The colistin MIC 90 and MIC 50 values obtained to *E. coli* were 0.25 μg/mL and 0.5 μg/mL, the MIC 90 and MIC 50 to *S. enterica* were 1 μg/mL and 8 μg/mL. Considering the importance of colistin in control of nosocomial human infections with Gram-negative multiresistant bacteria, and the large use of this drug in animal production, the colistin resistance prevalence in enterobacteriaceae of animal origin must be monitored more closely.

1. Introduction

Polymyxyns are a group of polypeptide antibiotics positively charged that derive from various species of *Paenibacillus (Bacillus) polymyxa*. Out of five polimixyns originally described, two have been used in the clinical setting, polimixyn B and polymyxyn E, also known as colistin [1].

Colistin was discovered in 1949 and was later cautiously used clinically because of reported high incidence of nephrotoxicity and neurotoxicity. There are two forms of colistin commercially available: colistin sulfate for oral and topical use and colistimethate sodium for parenteral use; both can be delivered by inhalation, but colistin sulfate, and not colistimethate sodium, should be used for susceptibility testing [2, 3].

Human Infections caused by multiresistant Gram-negative bacteria such as *Pseudomonas aeruginosa, Acinetobacter baumannii* and *Klebsiella pneumoniae* are increasing worldwide. In these cases, colistin has been attracting great interest because of its significant activity against these agents and low resistance rates to it [2].

In veterinary medicine, colistin sulfate is mainly used in oral preparations, due to its excellent activity against *Escherichia coli* and *Salmonella enterica*, low frequency of resistance, and poor absorption after oral administration, especially in pigs and poultry production, although in the last few years the *E. coli* resistant to colistin is becoming more common [4]. Mechanisms of acquired colistin resistance have been described in different Gram-negative bacteria, and, more extensively, in *A. baumannii* and *Salmonella* Typhimurium [1, 5].

The disk diffusion test that is largely used in veterinary laboratories does not seem to be a reliable method for detection of colistin resistance. A previous study [4] describes the use of a disk prediffusion method as a rapid test to determine susceptibility of pig *E. coli* isolates in Belgium, but occurrence of colistin resistance in *Salmonella enterica* strains from swine have not been described yet. In Brazil, there are no reports of colistin resistance in *E. coli* and *Salmonella enterica* of animal origin. The objective of this study is to evaluate colistin resistance in *E. coli* and *Salmonella enterica* isolated from pigs from commercial swine herds in Brazil.

2. Material and Methods

2.1. Collecting and Isolating Strains. One hundred and twenty-six *E. coli* strains isolated from pigs presenting either postweaning diarrhea or oedema disease were selected from ten different Brazilian swine herds. One hundred and twenty-four *Salmonella enterica* subspecies enterica strains were isolated from pigs presenting enterocolitis (45/124) from nine swine herds. Carcasses, feces, and lymph nodes of healthy pigs were examined at four Brazilian slaughterhouses representing eight different swine herds (79/124). There was no correlation between the properties or animals where the strains of *E. coli* and Salmonella enterica were isolated.

For *E. coli* isolation, feces and gut samples were inoculated on Columbia agar (Difco-BBL, Detroit, MIUSA) supplemented with 5% sheep blood and MacConkey Agar (Difco-BBL, Detroit, MI/USA), incubated for 24 h at 37°C.

S. enterica isolation protocol consisted in inoculation of feces, mesenteric lymph nodes, and carcass swabs into 100 mL of tetrathionate broth (Difco-BBL, Detroit, MI/USA) and incubation at 37°C for 48 h, subculturing 10 μL of the tetrathionate broth into 10 mL Rappaport Vassiliadis (RV) broth (Difco-BBL, Detroit, MI/USA) and incubation at 37°C for 24 h, then inoculating xylose-lysine-tergitol-4 (XLT4) agar plates with 10 μL of the RV broth, and incubation for 24 h at 37°C [6]. The isolates were identified as *E. coli* or *S. enterica* by colony morphology and standard biochemical methods [7].

2.2. Characterization of Strains. Isolates identified as *E. coli* were characterized using polymerase chain reaction (PCR) as previously described [8]. For this study one hundred and twenty-six ETEC strains positive to one or more virulence genes related to postweaning diarrhea or oedema disease as F18 and F4 fimbria and heat-labile LT, heat-stable STa, and Stx2e toxins were selected (data not shown).

Isolates identified as *S. enterica* through biochemical tests were submitted to serotyping with antigenic characterization based on the Kauffmann-White [9] at Fundação Instituto Oswaldo Cruz (Fiocruz, Rio de Janeiro).

2.3. Colistin Susceptibility Tests. Antimicrobial sensitivity testing was carried out using two different techniques: the agar dilution method [10] and the Kirby Bauer disk diffusion test (Oxoid Ltd., Cambridge/UK). Colistin sulfate powder was obtained from Sigma Chemical (St. Louis, Mo/EUA.) and all tests were performed in Mueller Hinton agar (Difco-BBL, Detroit, MI/USA).

The minimum inhibitory concentration (MIC) was determined as the lowest concentration that inhibited visible growth. The strains were considered to have acquired resistance when their MIC was higher than the wild type cut-off value (MIC > 2μg/mL) [4].

The disk diffusion test was performed with tablets of 10 μg (Oxoid Ltd., Cambridge/UK) according to the CLSI guidelines [10]. Growth inhibition zone diameters were measured manually. Interpretative criteria to determine clinical resistance were based upon breakpoints described previously [11]-resistant $\leq$ 11 mm and susceptible $\geq$ 14 mm. *E. coli* ATCC 25922 and *S.* Typhimurium ATCC 14024 were used as control strains in all performed tests [12].

3. Results

3.1. Escherichia coli Strains. Using the agar dilution method, eight *E. coli* strains (6.3%) were considered resistant to colistin (Table 1). MIC 50 and MIC 90 values observed were 0.25 μg/mL and 0.5 μg/mL, respectively. When evaluating the disk diffusion test results (Table 2), four strains classified as resistant (3.2%), 37 with intermediate susceptibility (29.4%) and 85 susceptible strains (67.4%) were observed.

3.2. Salmonella enterica Strains. From 124 *S. enterica* strains, 81 were classified as serotype Typhimurium, 13 as serotype London, 11 as serotype Anatum, eight classified as *S. enterica* subspecies *enterica* (O:4,5:-:1,2), seven as serotype Choleraesuis, three as serotype Infantis and one as serotype Bredeney. The distribution of resistant strains according to serotype is presented in Table 3. Using agar dilution method 26 (21%) *S. enterica* strains were considered resistant to colistin (Table 1). Observed MIC 50 and MIC 90 values were 1 μg/mL and 8 μg/mL, respectively. When analyzing disk diffusion test results (Table 2), five strains classified as resistant (4%), 29 with intermediate susceptibility (23.4%), and 90 susceptible strains (72.6%) were observed.

4. Discussion

The results obtained in this study confirm that the disk diffusion method is not the recommended test to monitor colistin resistance, since only 50% of *E. coli* and 20% of *S. enterica* colistin resistant strains were detected using this test. Poor results using the disk diffusion method to detect colistin resistance had been previously described [4].

Using the agar dilution test, which is considered the gold standard for colistin evaluation, 6.3% of *E. coli* and 21% of *S. enterica* tested strains resistant to colistin were detected. The frequency of *E. coli* resistant strains is similar to those described by Boyen et al. [4], who report 9.6% (15/157), and have also been reported before in *E. coli* of animal origin [13, 14].

Table 1: Distribution of MIC values of swine *E. coli* and *S. enterica* strains through agar dilution test against colistin.

Agar dilution	Number of strains with colistin MIC values (μg/mL)											
	≤0.125	0.25	0.5	1	2	4	8	16	32	64	128	256
E. coli	23	51	40	4	0	[0	2	4	2	0	0	0]
S. enterica	0	1	59	30	8	[13	13	0	0	0	0	0]

The values inside [] represent resistant strains.

Table 2: Distribution of inhibition zone diameters swine *E. coli* and *S. enterica* strains through disk diffusion test against colistin.

Disk difusion	Number of strains with colistin inhibition zone values (mm)											
	8	9	10	11	12	13	14	15	16	17	18	19
E. coli	[0	0	4	0]	34	3	74	2	8	0	1	0
S. enterica	[0	0	5	0]	17	12	69	4	12	0	5	0

The values inside [] represent resistant strains.

Table 3: Distribution of colistin resistant strains among different *Salmonella enterica* serotypes isolated from swine.

Serotype	Strains No (%)	Number of resistant strains: Agar dilution test	Disk diffusion test
S. Typhimurium	81 (65.3)	12	2
S. London	13 (10.5)	6	0
S. Anatum	11 (8.9)	3	0
S. enterica subsp. *enterica* (O:4,5:-:1,2)	8 (6.5)	4	3
S. Choleraesuis	7 (5.6)	0	0
S. Infantis	3 (2.4)	0	0
S. Bredeney	1 (0.8)	1	0
Total	124	26	5

Boyen et al. [4] described that the published MIC values for human use do not predict clinical efficiency of colistin when used in animal oral formulations. Following values calculated by Burch [15], for a feed concentration of 66 ppm of colistin, the antimicrobial will reach bactericidal concentration in the porcine jejunum for strains with a MIC of 8 μg/mL, but not for strains with an MIC of 16 μg/mL. The MIC values observed in this study in *E. coli* resistant strains were 8 μg/mL (2 strains), 16 μg/mL (4 strains), and 32 μg/mL (2 strains).

Salmonella Typhimurium resistance to colistin was described by Sun et al. [3], who assessed spontaneous mutations in *Pmr*A and *Pmr*B genes in *S.* Typhimurium LT2 that present reduced susceptibility to colistin. They report that the mutation rate to colistin resistance was 0.6×10^6 per cell generation, which was considered several times higher than mutations rates to other antibiotics, such as streptomycin, rifampicin, and nalidixic acid. The MIC values observed in these mutants (2.5 μg/mL to 4 μg/mL) increased 20 to 30 times comparing to susceptible strain (0,125 μg/mL). Reports of colistin resistance frequency in wild *S. enterica* strains of animal origin and reports of resistance detection in other serotypes different from Typhimurium were not found in the literature.

The MIC values identified in *S. enterica* resistant strains (4 μg/mL and 8 μg/mL) were lower than those observed in *E. coli*, but are still above the considered breakpoint and are 32 to 64 times higher than MIC observed in *S.* Typhimurium ATCC 14024 (0,125 μg/mL). In this study colistin resistance was detected in wild *Salmonella* strains from serotype Typhimurium, London, Anatum, Bredeney and *S. enterica* subsp. *enterica* (O:4,5:-:1,2), suggesting that the large use of colistin in swine herds from Brazil is selecting resistant strains independent of serotype. Part of these *Salmonella* resistant strains was isolated from carcasses, lymph nodes and feces of pigs at slaughterhouses.

Humans may obtain antimicrobial resistant bacteriaor resistance genes of animal origin directly via contact with animals, food of animal origin, or the environment. These bacteria may subsequently colonize humans or may transfer resistance genes to other bacteria during passage through the intestinal tract. The contribution of the animal reservoir to the burden of antimicrobial resistance in humans has not been quantified; however, the use of antimicrobial agents regarded as critically or highly important for use in humans should be avoided or minimized in food animals [16].

Considering the high use of colistin in animal production and the importance of this antimicrobial for the control of multiresistant Gramnegative nosocomial infections in humans, more intensive studies must be conducted to monitor the resistance in animal isolates and resistance mechanisms involved.

Acknowledgments

This study was sponsored by FAPESP (process: 2009/14906-6 and 2009/14939-1) and CAPES.

References

[1] D. Landman, C. Georgescu, D. A. Martin, and J. Quale, "Polymyxins revisited," *Clinical Microbiology Reviews*, vol. 21, no. 3, pp. 449–465, 2008.

[2] J. Li, R. L. Nation, J. D. Turnidge et al., "Colistin: the re-emerging antibiotic for multidrug-resistant Gram-negative bacterial infections," *Lancet Infectious Diseases*, vol. 6, no. 9, pp. 589–601, 2006.

[3] S. Sun, A. Negrea, M. Rhen, and D. I. Andersson, "Genetic analysis of colistin resistance in Salmonella enterica serovar typhimurium," *Antimicrobial Agents and Chemotherapy*, vol. 53, no. 6, pp. 2298–2305, 2009.

[4] F. Boyen, F. Vangroenweghe, P. Butaye et al., "Disk prediffusion is a reliable method for testing colistin susceptibility in porcine *E. coli* strains," *Veterinary Microbiology*, vol. 144, no. 3-4, pp. 359–362, 2010.

[5] J. H. Moffatt, M. Harper, B. Adler, R. L. Nation, J. Li, and J. D. Boyce, "Insertion sequence ISAba11 is involved in colistin resistance and loss of lipopolysaccharide in *Acinetobacter baumannii*," *Antimicrobial Agents and Chemotherapy*, vol. 55, no. 6, pp. 3022–3024, 2011.

[6] B. C. Love and M. H. Rostagno, "Comparison of five culture methods for *Salmonella* isolation from swine fecal samples of known infection status," *Journal of Veterinary Diagnostic Investigation*, vol. 20, no. 5, pp. 620–624, 2008.

[7] P. Quinn, M. Carter et al., *Clinical Veterinary Microbiology*, Mosby, Edinburgh, UK.

[8] W. Zhang, M. Zhao, L. Ruesch, A. Omot, and D. Francis, "Prevalence of virulence genes in *Escherichia coli* strains recently isolated from young pigs with diarrhea in the US," *Veterinary Microbiology*, vol. 123, no. 1–3, pp. 145–152, 2007.

[9] P. A. D. Grimont and F. X. Weill, "Antigenic formulae of the Salmonella serovars. *WHO* Collaborating Centre for Reference and Research on Salmonella," Institute Pasteur, France, Antigenic Formulae of the Salmonella Serovars, 9th edition, 2007, http://www.scacm.org/divc/.

[10] CLSI, "Performance standards for antimicrobial disk and dilution susceptibility tests for bacteria isolated from animals," Approved standard, 3rd ed., M31-A3. Clinical and Laboratory Standards Institute, Wayne, Pa, USA, 2008.

[11] A. C. Gales, A. O. Reis, and R. N. Jones, "Contemporary assessment of antimicrobial susceptibility testing methods for polymyxin B and colistin: review of available interpretative criteria and quality control guidelines," *Journal of Clinical Microbiology*, vol. 39, no. 1, pp. 183–190, 2001.

[12] R. N. Jones, T. R. Anderegg, and J. M. Swenson, "Quality control guidelines for testing gram-negative control strains with polymyxin B and colistin (polymyxin E) by standardized methods," *Journal of Clinical Microbiology*, vol. 43, no. 2, pp. 925–927, 2005.

[13] M. Kijima-Tanaka, K. Ishihara, A. Morioka et al., "A national surveillance of antimicrobial resistance in *Escherichia coli* isolated from food-producing animals in Japan," *Journal of Antimicrobial Chemotherapy*, vol. 51, no. 2, pp. 447–451, 2003.

[14] G. Q. Wang, C. M. Wu, X. D. Du et al., "Characterization of integrons-mediated antimicrobial resistance among *Escherichia coli* strains isolated from bovine mastitis," *Veterinary Microbiology*, vol. 127, no. 1-2, pp. 73–78, 2008.

[15] D. G. S. Burch, "Pharmacokinetics of antimicrobials at different levels of the intestinal tract and their relationship to *Escherichia coli* resistance patterns in the pig," *Pig Journal*, vol. 59, pp. 91–111, 2007.

[16] A. M. Hammerum and O. E. Heuer, "Human health hazards from antimicrobial-resistant *Escherichia coli* of animal origin," *Clinical Infectious Diseases*, vol. 48, no. 7, pp. 916–921, 2009.

2

Isolation and Identification of Sodium Fluoroacetate Degrading Bacteria from Caprine Rumen in Brazil

Expedito K. A. Camboim,[1] Arthur P. Almeida,[1] Michelle Z. Tadra-Sfeir,[2] Felício G. Junior,[1] Paulo P. Andrade,[3] Chris S. McSweeney,[4] Marcia A. Melo,[1] and Franklin Riet-Correa[1]

[1] *Unidade Acadêmica de Medicina Veterinária, Universidade Federal de Campina Grande, 58708 Patos, PB, Brazil*
[2] *Laboratório de Fixação Biológica de Nitrogênio, Departamento de Bioquímica e Biologia Molecular, Universidade Federal do Paraná, 80060 Curitiba, PR, Brazil*
[3] *Departamento de Genética, Universidade Federal de Pernambuco, 50670 Recife, PE, Brazil*
[4] *CSIRO Livestock Industries, Queensland Bioscience Precinct, St Lucia, QLD 4067, Australia*

Correspondence should be addressed to Marcia A. Melo, marcia.melo@pq.cnpq.br

Academic Editors: T. Ledon, S. F. Porcella, and B. I. Yoon

The objective of this paper was to report the isolation of two fluoroacetate degrading bacteria from the rumen of goats. The animals were adult goats, males, crossbred, with rumen fistula, fed with hay, and native pasture. The rumen fluid was obtained through the rumen fistula and immediately was inoculated 100 μL in mineral medium added with 20 mmol L^{-1} sodium fluoroacetate (SF), incubated at 39°C in an orbital shaker. *Pseudomonas fluorescens* (strain DSM 8341) was used as positive control for fluoroacetate dehalogenase activity. Two isolates were identified by 16S rRNA gene sequencing as *Pigmentiphaga kullae* (ECPB08) and *Ancylobacter dichloromethanicus* (ECPB09). These bacteria degraded sodium fluoroacetate, releasing 20 mmol L^{-1} of fluoride ion after 32 hours of incubation in Brunner medium containing 20 mmol L^{-1} of SF. There are no previous reports of fluoroacetate dehalogenase activity for *P. kullae* and *A. dichloromethanicus*. Control measures to prevent plant intoxication, including use of fences, herbicides, or other methods of eliminating poisonous plants, have been unsuccessful to avoid poisoning by fluoroacetate containing plants in Brazil. In this way, *P. kullae* and *A. dichloromethanicus* may be used to colonize the rumen of susceptible animals to avoid intoxication by fluoroacetate containing plants.

1. Introduction

The most important group of poisonous plants in Brazil is one that causes "sudden death" during physical effort, responsible for nearly 500 000 cattle deaths each year. It is composed of 13 species of plants, belonging to 3 families: Rubiaceae (*Palicourea marcgravii*, *P. aeneofusca*, *P. juruana*, and *P. grandiflora*); Bignoniaceae (*Pseudocalymma elegans*, *Arrabidaea bilabiata*, and *A. japurensis*); and Malpighiaceae (*Mascagnia rigida*, *M. elegans*, *M. pubiflora*, *M. aff. rigida*, *M. exotropica*, and *M. sepium*) [1–10]. *P. marcgravii* is the most important Brazilian toxic plant and *M. rigida* is the most important toxic plant in Northeastern Brazil [11]. Sodium fluoroacetate was identified as the active principle in *P. marcgravii*, *A. bilabiata* [12, 13], and *M. rigida* [14]. In the other plants the active principle has not been identified, but is probably also sodium fluoroacetate [15]; it disrupts the tricarboxylic acid cycle, being first converted to fluorocitrate, which in turn inhibits the enzymes aconitase and succinate dehydrogenase resulting in citrate accumulation in tissues and plasma, and ultimately causing energy deprivation, and death [16]. Microbial degradation of sodium fluoroacetate is catalyzed by a fluoroacetate dehalogenase, which cleaves the strong carbon-fluorine bond [17], but also cleaves, although less effectively, other bonds such as carbon-chlorine, carbon-bromine and carbon-iodine [18]. Sodium fluoroacetate can also be defluorinated by L-2 haloacid dehalogenases [19].

Several soil bacteria have the ability to degrade sodium fluoroacetate. In central Australia, seven fluoroacetate degrading bacteria genera including *Acinetobacter, Arthrobacter, Aureobacterium, Bacillus, Pseudomonas, Weeksella,* and *Streptomyces* were isolated [20]. Recently, seven bacterial strains isolated from Brazilian soil samples have been described, belonging to the genera *Ancylobacter, Burkholderia, Cupriavidus, Paenibacillus, Staphylococcus, Stenotrophomonas,* and *Ralstonia* [21]. However, a single ruminal bacterial isolate, belonging to the phylum Synergistetes, was reported as being able to degrade sodium fluoroacetate [22, 23]. As the result of our attempt to ascertain whether naturally-occurring fluoroacetate-degrading microorganisms exist in the gastrointestinal systems of animals, we report here the isolation of two new fluoroacetate degrading bacteria from goat rumen.

2. Material and Methods

2.1. Collection and Samples Processing. The animals were male adult goats, crossbred, with rumen fistula, and fed with hay, native pasture, and water *ad libitum*. They were housed in the Veterinary Hospital of the Universidade Federal de Campina Grande in the State of Paraíba, Northeastern Brazil, and had no access to areas with sodium fluoroacetate-containing toxic plants.

The rumen fluid was obtained through the rumen fistula and immediately inoculated in test tubes.

2.2. Bacterial Isolation. Bacterial isolation started by the inoculation of 100 μL of rumen fluid in tubes containing 9 mL of mineral medium (Brunner) added with vitamins (http://www.dsmz.de/microorganisms/medium/pdf/DSMZ_Medium457.pdf) and 20 mmol L^{-1} sodium fluoroacetate (SF) (Sigma-Fluka) as single carbon source. This medium will be here designated as Brunner medium. Samples were incubated at 39°C in an orbital shaker. After 48 hours, 1 mL of the first growth was transferred to test tubes containing 9 mL of Brunner medium and incubated under the same conditions described above.

The SF defluorination was measured with a F^- selective electrode (Thermo Electron Corporation) in 24-well plates containing 500 μL of culture and 500 μL of Total Ionic Strength Adjustment Buffer-TISAB (Diaminocyclohexane, sodium chloride, and glacial acetic acid, pH 5.5). The fluoride ion released by the microbial SF degradation was expressed in millimoles, the defluorination rate of 20 mmol L^{-1} corresponding to the release of 20 mmol L^{-1} F^-.

Samples presenting SF defluorination were cultivated in serial dilutions from 10^{-1} to 10^{-9}. To obtain pure colonies the highest dilution that presented SF defluorination was plated on Brunner agar (Brunner medium with agar 1%) and incubated at 39°C for 72 hours. Subsequently, each colony was used to inoculate three test tubes containing 9 mL of Brunner medium, which were monitored for SF defluorination. *Pseudomonas fluorescens* (strain DSM 8341) was used as positive control for fluoroacetate dehalogenase activity, cultivated under the same conditions except that the incubation was at 28°C [24]. Nine mL of Brunner medium without bacteria were incubated under the same conditions to evaluate the sodium fluoroacetate degradation background.

2.3. 16S rRNA Gene Sequence Identification. Genus identification for bacteria displaying defluorination activity was done by polymerase chain reaction (PCR) amplification and sequencing of the 16S rRNA gene. DNA extraction was performed with Brazol (LGC Biotechnology) according to the manufacturer's specifications. 16S rRNA gene was amplified in buffer containing 0.5 μM of 27f and 1492r universal primers [25], 2U of Taq DNA polymerase, 0.2 mM of dNTP and 100 ng of DNA and ultrapure water to a final volume of 20 μL. In the negative control, the DNA volume was substituted by ultrapure water. The amplified products were applied into 1% agarose gel and submitted to electrophoresis. DNA was stained with ethidium bromide and bands visualized with an imaging system (UVP-Bioimaging Systems).

The sequencing reaction was performed with BigDye kit according to manufacturer's recommendations (Applied Biosystems) and the product sequenced in the Genetic Analyzer 3500 XL sequencer (Applied Biosystems).

2.4. Sequence Analysis and Phylogram. 16S rRNA gene sequences were assembled with the CAP3 Sequence Assembly Program (http://pbil.univ-lyon1.fr/cap3.php). DNA sequences were analyzed by basic local alignment search tool (BLAST) available on the website of the National Center for Biotechnology Information (NCB—http://www.ncbi.nlm.nih.gov/BLAST). Species identification was based on maximum score, identity and coverage values. The Greengenes database and workbench were used to corroborate species identification (http://greengenes.lbl.gov). The Bootstrap consensus tree was generated with MEGA5 software using the neighbor-joining statistical method (http://www.megasoftware.net/mega.php) [26].

3. Results and Discussion

The 16S rRNA gene sequences from the two fluoroacetate degrading isolates ECPB08 (JQ345720) and ECPB09 (JQ345721) were similar to the 16S rRNA genes from *Pigmentiphaga* and *Ancylobacter* species, respectively (Table 1). On the basis of score value alone, the *P. kullae* sequence was the most similar (score = 2237) to ECPB08, although other 16S rRNA sequences had the same coverage and identity parameter values. Similarly, the 16S rRNA sequences from *Ancylobacter vacuolatus* and *Ancylobacter sp.* strain WPCB135 were the most similar (score 2388) to ECPB09, but the differences in alignment parameters for other *Ancylobacter* 16S rRNA sequences were only marginal. Consequently, it was not possible to infer from the score values which species would be phylogenetically the closest to ECPB09 (JQ345721).

Comparative sequence analysis using global alignment confirmed that the isolates ECPB08 (JQ345720) and ECPB09

Table 1: Local alignment results for fluoroacetate-degrading bacterial isolates 16S rRNA sequences. Sequences were compared to those deposited at the National Center for Biotechnology Information using the regular BlastN algorithm available at http://www.ncbi.nlm.nih.gov/BLAST. Organisms with sequences similar to those of isolates ECPB08 (JQ345720) and ECPB09 (JQ345721) are listed on the second column. Values for the parameters total score, query coverage, and maximum identity are displayed in columns 3 to 5. GenBank access codes are displayed in parentheses.

Isolate (acc. no.)	Species/strain (accession no.)	Total score	Query coverage (%)	Max identity (%)
ECPB08 (JQ345720)	*Pigmentiphaga kullae* strain K24 (NR_025112.1)	2237	100	98
	Pigmentiphaga daeguensis strain K110 (NR_044082.1)	2215	100	98
	Pigmentiphaga daeguensis strain NML080357 (JN585327.1)	2197	100	97
	Pigmentiphaga litoralis strain JSM 061001 (NR_044530.1)	2152	99	97
ECPB09 (JQ345721)	*Ancylobacter* sp. WPCB135 (FJ006900.1)	2388	99	99
	Ancylobacter vacuolatus strain DSM 1277 (NR_042794.1)	2388	99	99
	Ancylobacter dichloromethanicus strain DM16 (EU589386.1)	2387	99	99
	Ancylobacter polymorphus strain DSM 2457 (NR_042795.1)	2372	99	99
	Ancylobacter rudongensis strain AS1.1761 (NR_029047.1)	2370	99	99
	Ancylobacter polymorphus T10AII (GQ921957.1)	2358	98	99
	Ancylobacter aquaticus (NR_044737.1)	2351	99	98
	Ancylobacter oerskovii strain NS05 (NR_042655.1)	2341	99	98

(JQ345721) were phylogenetically closely related to the genera *Pigmentiphaga* and *Ancylobacter*, respectively (Figure 1). Indeed, the global alignment corroborates the taxonomic inference based on the 16S rRNA local alignment results for ECPB08 (JQ345720), indicating that this isolate is closely related to *P. kullae* strain K24 (Figure 1(a)), and is supported by previous results on the taxonomy of this genus [27, 28]. Moreover, the global alignment allowed a better estimative of taxon position for ECPB09 (JQ345721), suggesting its close relationship with *A. polymorphus* (Figure 1(b)). Although the upper part of the tree in Figure 1(b) has low bootstrap values, the whole dendrogram is consistent with the results presented by Firsova et al. [29] for the genus *Ancylobacter*.

The genus *Pigmentiphaga* was initially proposed by Blümel et al. [30] with *Pigmentiphaga kullae* (strain K24) as its unique specie, which degrades xenobiotic compounds. In 2007, Yoon et al. [31] described a new member of the genus, *Pigmentiphaga daeguensis* (strain K110T), isolated from wastewater collected from a dye works in Korea. Later, Chen et al. [27] and Lee et al. [28] isolated *Pigmentiphaga litoralis* (strain JSM 061001) and *P. soli* from a tidal flat sample in the South China Sea and from soil in South Korea, respectively.

Raj and Maloy [32] proposed the replacement of the genus name *Microcyclus* by *Ancylobacter*, with a single species, *A. aquaticus* [33]. Since then, five new species have been described, the latest being *Ancylobacter dichloromethanicus* (strain DM16), isolated from contaminated soil [29]. This species uses dichloromethane, methanol, formate, and formaldehyde polycarbonate compounds as carbon and energy sources. Enzymatic analysis showed that it contains a GSH-dependent dichloromethane dehalogenase.

Both ECPB08 (JQ345720) and ECPB09 (JQ345721) grew in culture medium containing SF as the sole carbon source. These bacteria displayed SF degradation activity, releasing 20 mmol L^{-1} of fluoride ion after 32 hours of incubation in Brunner medium with 20 mmol L^{-1} of SF (Figure 2). These results are similar to those reported by Davis et al. [34] for *Burkholderia* sp. The *Pseudomonas fluorescens* control strain (DSM 8341) reached the same level of defluorination, and there was no release of fluoride ions when the Brunner medium was incubated without bacteria, due to the stability of the strong carbon-fluorine bond in the fluoroacetate [17]. There are no previous reports of fluoroacetate dehalogenase activity for any *Pigmentiphaga* or *Ancylobacter* species.

The defluorination ability of both isolates can be due to the expression of a fluoroacetate dehalogenase gene or to another unspecific dehalogenase. Although for *Pigmentiphaga* no dehalogenase gene has yet been described, a dichloromethane dehalogenase sequence from *A. dichloromethanicus* is deposited in GenBank [29]. Liu et al. [35] confirmed that fluoroacetate dehalogenase degrades other halogenated compounds such as chloroacetate, bromoacetate, iodoacetate, and dichloroacetate, by a cross-adaptation mechanism [36]. Similar results were obtained by Donnelly and Murphy [24] who found a fluoroacetate dehalogenase able to degrade chloroacetate, bromoacetate, and ethyl fluoroacetate. Alternatively, sodium fluoroacetate was defluorinated by L-2 haloacid dehalogenase [18].

Sodium fluoroacetate degrading bacteria, mostly *Bacillus* and *Flavobacterium* species, were isolated from soil in Australia, even in the absence of sodium fluoroacetate in the environment [37]. In this study, two *Pigmentiphaga* and *Ancylobacter* species were isolated from goat rumen, although the animals were not fed plants that produce this component. This finding suggests that the fluoroacetate dehalogenase gene is rather ubiquitous and that its expression may represent a selective advantage for microorganism, possible due to the ability of the enzyme to degrade other related compounds, as mentioned before.

On the other hand, it has been reported that animals grazing in areas where *Mascagnia rigida* is present are more resistant to poisoning than those kept in areas without these

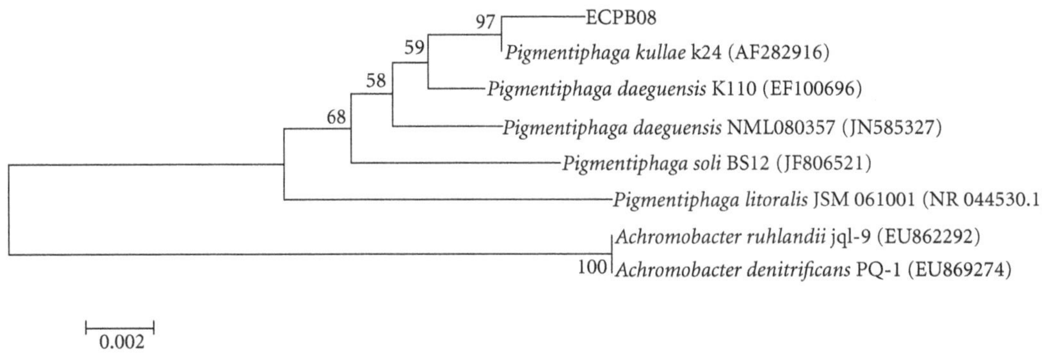

(a)

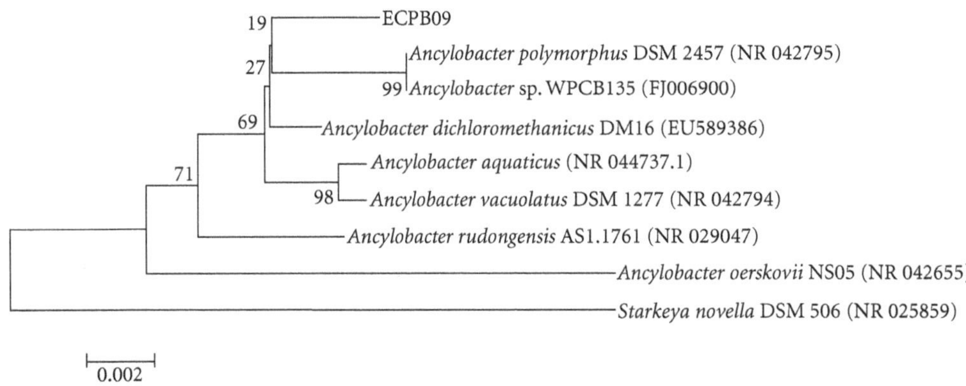

(b)

Figure 1: Phylogenetic tree based on 16S rRNA sequences by Maximum Parsimony analysis. ECPB08 (JQ345720) and ECPB09 (JQ345721) are the codes for the isolates. In parentheses are the GenBank codes. The relationship between ECPB08 (JQ345720) (a), ECPB09 (JQ345721) (b) related taxa, and the outgroups *Achromobacter ruhlandii, A. denitrificans,* and *Starkeya novella* is shown. The bootstrap consensus tree inferred from 1000 replicates is taken to represent the evolutionary history of the taxa analyzed. Scale of 0.002: evolutionary distance.

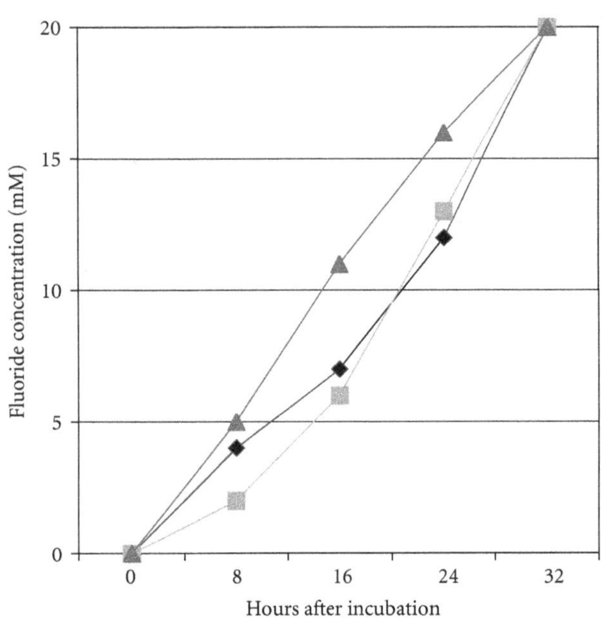

Figure 2: Sodium fluoroacetate degradation rate by bacteria isolated from caprine rumen. Isolate ECPB08 (light grey square), isolate ECPB09 (black rhombus), and *P. fluorescens* (dark grey triangle, positive control).

plants [6]. Recent results of our research group demonstrated that resistance to *M. rigida* poisoning can be induced by the administration of repeated low nontoxic doses of the plant or by transfaunation of rumen fauna from resistant to susceptible animals (unpublished data). These results suggest that either changes in rumen microflora or sustained high expression levels of the SF dehalogenase gene from the endogenous rumen microbiota are responsible for this tolerance.

Control measures to prevent plant intoxication, including use of fences, herbicides, or other methods of eliminating poisonous plants, have been unsuccessful to avoid poisoning by fluoroacetate containing plants in Brazil [38]. An alternative way would be the microbial detoxification of plants by inoculation of fluoroacetate degrading bacteria into the rumen. This strategy was used by Gregg et al. [39] who inoculated in the rumen a genetically modified strain of *Butyrivibrio fibrisolvens* with a gene encoding fluoroacetate dehalogenase from *Moraxella* species, which was efficient to prevent fluoroacetate poisoning in sheep. In an alternative approach, the two isolates, *Pigmentiphaga* sp. and *Ancylobacter* sp. are candidates to be used in colonizing the rumen to avoid intoxication by fluoroacetate containing plants.

Acknowledgment

This work was supported by the INCT for the control of plant poisonings, Grant no.: 573534/2008-0.

References

[1] A. Gava, J. Cristani, J. V. Branco, D. S. Neves, A. J. Mondadori, and R. S. Sousa, "Sudden death in cattle by *Mascagnia* sp (Malpighiaceae) in the State of Santa Catarina, Brazil," *Pesquisa Veterinaria Brasileira*, vol. 18, no. 1, pp. 16–20, 1998.

[2] M. A. Helayel, T. N. França, J. N. Seixas, V. A. Nogueira, S. A. Caldas, and P. V. Peixoto, "Sudden death in cattle caused by ingestion of *Pseudocalymma elegans* (Bignoniaceae) in the county of Rio Bonito, Rio de Janeiro," *Pesquisa Veterinaria Brasileira*, vol. 29, no. 7, pp. 498–508, 2009.

[3] R. M. T. Medeiros, S. A. Geraldo Neto, R. C. Barbosa, E. F. Lima, and F. Riet-Correa, "Sudden bovine death from *Mascagnia rigida* in Northeastern Brazil," *Veterinary and Human Toxicology*, vol. 44, no. 5, pp. 286–288, 2002.

[4] S. P. Pavarini, M. P. Soares, P. M. Bandarra et al., "Sudden death in cattle due to the consumption of *Amorimia exotropica* (Malpighiaceae) in Rio Grande do Sul, Brazil," *Pesquisa Veterinaria Brasileira*, vol. 31, no. 4, pp. 291–296, 2011.

[5] B. Soto-Blanco, M. Haraguchi, J. A. Silva, and Górniak, "Intoxicação natural de caprinos e ovinos por *Palicourea marcgravii* St. Hil. (Rubiaceae)," *Caatinga*, no. 1, pp. 52–56, 2004.

[6] I. P. Silva, R. A. Lira, R. R. Barbosa, J. S. Batista, and B. Soto-Blanco, "Intoxicação natural pelas folhas de *Mascagnia rigida* (Malpighiaceae) em ovinos," *Arquivos do Instituto Biologico*, vol. 75, no. 2, pp. 229–233, 2008.

[7] S. V. Schons, T. L. de Mello, F. Riet-Correa, and A. L. Schild, "Poisoning by *Amorimia (Mascagnia) sepium* in sheep in Northern Brazil," *Toxicon*, vol. 57, no. 5, pp. 781–786, 2011.

[8] C. H. Tokarnia, J. Döbereiner, and P. V. Peixoto, *Plantas Tóxicas do Brasil*, Editora Helianthus, Rio de Janeiro, Brazil, 2000.

[9] J. S. Vasconcelos, F. Riet-Correa, A. F. M. Dantas et al., "Poisoning by *Mascagnia rigida* (Malpighiaceae) in sheep and goats," *Pesquisa Veterinaria Brasileira*, vol. 28, no. 10, pp. 521–526, 2008.

[10] J. S. Vasconcelos, F. Riet-Correa, A. F. M. Dantas, R. M. T. Medeiros, and A. J. A. Dantas, "Sudden deaths caused by *Palicourea aeneofusca* (Rubiaceae) and *Mascagnia rigida* (Malpighiaceae) in cattle in the Zona da Mata of Paraíba," *Pesquisa Veterinaria Brasileira*, vol. 28, no. 10, pp. 457–460, 2008.

[11] C. H. Tokarnia, P. V. Peixoto, and J. Dobereiner, "Poisonous plants affecting heart funtions of cattle in Brazil," *Pesquisa Agropecuária Brasileira*, vol. 10, pp. 1–10, 1990.

[12] M. M. de Oliveira, "Chromatographic isolation of monofluoroacetic acid from *Palicourea marcgravii* St. Hil," *Experientia*, vol. 19, no. 11, pp. 586–587, 1963.

[13] H. C. Krebs, W. Kemmerling, and G. Habermehl, "Qualitative and quantitative determination of fluoroacetic acid in *Arrabidea bilabiata* and *Palicourea marcgravii* by 19F-NMR spectroscopy," *Toxicon*, vol. 32, no. 8, pp. 909–913, 1994.

[14] L. C. Cunha, S. L. Gorniak, M. Haraguchi, F. Riet-Correa, F. G. Xavier, and J. C. Florio, "*Palicourea marcgravii* e *Mascagnia rigida*: um estudo por cromatografia em camada delgada (CCD)," in *Proceedings of the II Simpósio de Pós-Graduação and XV Semana Científica*, Prof. Dr. Benjamin Eurico Malucelli, São Paulo, Brazil, 2006.

[15] F. Riet-Correa and M. C. Méndez, "Intoxicações por plantas e micotoxinas," in *Doenças de Ruminantes e Eqüídeos*, F. Riet-Correa, A. L. Schild, R. A. A. Lemos, and J. R. J. Borges, Eds., vol. 2, Editora Pallotti, Santa Maria, RS, Brasil, 2007.

[16] P. A. Mayes, "O ciclo do ácido cítrico: o catabolismo da Acetil-coA," in *Harper: Bioquímica*, K. R. Murray, Ed., pp. 182–189, Atheneu, São Paulo, Brazil, 9th edition, 2002.

[17] S. Fetzner and F. Lingens, "Bacterial dehalogenases: biochemistry, genetics, and biotechnological applications," *Microbiological Reviews*, vol. 58, no. 4, pp. 641–685, 1994.

[18] T. Kurihara, T. Yamauchi, S. Ichiyama, H. Takahata, and N. Esaki, "Purification, characterization, and gene cloning of a novel fluoroacetate dehalogenase from *Burkholderia* sp. FA1," *Journal of Molecular Catalysis B*, vol. 23, no. 2–6, pp. 347–355, 2003.

[19] W. Y. Chan, M. Wong, J. Guthrie et al., "Sequence- and activity-based screening of microbial genomes for novel dehalogenases," *Microbial Biotechnology*, vol. 3, no. 1, pp. 107–120, 2010.

[20] L. E. Twigg and L. V. Socha, "Defluorination of sodium monofluoroacetate by soil microorganisms from central Australia," *Soil Biology and Biochemistry*, vol. 33, no. 2, pp. 227–234, 2001.

[21] E. K. A. Camboim, M. Z. Tadra-Sfeir, E. M. Souza et al., "Defluorination of sodium fluoroacetate by bacteria from soil and plants in Brazil," *The Scientific World Journal*, vol. 2012, Article ID 149893, 5 pages, 2012.

[22] C. Davis, *Investigations on the microbial degradation of fluoroacetate [Ph.D. thesis]*, School of Chemistry and Molecular Bioscience. The University of Queensland, Australia, 2011.

[23] L. E. X. Leong, S. E. Denman, C. K. Davis, T. Huber, and C. S. McSweeney, "Peptide utilization of the novel fluoracetate-degrading ruminal bacterium," *Proceedings of the Australian Society of Animal Production*, vol. 28, p. 64, 2010.

[24] C. Donnelly and C. D. Murphy, "Purification and properties of fluoroacetate dehalogenase from *Pseudomonas fluorescens* DSM 8341," *Biotechnology Letters*, vol. 31, no. 2, pp. 245–250, 2009.

[25] W. G. Weisburg, S. M. Barns, D. A. Pelletier, and D. J. Lane, "16S ribosomal DNA amplification for phylogenetic study," *Journal of Bacteriology*, vol. 173, no. 2, pp. 697–703, 1991.

[26] K. Tamura, D. Peterson, N. Peterson, G. Stecher, M. Nei, and S. Kumar, "MEGA5: molecular evolutionary genetics analysis using maximum likelihood, evolutionary distance, and maximum parsimony methods," *Molecular Biology and Evolution*, vol. 28, no. 10, pp. 2731–2739, 2011.

[27] Y. G. Chen, Y. Q. Zhang, K. Huang et al., "*Pigmentiphaga litoralis* sp. nov., a facultatively anaerobic bacterium isolated from a tidal flat sediment," *International Journal of Systematic and Evolutionary Microbiology*, vol. 59, no. 3, pp. 521–525, 2009.

[28] J. J. Lee, S. Srinivasan, and M. K. Kim, "*Pigmentiphaga soli* sp. nov., a bacterium isolated from soil," *J. Microbiol*, vol. 49, no. 5, pp. 857–861, 2011.

[29] J. Firsova, N. Doronina, E. Lang, C. Spröer, S. Vuilleumier, and Y. Trotsenko, "*Ancylobacter dichloromethanicus* sp. nov.—a new aerobic facultatively methylotrophic bacterium utilizing dichloromethane," *Systematic and Applied Microbiology*, vol. 32, no. 4, pp. 227–232, 2009.

[30] S. Blümel, B. Mark, H. J. Busse, P. Kämpfer, and A. Stolz, "*Pigmentiphaga kullae* gen. nov., sp. nov., a novel member of the family Alcaligenaceae with the ability to decolorize azo dyes aerobically," *International Journal of Systematic and Evolutionary Microbiology*, vol. 51, no. 5, pp. 1867–1871, 2001.

[31] J. H. Yoon, S. J. Kang, W. Kim, and T. K. Oh, "*Pigmentiphaga daeguensis* sp. nov., isolated from wastewater of a dye works, and emended description of the genus *Pigmentiphaga*," *International Journal of Systematic and Evolutionary Microbiology*, vol. 57, no. 6, pp. 1188–1191, 2007.
[32] H. D. Raj and S. R. Maloy, "Family Spirosomaceae: gram-negative ring-forming aerobic bacteria," *Critical Reviews in Microbiology*, vol. 17, no. 5, pp. 329–364, 1990.
[33] J. Orskov, "Beschreibung eines neuen Microben, Microcyclus aquaticus, mit eigentiimlicher Morphologie," *Zentralblatt fur Bakteriologie, Parasitenkunde, Infektionskrankheiten und Hygiene*, vol. 107, pp. 180–184, 1923.
[34] C. K. Davis, S. E. Denman, L. I. Sly, and C. S. McSweeney, "Development of a colorimetric colony-screening assay for detection of defluorination by micro-organisms," *Applied Microbiology*, vol. 53, no. 4, pp. 417–423, 2011.
[35] J. Q. Liu, T. Kurihara, S. Ichiyama et al., "Reaction mechanism of fluoroacetate dehalogenase from *Moraxella* sp. B," *Journal of Biological Chemistry*, vol. 273, no. 47, pp. 30897–30902, 1998.
[36] I. S. Melo and J. L. Azevedo, "Como isolar microrganismos degradadores de moléculas xenobióticas," in *Microbiologia Ambiental*, I. S. Melo and L. J. Azevedo, Eds., pp. 167–183, EMBRAPA-CNPMA, Jaguariuna, Brazil, 1997.
[37] D. H. Wong, W. E. Kirkpatrick, D. R. King, and J. E. Kinnear, "Defluorination of sodium monofluoroacetate (1080) by microorganisms isolated from western Australian soils," *Soil Biology and Biochemistry*, vol. 24, no. 9, pp. 833–838, 1992.
[38] F. Riet-Correa and R. M. T. Medeiros, "Intoxicações por plantas em ruminantes no Brasil e no Uruguai: importância econômica, controle e riscos para a saúde pública," *Pesquisa Veterinaria Brasileira*, vol. 21, no. 1, pp. 38–42, 2001.
[39] K. Gregg, B. Hamdorf, K. Henderson, J. Kopecny, and C. Wong, "Genetically modified ruminal bacteria protect sheep from fluoroacetate poisoning," *Applied and Environmental Microbiology*, vol. 64, no. 9, pp. 3496–3498, 1998.

3

Thermographic Imaging of the Superficial Temperature in Racing Greyhounds before and after the Race

Mari Vainionpää,[1] Esa-Pekka Tienhaara,[2] Marja Raekallio,[1] Jouni Junnila,[3] Marjatta Snellman,[1] and Outi Vainio[1]

[1] *Department of Equine and Small Animal Medicine, Pharmacology and Toxicology, Faculty of Veterinary Medicine, University of Helsinki, Koetilantie 7, 00014 Helsinki, Finland*
[2] *Kosonkuja 3, 04370 Rusutjärvi, Finland*
[3] *4Pharma Ltd, 02130 Espoo, Finland*

Correspondence should be addressed to Mari Vainionpää, mari.vainionpaa@helsinki.fi

Academic Editors: L. Kratochvil, M. F. Landoni, and G. T. Pharr

A total of 47 racing greyhounds were enrolled in this study on two race days (in July and September, resp.) at a racetrack. Twelve of the dogs participated in the study on both days. Thermographic images were taken before and after each race. From the images, superficial temperature points of selected sites (*tendo calcaneus, musculus gastrocnemius, musculus gracilis,* and *musculus biceps femoris portio caudalis*) were taken and used to investigate the differences in superficial temperatures before and after the race. The thermographic images were compared between the right and left legs of a dog, between the raced distances, and between the two race days. The theoretical heat capacity of a racing greyhound was calculated. With regard to all distances raced, the superficial temperatures measured from the *musculus gastrocnemius* were significantly higher after the race than at baseline. No significant differences were found between the left and right legs of a dog after completing any of the distances. Significant difference was found between the two race days. The heat loss mechanisms of racing greyhounds during the race through forced conduction, radiation, evaporation, and panting can be considered adequate when observing the calculated heat capacity of the dogs.

1. Introduction

Racing greyhounds have been bred for the purpose of competitive racing for centuries [1]. This selective breeding has influenced the biochemical properties of racing greyhounds as well as their musculature and appearance [1, 2]. Due to their unique ability to run fast, the dogs also have different energy requirements especially for race performance [3]. The efficiency of the physical exertion with the muscles is a measure of the body's effectiveness in converting nutrients' energy into external muscle work [1, 2]. In humans, the efficiency of muscle work has been studied and estimated to be 24.4%–34.0% [4, 5]. Similar data is not readily available for racing greyhounds.

Running speed has yielded a wind effect during the race and influences the convection of body heat. Furthermore, the vasodilation of the peripheral vascular system is an important way of releasing heat from the body [6]. Other ways for the heat of the body to escape are radiation, evaporation, conduction, and panting [6–8].

Thermographic imaging (also known as thermography, infrared thermography, and infrared imaging) can be used to measure superficial temperature changes in the body [9]. Compared to other commonly used diagnostic methods, thermographic imaging is a noninvasive and safe method of detecting and visualizing changes in superficial temperature in animals [10–14]. A change in superficial temperature due to changes in peripheral blood flow can be measured feasibly with thermography [9]. The method has been used to study dogs [15–17], horses [10, 11, 13], farm animals [12], and humans [18–20]. Thermography can be used to detect, for example, muscle injuries in dogs [21] since such injuries cause a change in peripheral blood flow.

Studies on humans suggest that in healthy individuals, the difference in the symmetry of superficial temperatures between the left and right side is approximately 0.4°C ± 0.3°C [22]. Differences greater than those found in healthy humans could be considered abnormal. No similar studies have been done on animals, but we hypothesized that asymmetry in the superficial temperatures detected by means of thermography may be indicative of adverse events during the race, such as asymmetric strain on the legs or trauma in racing greyhounds. Our secondary hypothesis was that thermography can also be used to detect exercise-induced vasodilatation and increased heat production in racing greyhounds. To our knowledge, thermographic imaging has not been applied before to study the heat balance of healthy racing greyhounds.

The aim of this study was to investigate the differences in superficial temperature on selected points of the muscles and tendons in racing greyhound before and after the race by means of thermographic imaging. The secondary aim was to compare the thermographic images between the right and left legs of individual dogs, as well as between the raced distances and between the two race days. Additional aims were to calculate the theoretical heat capacity of a racing greyhound and measure the relationships between the two race days as well as between the left and right legs with two predetermined factors (kinetic energy and rank) by using the data obtained from the thermographic images and the race records. Our hypotheses were that the superficial temperature measured by thermographic imaging would change due to exercise and that change between the right and left legs would be minor. The superficial temperature difference before and after the race is an important indicator of the well-being of the racing greyhound.

2. Materials and Methods

2.1. The Dogs. Forty-eight racing greyhounds were enrolled in this study at two races, in July and in September, respectively. The owners of the dogs were asked for consent to participate before enrolment. The dogs were between 15 months and 8 years of age and weighted, on average, 32.4 kg, range 24.7–39.5 kg. All the dogs were preliminarily considered to be healthy since they were participating in a race. The dogs also had to go through a health check performed by a veterinarian before being cleared to race. The dogs and runs with notably incomplete data from the race records or thermographic images were excluded ($n = 1$ and $n = 8$, resp.) from the study, thus leaving a total of 47 dogs and 59 races used in the statistical calculations. Twelve of the 47 dogs participated in the study on both days.

2.2. Thermographic Imaging. All the thermographic images were taken with a thermal camera with a resolution of 320 by 240 pixels (T425, FLIR Systems Inc., Danderyd, Sweden). The high-rainbow Color Palette was chosen for taking and displaying the images. The emissivity of one ($e = 1$) was set for the imaging. The thermographic images from the caudal part of the dog, one distally and one proximally (Figure 1), were taken before the veterinary checkup outside with no shelter from the wind or sun due to the lack of a covered space in the area and again within 5 minutes after the race in a large tent set up beside the racetrack near the gate where the racing dogs exited after the race.

2.3. Racetrack and Racing Distances. The thermographic imaging was carried out at a racetrack in Turku, Finland. The track is 475 metres long and has a diameter of the curve of 104 metres.

The dogs in this study were racing in four different distances: 325, 495, 560, and 785 metres. For the 325-metre sprint, there were a total of 27 runs, and for the 495, 560, and 785-metre sprints, 17, 9, and 6 runs, respectively.

2.4. Data Analysis. The freeware FLIR QuickReport 2.1. [23] was applied to interpret the thermographic images. One veterinarian blinded to the dog in question analysed all the images. From the images, four superficial temperature measurement points were selected: *tendo calcaneus, musculus gastrocnemius, musculus gracilis,* and *musculus biceps femoris portio caudalis.* The thermal symmetry was studied from the thermographic images by means of calculating the superficial temperatures of the *tendo calcaneus* and the *musculus gastrocnemius* as well as the *musculus gracilis* and *musculus biceps femoris portio caudalis* before and after the race (Figure 1). The measurement sites were chosen because the areas of interest are affected by physical exercise and they are easily accessed and seen with thermal imaging.

The ambient temperature was measured with a reference thermometer (Fluke T524, Fluke corporation, USA) when available. In July, this measurement device was not available to us, and the ambient temperature was measured from the thermal images by determining the coldest spots in the background temperatures in the four images taken from a specific dog, after which the warmest of these cold spots was selected for calculations. The average ambient temperature on the first race day in July was 18.3°C (13.1–23.3°C) and on the second race day in September 15.7°C (14.5–16.1°C).

The velocity of the sprint was calculated using the formula $v = s/t$, where s = distance (metres), t = time (seconds). Kinetic energy was calculated using the formula $(1/2)\ m * v^2$, where m = mass (kilograms), v = velocity (metres/second). Heat capacity was calculated using the formula C*m, where C = 4,186 J/(kg*K) = constant (heat capacity of water), m = dog weight (kilograms). The efficiency of muscle work was estimated to be 30% for the calculations [4, 5].

2.5. Statistical Analysis. Descriptive statistics were constructed for superficial temperatures based on the thermographic images by time point (before race versus after race), leg, day, and distance for each site (*tendo calcaneus, musculus gastrocnemius, musculus gracilis,* and *musculus biceps femoris portio caudalis*). The differences between the time points, legs, and days in the superficial temperatures based on the thermographic images were evaluated with analysis of variance for repeated measures (RM ANOVA) separately for each measurement point. As two of the different distances had data from only one day and two of the distances from two days, the effects of day and distance were confounded.

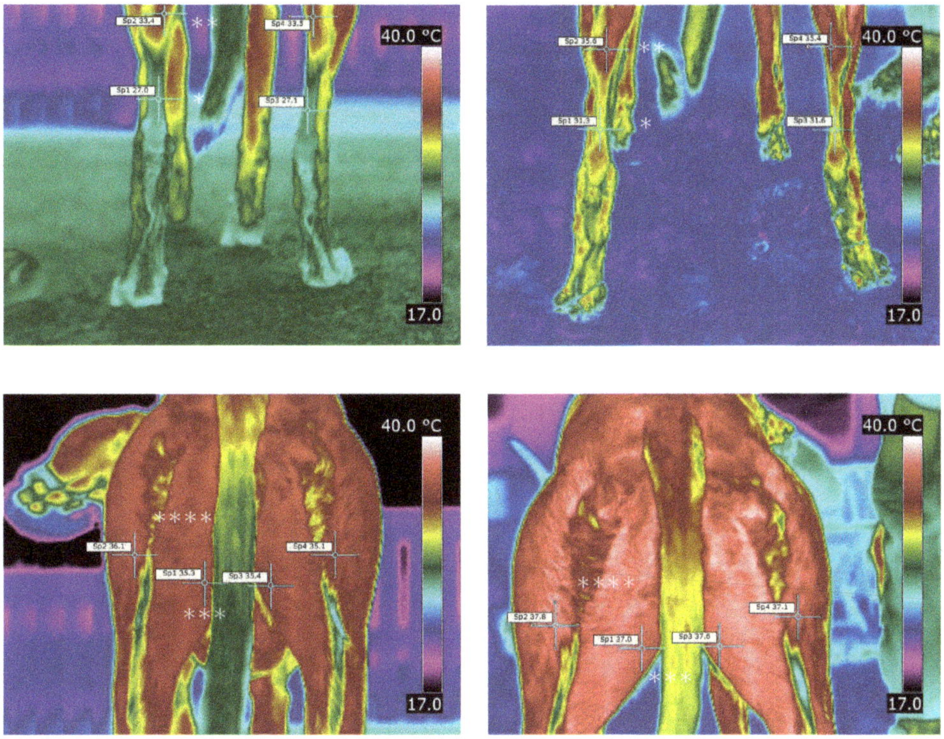

(a) (b)

Figure 1: Thermographic images before (a) and after (b) the race, showing the four measurement points of the *tendo calcaneus* (*), *musculus gastrocnemius* (**), *musculus gracilis* (***), and *musculus biceps femoris portio caudalis* (****).

Therefore, the modelling had to be performed separately for each distance. With the two shortest distances (325 and 495 metres), the statistical model included time point, leg, day, and an interaction term of time point and leg as fixed effects and dog as a random effect. With the two longer distances (560 and 785 metres), the model was the same, excluding the effect of day.

The relationship between the difference between the prerace and postrace superficial temperatures and the predetermined explaining factors was assessed with ANOVA models separately for each measurement point. Based on the primary models, the difference between the legs was negligible with all locations and distances. Therefore, this analysis was only conducted for the difference between time points. The response variable was the mean change in the superficial temperature (before and after) of the two thermographically imaged legs of the dog. The fitted statistical model included (for the two shortest distances) day, rank, and kinetic energy as fixed effects. For the 560 metre distance, the model was the same, excluding the effect of day. For the longest distance, there was not enough data available on the different starts for the evaluation of the effect of rank. Therefore, the model for the longest distance included only the effect of kinetic energy.

All statistical analyses were carried out using the SAS System for Windows, version 9.3 (SAS Institute Inc., Cary, NC, USA).

This study was approved by the Ethical Committee of the Viikki Campus at the University of Helsinki.

3. Results

After all of the distances raced, the superficial temperatures were significantly higher than those at baseline in *musculus gastrocnemius* (Table 1). The superficial temperature differences measured from other points before and after the race varied depending on the measurement point (Table 1). The estimates of the superficial temperature difference varied from 0.6 to 2.1 degrees depending on the distance raced. The superficial temperature differences between left and right leg varied between 0.0 and 4.0 degrees. No significant differences were found between the two thermographically imaged legs of the dog after any of the distances and measurement points. No clinical signs of obvious injuries were detected by the veterinarian responsible for the racing dogs during or after the race.

After the 325- and 495-metre sprints, a significant difference was found between the two race days with all of the measurement points, excluding the 325-metre sprint from *musculus biceps femoris portio caudalis*. No significant differences were detected between rank and kinetic energy when compared to the pre- and postrace superficial temperatures for any of the distances or any of the measurement points. The calculated heat capacity values were similar for all of the distances run and both race days. Data on the dogs, race,

Table 1: Averages ± SD as well as minimum (min) and maximum (max) superficial temperatures obtained from the thermographic images. Measurement points (MPs) for the left and right leg: (1) *musculus gastrocnemius*, (2) *tendo calcaneus*, (3) *musculus biceps femoris portio caudalis*, and (4) *musculus gracilis*. *P* values are for differences before and after the race for each measurement point and distance estimated from the primary statistical models.

Day	Meters	MP	Thermographic images (t°C) Before race Left leg Mean ± SD (min, max)	Before race Right leg Mean ± SD (min, max)	After race Left leg Mean ± SD (min, max)	After race Right leg Mean ± SD (min, max)	*P* value
July	325	1	33.8 ± 1.2 (32.2, 35.6)	33.8 ± 1.3 (31.9, 35.5)	34.5 ± 1.7 (31.6, 37.4)	34.5 ± 1.7 (31.0, 37.7)	
Sep.	325	1	31.6 ± 1.9 (26.2, 33.8)	31.5 ± 2.0 (25.7, 33.4)	32.0 ± 1.4 (29.3, 34.8)	33.1 ± 1.1 (31.6, 35.0)	0.002
July	325	2	30.6 ± 2.1 (26.6, 33.1)	30.7 ± 2.2 (26.9, 33.9)	29.5 ± 2.3 (26.8, 33.2)	29.6 ± 2.3 (26.3, 34.4)	
Sep.	325	2	24.7 ± 4.3 (18.1, 32.6)	24.1 ± 4.4 (14.8, 31.0)	26.3 ± 3.0 (18.4, 29.8)	27.1 ± 3.3 (18.6, 30.4)	0.285
July	325	3	33.2 ± 2.5 (28.4, 36.2)	33.3 ± 2.4 (28.9, 36.6)	32.8 ± 3.7 (26.4, 37.9)	33.3 ± 3.8 (26.2, 38.7)	
Sep.	325	3	29.9 ± 3.7 (23.4, 35.1)	29.8 ± 3.4 (22.9, 35.7)	31.6 ± 3.3 (25.9, 36.8)	31.5 ± 3.1 (25.3, 36.0)	0.043
July	325	4	35.6 ± 0.8 (34.0, 36.8)	35.5 ± 1.0 (32.7, 36.9)	36.6 ± 1.1 (35.1, 38.3)	36.6 ± 0.9 (35.5, 38.4)	
Sep.	325	4	32.8 ± 3.1 (25.2, 35.9)	32.9 ± 2.6 (27.7, 35.9)	34.7 ± 1.4 (31.2, 36.4)	34.3 ± 1.1 (31.6, 35.9)	<0.001
July	495	1	34.6 ± 1.1 (32.5, 36.2)	34.4 ± 1.0 (32.7, 35.8)	34.9 ± 1.0 (33.4, 36.5)	35.2 ± 0.9 (33.6, 36.4)	
Sep.	495	1	31.1 ± 0.8 (29.9, 31.5)	31.5 ± 0.6 (31.0, 32.4)	31.2 ± 1.3 (29.4, 32.6)	32.7 ± 0.9 (31.6, 33.8)	0.003
July	495	2	30.6 ± 2.1 (27.0, 34.0)	31.2 ± 2.5 (27.1, 35.1)	28.9 ± 1.7 (25.4, 31.7)	29.8 ± 1.8 (26.1, 32.5)	
Sep.	495	2	24.5 ± 3.6 (20.7, 29.0)	24.6 ± 3.3 (21.5, 27.9)	23.2 ± 4.1 (18.5, 28.6)	24.8 ± 4.0 (21.3, 30.6)	0.003
July	495	3	34.9 ± 1.4 (31.1, 36.6)	35.0 ± 1.2 (32.0, 36.6)	34.7 ± 2.1 (29.7, 37.8)	34.9 ± 1.7 (31.7, 38.2)	
Sep.	495	3	30.3 ± 2.7 (27.7, 34.0)	28.4 ± 2.5 (26.4, 31.8)	31.5 ± 2.3 (29.8, 34.9)	29.5 ± 3.7 (25.6, 34.5)	0.629
July	495	4	35.7 ± 0.4 (34.8, 36.4)	35.8 ± 0.3 (35.3, 36.2)	36.7 ± 0.8 (35.7, 38.3)	37.0 ± 0.9 (35.7, 38.7)	
Sep.	495	4	34.1 ± 0.7 (32.6, 34.2)	33.9 ± 0.6 (33.2, 34.4)	34.9 ± 2.2 (29.9, 34.4)	34.8 ± 0.4 (33.6, 34.5)	<0.001
July	560	1	33.5 ± 1.2 (31.8, 34.9)	33.7 ± 1.4 (31.4, 35.8)	34.3 ± 1.5 (32.1, 36.4)	34.7 ± 1.3 (32.5, 36.5)	0.005
July	560	2	28.3 ± 1.1 (27.2, 29.8)	28.4 ± 1.0 (27.4, 30.3)	29.4 ± 2.4 (25.6, 32.6)	28.1 ± 4.7 (17.8, 33.4)	0.683
July	560	3	34.7 ± 1.5 (31.1, 35.9)	34.7 ± 1.6 (30.9, 36.2)	34.3 ± 2.9 (30.4, 37.4)	34.3 ± 2.1 (30.5, 36.6)	0.447
July	560	4	35.5 ± 1.3 (33.1, 37.0)	35.3 ± 1.2 (32.6, 37.1)	35.7 ± 1.3 (33.0, 36.8)	36.1 ± 1.4 (33.6, 37.7)	0.115
Sep.	785	1	30.6 ± 1.0 (29.1, 32.2)	30.4 ± 1.0 (29.1, 31.6)	32.6 ± 0.9 (31.4, 33.8)	32.5 ± 0.9 (31.5, 33.4)	<0.001
Sep.	785	2	21.8 ± 3.4 (18.3, 28.3)	22.8 ± 3.2 (18.1, 28.2)	23.9 ± 2.6 (20.5, 28.4)	24.3 ± 3.0 (20.7, 29.4)	0.153
Sep.	785	3	31.9 ± 2.0 (28.9, 34.5)	32.0 ± 1.6 (29.4, 33.6)	33.9 ± 2.2 (31.9, 37.6)	33.1 ± 3.2 (27.9, 37.4)	0.053
Sep.	785	4	33.4 ± 1.4 (31.6, 35.2)	33.4 ± 1.2 (32.1, 35.4)	35.4 ± 1.1 (34.3, 37.1)	35.6 ± 1.2 (34.0, 36.9)	0.005

velocity, kinetic energy, and heat loss calculations are shown in Table 2.

4. Discussion

After the race, the superficial temperatures of the greyhounds, as evaluated by means of thermographic images, were significantly higher than those before the race for all the distances raced on the *musculus gastrocnemius*, and after some of the distances also on the other measurement points. The superficial temperature change was predictable since the muscle work during the race generated a considerable amount of heat as seen in the heat capacity calculations. Furthermore, the subsequent vasodilation of the superficial vasculature and the distribution of the blood have an effect. However, the circumstantial factors on the day of the race also seemed to be important in explaining the change in the superficial temperatures. On the race day in July, the ambient temperature was higher than that on race day in September.

The amount of heat generated during the run (heat capacity) was calculated based on known constants (C), the body weight of the dog, and the calculated kinetic energy. Although this was a theoretical count, it indicated that heat production during the race was considerable and would have led to hyperthermia without proper cooling systems in the dog. It has been shown in previous studies that dogs lose heat *via* conductance through the tissue [6] and respiratory evaporation [8]. Our findings indicate that these methods of heat loss are most likely not sufficient but, additionally, that heat is lost *via* convection and the wind effect generated by the velocity of the dog, a forced convection. The small amount of body fat in racing greyhounds [2] and the lack

Table 2: Data on the races as well as energy and heat capacity calculations for each dog, distance and race day.

Day	Running distance (m)	Number of dogs	Body mass (kg) Ave. ± SD (min, max)	Running time (s) Ave. ± SD (min, max)	Velocity (m/s) Ave. ± SD (min, max)	Kinetic energy (kJ) Ave. ± SD (min, max)	Heat capacity (kJ) Ave. ± SD (min, max)
July	325	14	33.7 ± 3.3 (29.2, 38.6)	19.6 ± 0.3 (19.3, 20.4)	16.6 ± 0.2 (15.9, 16.7)	4.6 ± 0.5 (4.0, 5.5)	141.4 ± 14.0 (122.4, 161.7)
Sep	325	13	32.9 ± 3.6 (26.9, 39.5)	19.2 ± 0.3 (18.9, 19.7)	16.9 ± 0.2 (16.5, 17.2)	4.7 ± 0.5 (3.8, 5.7)	137.9 ± 15.0 (112.3, 165.5)
July	495	13	31.0 ± 4.1 (25.3, 38.4)	29.6 ± 0.3 (29.3, 30.2)	16.7 ± 0.2 (16.4, 16.9)	4.3 ± 0.6 (3.4, 5.4)	129.8 ± 17.3 (106.0, 160.9)
Sep	495	4	31.5 ± 5.0 (26.1, 35.9)	29.6 ± 0.3 (29.2, 29.9)	16.7 ± 0.2 (16.6, 16.9)	4.4 ± 0.7 (3.7, 5.0)	131.9 ± 20.8 (109.4, 150.4)
July	560	9	32.1 ± 3.9 (25.1, 36.6)	33.4 ± 0.6 (32.5, 33.8)	16.8 ± 0.3 (16.6, 17.3)	4.5 ± 0.6 (3.6, 5.5)	134.4 ± 16.5 (105.2, 153.4)
Sep	785	6	31.8 ± 5.8 (24.7, 38.4)	48.6 ± 0.3 (48.4, 49.1)	16.2 ± 0.1 (16.0, 16.3)	4.1 ± 0.7 (3.2, 4.9)	133.3 ± 22.0 (103.5, 160.9)

of or very thin hair coat over the whole abdomen and hind legs contribute to the heat loss, since it is known that the thickness of the hair coat has an effect on the insulation capacity [7]. Since the dogs did not show any signs of hyperthermia after the race, the heat loss during the race was probably adequate in the ambient temperatures of the present study. The dogs expressed no signs of greater discomfort on the warmer race day in July when compared to the race day in September. This also suggests that the cooling mechanisms of racing greyhounds are functional regardless of the ambient temperature. The ambient temperatures on the two race days were low compared to those in many other countries. Despite the warmer ambient temperatures, racing greyhounds are known to complete the race without severe hyperthermia.

No significant differences were detected in the means of the superficial temperatures between the right and left legs of the dogs, despite of the effects of the counterclockwise race direction, suggesting that in general the dogs had been running in a balanced manner. Unilateral injuries can be seen in superficial temperature differences between the left and right sides in thermographic images [11, 22]. However, superficial temperature differences up to 4.0 degrees were detected between right and left legs after the race without any obvious sign of injury. Unbalanced use of the muscles can also be seen as superficial temperature differences between the sides. The characteristics of the racetrack have an effect on injuries occurring during the races, and the speed of the dog and the raced distance are also known to influence the injury rate [24]. However, we could not evaluate such associations due to the low incidence of injuries detected by means of thermographic imaging in our material.

As the current data was not balanced (data on some distances obtained from two days and on others from just one day), a full evaluation of the differences between the distances could not be conducted. Another limitation of the present study was the rather low number of dogs, decreasing the statistical power, especially when analysing the data for the two longest distances. The low number of dogs also affected the evaluation of the effects of the explanatory variables, rank and kinetic energy. The fact that this study was conducted during an actual race with racing dogs may have caused some minor bias due to the uncontrolled environment. For example, the amount of warm-up exercise before the first thermographic imaging was not known due to the individual and private training protocols of the dogs. Even though the amount of warm-up exercise before the first thermographic imaging was not known, the dogs were queuing for at least 10 minutes before the health check, during which time the thermographic images were taken. This waiting period before the imaging most likely levels out the differences between the dogs.

In conclusion, thermographic imaging appears to be a useful tool for measuring superficial temperatures in racing greyhounds in the race setting. Increases in the superficial temperatures induced by racing could be detected by thermographic imaging. This result was predictable since the muscle work during the race generates heat. No differences were seen in the superficial temperature between the left and right legs after the race, suggesting balanced muscle work and an appropriate racetrack for racing greyhounds. The calculated heat capacity was similar for all distances raced and for both race days. In spite of the amount of heat generated during the race, the dogs did not develop signs of severe hyperthermia, which suggests that the heat loss during the race through forced convection, conduction, radiation, evaporation, and panting was adequate. Our result suggests that thermographic imaging can be used to monitor heat-balance-related well-being of the racing greyhound. However, the method of thermographic imaging needs to be studied further for more advanced applications for racing greyhounds.

Acknowledgments

The authors wish to thank Flir Sweden for providing the thermal camera for executing this study; Jouni Niemi, DVM, for the help in organizing the study; all the dogs and their owners for their contribution to the study. None of the authors of this paper have any financial or personal relationships that could inappropriately influence or bias the content of the paper.

References

[1] G. P. Dobson, W. S. Parkhouse, J. M. Weber et al., "Metabolic changes in skeletal muscle and blood of greyhounds during 800-m track sprint," *American Journal of Physiology*, vol. 255, no. 3, pp. R513–R519, 1988.

[2] S. Zaldívar-López, L. M. Lopez, M. C. Iazbik, N. Westendorf-Stingle, S. Hensley, and C. G. Couto, "Clinical pathology of Greyhounds and other sighthounds," *Veterinary Clinical Pathology*, vol. 40, no. 4, pp. 414–425, 2011.

[3] R. C. Hill, M. S. Bloomberg, V. Legrand-Defretin et al., "Maintenance energy requirements and the effect of diet on performance of racing Greyhounds," *American Journal of Veterinary Research*, vol. 61, no. 12, pp. 1566–1573, 2000.

[4] G. A. Gaesser and G. A. Brooks, "Muscular efficiency during steady rate exercise: effects of speed and work rate," *Journal of Applied Physiology*, vol. 38, no. 6, pp. 1132–1139, 1975.

[5] M. Mogensen, M. Bagger, P. K. Pedersen, M. Fernström, and K. Sahlin, "Cycling efficiency in humans is related to low UCP3 content and to type I fibres but not to mitochondrial efficiency," *Journal of Physiology*, vol. 571, no. 3, pp. 669–681, 2006.

[6] H. T. Hammel, C. H. Wyndham, and J. D. Hardy, "Heat production and heat loss in the dog at 8–36°C environmental temperature," *American Journal of Physiology*, vol. 194, no. 1, pp. 99–108, 1958.

[7] H. T. Hammel, "Thermal properties of fur," *The American Journal of Physiology*, vol. 182, no. 2, pp. 369–376, 1955.

[8] C. R. Taylor, K. Schmidt-Nielsen, R. Dmi'el, and M. Fedak, "Effect of hyperthermia on heat balance during running in the African hunting dog," *The American Journal of Physiology*, vol. 220, no. 3, pp. 823–827, 1971.

[9] M. Stewart, J. R. Webster, G. A. Verkerk, A. L. Schaefer, J. J. Colyn, and K. J. Stafford, "Non-invasive measurement of stress in dairy cows using infrared thermography," *Physiology and Behavior*, vol. 92, no. 3, pp. 520–525, 2007.

[10] D. Graf von Schweinitz, "Thermographic diagnostics in equine back pain," *The Veterinary Clinics of North America Equine Practice*, vol. 15, no. 1, pp. 161–177, 1999.

[11] T. A. Turner, "Diagnostic thermography," *The Veterinary Cof North America Equine Practice*, vol. 17, no. 1, pp. 95–113, 2001.

[12] I. Kízková and P. Kunc, "Applications of infrared thermography in animal production," *Journal of Faculty of Agriculture*, vol. 22, no. 3, pp. 329–336, 2007.

[13] T. Levet, A. Martens, L. Devisscher, L. Duchateau, L. Bogaert, and L. Vlaminck, "Distal limb cast sores in horses: risk factors and early detection using thermography," *Equine Veterinary Journal*, vol. 41, no. 1, pp. 18–23, 2009.

[14] M. H. Vainionpää, K. Salla, F. Restitutti et al., "Thermographic imaging of superficial temperature in dogs sedated with medetomidine and butorphanol with and without MK-467 (L-659'066)," *Journal of Veterinary Anaesthesia and Analgesia*. In press.

[15] C. A. Loughin and D. J. Marino, "Evaluation of thermographic imaging of the limbs of healthy dogs," *American Journal of Veterinary Research*, vol. 68, no. 10, pp. 1064–1069, 2007.

[16] T. Infernuso, C. A. Loughin, D. J. Marino, S. E. Umbaugh, and P. S. Solt, "Thermal imaging of normal and cranial cruciate ligament-deficient stifles in dogs," *Veterinary Surgery*, vol. 39, no. 4, pp. 410–417, 2010.

[17] D. J. Marino and C. A. Loughin, "Diagnostic imaging of the canine stifle: a review," *Veterinary Surgery*, vol. 39, no. 3, pp. 284–295, 2010.

[18] G. Varjú, C. F. Pieper, J. B. Renner, and V. B. Kraus, "Assessment of hand osteoarthritis: correlation between thermographic and radiographic methods," *Rheumatology*, vol. 43, no. 7, pp. 915–919, 2004.

[19] E. Y. K. Ng and E. C. Kee, "Advanced integrated technique in breast cancer thermography," *Journal of Medical Engineering and Technology*, vol. 32, no. 2, pp. 103–114, 2008.

[20] J. H. Tan, E. Y. K. Ng, U. Rajendra Acharya, and C. Chee, "Infrared thermography on ocular surface temperature: a review," *Infrared Physics and Technology*, vol. 52, no. 4, pp. 97–108, 2009.

[21] J. E. Steiss, "Muscle disorders and rehabilitation in canine athletes," *Veterinary Clinics of North America*, vol. 32, no. 1, pp. 267–285, 2002.

[22] R. Vardasca, F. Ring, P. Plassmann, and C. Jones, "Termal symmetry of the upper and lower extremities in healthy subjects," *Thermology International*, vol. 22, no. 2, pp. 53–60, 2012.

[23] FLIR Systems, Inc. 1999–2012, http://www.flir.com/cs/emea/en/view/?id=42406.

[24] G. K. Sicard, K. Short, and P. A. Manley, "A survey of injuries at five greyhound racing tracks," *Journal of Small Animal Practice*, vol. 40, no. 9, pp. 428–432, 1999.

4

High Prevalence of *Candida* Yeast in Milk Samples from Cows Suffering from Mastitis in Poland

Bozena Dworecka-Kaszak,[1] Alicja Krutkiewicz,[1] Daniel Szopa,[2] Miroslaw Kleczkowski,[3] and Malgorzata Biegańska[1]

[1] *Mycology Division, Preclinical Science Department, Faculty of Veterinary Medicine, Warsaw University of Life Sciences, Ciszewskiego 8, 02-789 Warsaw, Poland*
[2] *Molecular Genetic Division, Mother and Child institute, Kasprzaka 17a, 01-211 Warsaw, Poland*
[3] *Division of Laboratory Diagnostics, Department of Pathology and Veterinary Diagnostics, Faculty of Veterinary Medicine, Warsaw University of Life Sciences, Nowoursynowska 159, 02-776 Warsaw, Poland*

Correspondence should be addressed to Bozena Dworecka-Kaszak, bozena_kaszak@sggw.pl

Academic Editor: Lawrence W. Svenson

Mastitis is an economically important disease in which fungi belonging to the genus *Candida* may participate as etiological agents. This study focused on determining the frequency of fungal isolation and differentiation of fungal species isolated from milk of mastitic cows. Sixty-six milk samples from mastitic cows were studied, and 55 strains of fungi were isolated. Seven different species classified as *Candida* were identified basing on phenotypic properties, and the dominating species was *C. parapsilosis*. Genomic DNA was isolated and amplified in PCR with ITS1 and NL2 primers. Amplification products were digested with restriction enzymes *Hpa*II and *Eco*RI. Amplification of DNA with ITS1 and NL2 primers resulted in products of different sizes. Comparison of product sizes in restriction fragment PCR REA confirmed differences among species. Strains grouped together on the basis of phenotype characteristics differed in restriction fragment profiles. None of the investigated species showed similar genetic profiles.

1. Introduction

Mastitis in dairy cattle is an inflammatory reaction of the udder. Infection of the mammary gland is the most common and most costly disease in the dairy industry. The symptoms of mastitis include abnormalities such as a watery appearance of milk, flakes, clots, or pus in milk [1–3]. Mastitis leads to a decline in potassium, lactoferrin, and casein content in milk. Because calcium in milk is associated with casein, the disruption of casein synthesis contributes to lower levels of calcium in milk. Milk from cows with mastitis also has a higher somatic cell count which lowers the quality of milk. Mastitis occurs when leucocytes are released into the mammary gland, usually in response to invasion by microorganisms through the teat canal. This disease can be identified by external symptoms such as swelling, heat, redness, hardness, or pain of the udder. There are many bacteria known to cause mastitis which include *Pseudomonas aeruginosa, Staphylococcus aureus, Staphylococcus epidermidis, Streptococcus agalactiae, Brucella melitensis, Corynebacterium bovis, Mycoplasma sp., Escherichia coli, Klebsiella pneumoniae, Klebsiella oxytoca, Enterobacter aerogenes, Pasteurella sp., Arcanobacterium pyogenes, Proteus sp.,* and *Prototheca sp.* (algae) [1–3]. Several species of yeast or yeast-like microorganisms have been reported to cause bovine mastitis [4, 5]. *Cryptococcus neoformans* and *Candida albicans* are by far the most common causes, but other *Candida* species have also been associated with bovine mastitis. Mastitis is usually transmitted through contaminated milking machines and milker's hands or other materials. Treatment is possible with long-acting antibiotics, but milk from such cows is not marketable until drug residues have left the cow's system. Antibiotics may be administered systemically, or they may be applied locally by upward force through the teat canal. Antibiotic therapy, without identifying the mastitis-causing organisms, is frequently the veterinarian and dairy farmer's first choice of treatment for diseased cows. As a result, cases of mastitis (including fungal mastitis) that are refractory to any type of treatment occur frequently.

The incidence of mastitis due to yeast is usually low in dairy herds, but it has significantly increased during the last decade. Fungal mastitis has been described as related to treatment directed against other pathogens using contaminated syringes, canulars, or contaminated antibiotic preparations. Teat injuries may predispose to establishment of a yeast infection. Yeast intramammary infections have been reported to be responsible for at least 10% of all clinical cases seen in veterinary practice [1–3], and the majority of the cases are usually mild. Although antimycotic drugs have been used for treatment of yeast mastitis, there is no clear evidence of the effectiveness of this therapy [1–5].

The aim of the present study was to isolate, identify, and determine the prevalence of yeast in milk samples from cows suffering from mastitis in Poland.

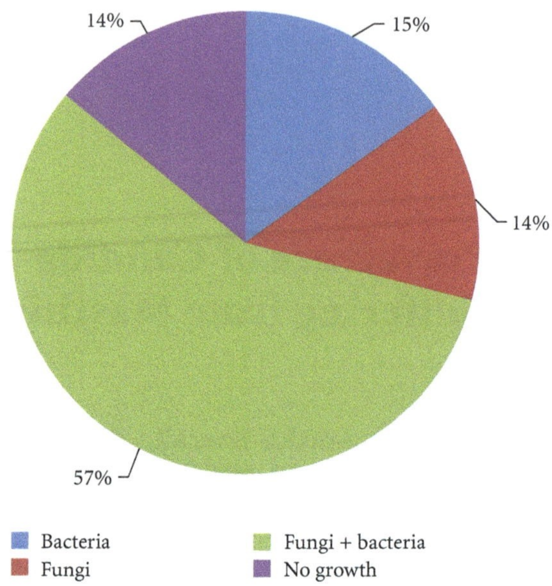

FIGURE 1: Cultivation results of milk samples from cows suffering from mastitis.

2. Materials and Methods

Sixty-six quarter-milk samples were collected from 44 cows with clinical or subclinical mastitis on small farms in the North of Poland (Łomża) or near Warsaw. Samples were plated onto Blood Agar, Macconkey Agar, and Sabouraud Dextrose Agar and incubated at 37°C for 72 h for bacteria growth and for 2 weeks for yeast. Fungi were identified phenotypically, and selected species were also identified genotypically. The genera and species of yeast were identified by API *Candida* (API C), API ID32C tests (bioMerieux), and germ tube test. Bacteria were identified and classified according to Bergey's Manual of Systematic Bacteriology [6], using morphological and biochemical characteristics and by API strip tests (API20E, API Staph, API Coryne, and API Strept).

2.1. Isolation and Amplification of Candida DNA. A PCR-based method was used to verify the identity of 20 *Candida* strains. Genomic DNA was isolated with Genomic Mini-AX Yeast Kit (DNA-Gdańsk) according to the manufacturer's protocol. DNA isolation was verified by separation on 0.8% agarose gel with ethidium bromide in TBE buffer. Electrophoresis was performed for 1 h at 100 V, and the gels were analysed in VersaDoc (BioRad) gel documentation system and quantified by Quantity One software (BioRad). To further identify the species, a 629 bp DNA fragment containing the gene encoding 5,8S rRNA and ITS sequence was amplified with 2 primers as described by Skała et al. [7], with a slight modification

ITS1 5′-TCCGTAGGTGAACCTGCGG-3′

NL2 5′-CTCTCTTTTCAAGTGCTTTTCATCT-3′.

Primers were produced by DNA IBB, PAN, Poland. The reaction mixture (50 μL) contained 50 ng yeast genomic DNA, 1 U *Taq* polymerase (Fermentas), buffer for *Taq* polymerase (Fermentas), 2 mM of each dNTP (Fermentas), 20 mM $MgCl_2$, and 1 mM each primer. Amplification was performed in Mastercycler thermal cycler according to the following protocol: denaturation at 95°C for 5 min., then 25 cycles containing denaturation at 95°C for 45 sec., annealing at 50°C for 45 sec., first extention/elongation at 72°C for 90 sec., and final elongation at 72°C for 15 min. To separate amplicons, gel electrophoresis was performed (1 h/80 V). Gels were read in VersaDoc (BioRad) by Quantity One program.

2.2. Restriction Endonuclease Analysis. To compare *Candida* isolates within the genus, amplification products were digested by 2 restriction endonucleases: *Hpa*II and *Eco*RI (Fermentas) [8, 9]. For this purpose, 10 μL of the PCR product, 2 μL of restriction enzyme, and 6 μL of buffer were mixed and incubated for 2 h at 37°C and then heated at 65°C for 20 min to inactivate the enzymes. Restriction fragments were resolved by agarose gel electrophoresis (2 h/90 V) and analyzed by Quantity One software.

3. Results

Fifty-five *isolates belonging to Candida* genus were cultured from 66 milk samples examined (Figures 1 and 2). 25 were *Candida parapsilosis,* 15 were *Candida krusei,* 5 were *Candida lusitaniae,* 5 were *Candida famata,* 3 were *Candida guilliermondii,* 1 was *Candida tropicalis,* and 1 was *Candida albicans* (Figure 3). Additionally, 27 other fungi were isolated, among which 9 were *Cryptococcus* genus, 7 were *Trichosporon* genus, 5 were isolates of *Saccharomyces* genus, 3 were isolates of *Geotrichum* genus, and 3 were *Rhodotorula* genus. Growth of mycelial fungi was treated as contamination. Bacteria typical for mastitis were also isolated. Results are shown in Table 1.

Genomic DNA was isolated from 20 randomly chosen fungal isolates identified as members of *Candida* genus and amplified with ITS1 and NL2 primers. The investigated isolates were classified into seven different species (on the base of their phenotypic properties with assistance of striped

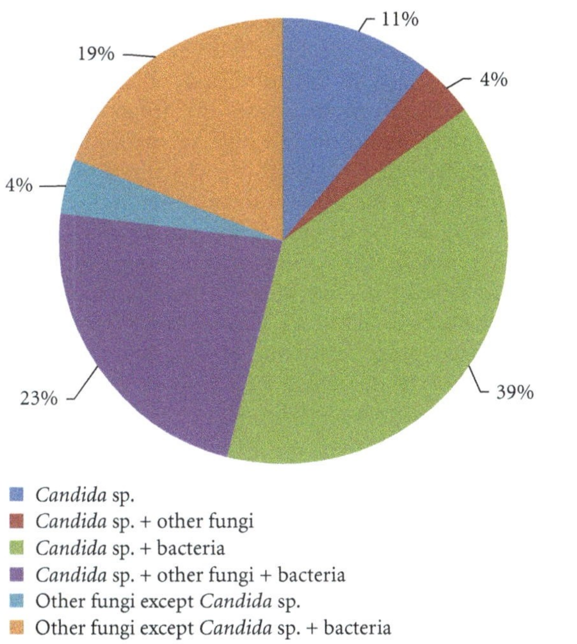

Figure 2: Percentage distribution of different mastitis aetiological agents isolated from milk samples.

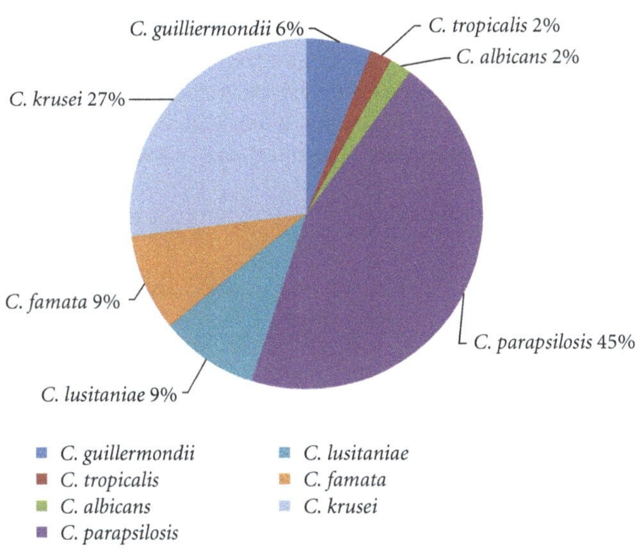

Figure 3: Proportion of *Candida* species isolated from milk samples of cows suffering from mastitis.

test evaluated API *Candida* and API ID 32C bioMerieux): 3 isolates of *C. krusei*, 3 isolates of *C. parapsilosis*, 5 isolates of *C. famata*, 3 isolates of *C. guilliermondii*, 4 isolates of *C. lusitaniae*, 1 of *C. albicans*, and 1 isolate of *C. tropicalis*. Amplification of DNA fragments with ITS1 and NL2 primers revealed products of different sizes, ranging from 700 to 1000 bp dependent on species from which genetic material was isolated (Table 2).

PCR amplification products were digested by restriction enzymes *Hpa*II and *Eco*RI (Table 3). Comparison of restriction fragments confirmed differences among species

Table 1: Bacteria isolated from milk samples of mastitic cows.

Species	Number of isolates
Streptococcus agalactiae	5
Streptococcus α-hemolytic	7
Staphylococcus coagulase-negative	3
Staphylococcus aureus	6
Escherichia coli	15
Proteus sp.	8
Corynebacterium sp.	2
Total	46

Table 2: PCR products of *Candida* of genomic DNA generated with the ITS1 and NL2 primers. Black bold type fonts shows Warsaw isolates.

Species	Strains	Product size [bp]
C. famata	1	950
	2	950
	3	750
	4	750
	5	**1050**
C. krusei	1	700
	2	650
	3	650
C. parapsilosis	1	950
	2	840
	3	700
C. guilliermondii	1	**800**
	2	700
	3	700
C. lusitaniae	1	800
	2	850
	3	1000
	4	1000
C. tropicalis	1	1000
C. albicans	1	900

(Table 3). However, isolates qualified on the base of phenotype into one species differed greatly in restriction fragment profiles. None of the investigated species revealed a characteristically similar genetic profile. Results reported here indicate that isolates of fungi phenotypically similar, such as *Candida* species, may exhibit a differentiated genotype regarding location of restriction sites of the same restriction enzyme.

4. Discussion

The fungi of *Candida* sp. generally grow well on Sabouraud Agar at 37°C, usually forming colonies within 24–48 h. Colonies are opaque, often white or yellowish, and at first usually smooth. Their texture is creamy or pasty, and in a microscopic smear it appears to consist solely of oval to round budding blastospores. In our examination, we noted that yeast from milk of mastitic cows required more

TABLE 3: Restriction endonuclease analysis of PCR products digested with *Hpa*II and *EcoR*I. Black bold type fonts shows Warsaw isolates.

Size of products after digestion with restriction enzymes [bp] *Hpa*II	*EcoR*I	Strains	Species
950	950	1	*C. famata*
950	950	2	
420 330	750	3	
420 330	750	4	
600 450	**>1000**	5	
410 400	**800**	1	*C. guilliermondii*
400 300	600 100	2	
400 300	600 100	3	
1000	1000	1	*C. tropicalis*
450 450	900	1	*C. albicans*
700	700	1	*C. krusei*
400 250	650	2	
400 250	650	3	
330	800	1	*C. lusitaniae*
350 300 200	850	2	
1000	1000	3	
1000	1000	4	
950	950	1	*C. parapsilosis*
350 250 240	840	2	
400 300	700	3	

time to form colonies during cultivation. Most colonies appeared at 48–72 h after the milk samples were plated, but some strains needed almost one week to grow on the medium. In our opinion, the delayed growth could have been a result of abnormal conditions previously found in the milk (acidic pH, lack of proteins, etc.) such that the fungi needed more time to adapt to growth in a new environment. This observation suggests that fungal growth may be underestimated if growth observation is terminated early.

Our investigation shows a high frequency of bacterial-fungal infections, approximately 57% of all examined samples. Bacteria or fungi as sole etiological agents were found in 15% and 14%, respectively, of investigated samples. *Candida* yeast was isolated from 39% of the mixed infections, and in 11% of these cases, it was a sole infectious agent.

Krukowski et al. [10] isolated fungi as pure cultures from 9.6% of investigated milk samples in the Lublin region in Poland, a result much similar to ours. According to Casia dos Santos and Mo acir Marin [11], the percentage of fungal isolation in surveys carried out in many countries varies considerably, with 6,1% rates described in Egypt [12], 1,3% in Denmark [13], and 12,07% in Brazil [14]. Casia dos Santos and Moacir Marin [11] isolated fungi in 32% of the cases, and 17.3% of these were *Candida* spp.

Candida is commonly viewed as an opportunistic yeast pathogen, and the source of infection may be skin of the udder, milker's hands, milking machines, floors, straw, feed, medications, sanitary agents, and other equipment [15, 16]. Under immunosuppressive conditions, the population size balance may be disrupted, and the fungi together with the other microorganisms are able to overcome the udder defense mechanisms. Although the distribution of *Candida* species shows diversity in several countries, it is important to note the increase in number of mammary gland infections caused by *Candida* species in the recent years. Krukowski et al. [10] reported that the most frequently isolated species in Poland were *C. kefyr, C. cirferi,* and *C. krusei.* In the other reports, more frequent were *C. krusei, C. rugosa,* and *C. albicans,* as described by Costa et al. [2, 14, 16] or Şeker [15]. In our investigation, the most frequently isolated species was *C. parapsilosis* (25 strains) followed by *C. krusei* (15 strains). *Candida albicans* was isolated only from one sample (confirmed by positive germ tube test). In our experiments, *Candida* strains were first identified phenotypically by API *Candida* (API C) and API ID 32C tests (bioMerieux) and germ tube test and then confirmed by genotypic methods. Comparison of PCR product size confirmed differences between species. However, isolates qualified into one species on the basis of phenotypic characteristics alone differed genotypically. We did not generate comparable genetic profiles in any of the species investigated, particularly in the strains originating from the North of Poland and the Warsaw area. Our results indicate that strains of fungi phenotypically classified as the same *Candida* species can have different genotypes generated by restriction endonuclease analysis. This high interspecies heterogeneity may suggest large environmental adaptive properties of *Candida* strains.

References

[1] H. Krukowski, "Mycotic mastitis in cows," *Medycyna Weterynaryjna*, vol. 57, no. 1, pp. 18–20, 2001.

[2] E. O. Costa, A. R. Ribeiro, E. T. Watanabe, and P. A. Melville, "Infectious bovine mastitis caused by environmental organisms," *Journal of Veterinary Medicine Series B*, vol. 45, no. 2, pp. 65–71, 1998.

[3] G. M. Jones, "Understanding the Basics of Mastitis," http://pubs.ext.vt.edu/404/404-233/404-233.html.

[4] Z. Staroniewicz, A. Włodarczak, M. Florek, and J. Król, "Fungal flora in cows with mastitis and its susceptibility to antimycotics," *Mikologia Lekarska*, vol. 14, no. 4, pp. 257–259, 2007.

[5] A. Sheena and L. Sigler, "*Candida krusei* isolated from a sporadic case of bovine mastitis," *Canadian Veterinary Journal*, vol. 36, no. 6, p. 365, 1995.

[6] *Bergey's Manual of Determinative Bacteriology*, Wiliams and Wilkins, Baltimore, Md, USA, 9th edition, 1994.

[7] J. Skała, N. Potocka, M. Bortniczuk et al., "Molecular identification strains from *Candida, Cryptococcus, Hansenula, Rhodotorula* and *Trichosporon* genus," in *Proceedings of the Materiały Naukowe 9 Konferencji Biologia Molekularna w Diagnostyce Chorób Zakaźnych i Biotechnologii*, pp. 143–146, Warszawa, Poland, 2006.

[8] J. Campos De Pinho Resende, G. R. Franco, C. A. Rosa, R. C. Hahn, and J. Soares Hamdan, "Phenotypic and genotypic identification of *Candida* spp. isolated from hospitalized

patients," *Revista Iberoamericana de Micologia*, vol. 21, no. 1, pp. 24–28, 2004.

[9] I. Mecler and U. Nawrot, "Molecular methods of *Candida* identifiction," *Mikologia Lekarska*, vol. 15, no. 2, pp. 99–103, 2008.

[10] H. Krukowski, M. Tietze, T. Majewski, and P. Różański, "Survey of yeast mastitis in dairy herds of small-type farms in the Lublin region, Poland," *Mycopathologia*, vol. 150, no. 1, pp. 5–7, 2001.

[11] R. De Casia Dos Santos and J. M. Marin, "Isolation of *Candida* spp. from mastitic bovine milk in Brazil," *Mycopathologia*, vol. 159, no. 2, pp. 251–253, 2005.

[12] F. I. Awad, A. El Molla, A. Fayed, M. Abd el-Halim, and M. Refai, "Studies of mycotic mastitis in Egypt," *Journal of Egyptian Veterinary Medical Association*, vol. 40, no. 3, pp. 35–41, 1980.

[13] B. Aalbek, J. Stenderup, H. E. Jensen, J. Valbak, B. Nylin, and A. Huda, "Mycotic and algal bovine mastitis in Denmark," *Acta Pathologica, Microbiologica et Immunologica*, vol. 102, no. 6, pp. 451–456, 1994.

[14] E. O. Costa, C. R. Gandra, M. F. Pires, S. D. Coutinho, W. Castilho, and C. M. Teixeira, "Survey of bovine mycotic mastitis in dairy herds in the State of São Paulo, Brazil," *Mycopathologia*, vol. 124, no. 1, pp. 13–17, 1993.

[15] E. Şeker, "Identification of *Candida* species isolated from bovine mastitic milk and their in vitro hemolytic activity in western Turkey," *Mycopathologia*, vol. 169, no. 4, pp. 303–308, 2010.

[16] E. O. Da Costa, M. Ribeiro, A. R. Ribeiro, N. S. Rocha, and G. D. N. Júnior, "Diagnosis of clinical bovine mastitis by fine needle aspiration followed by staining and scanning electron microscopy in a Prototheca zopfii outbreak," *Mycopathologia*, vol. 158, no. 1, pp. 81–85, 2004.

Effect of Dietary Supplements in Reducing Probability of Death for Uremic Crises in Dogs Affected by Chronic Kidney Disease (Masked RCCT)

Andrea Zatelli,[1] Marco Pierantozzi,[1] Paola D'Ippolito,[1] Mauro Bigliati,[2] and Eric Zini[3,4]

[1] *Clinica Veterinaria Pirani, Nephrology and Urology Division, Via Majakowski 2/L,M,N, 42124 Reggio Emilia, Italy*
[2] *Istituto Farmaceutico Candioli, Via Manzoni 2, 10192 Beinasco, Italy*
[3] *Istituto Veterinario di Novara, S.P. 9, 28060 Granozzo con Monticello, Italy*
[4] *Department of Veterinary Clinical Sciences, University of Padua, 35020 Agripolis, Legnaro, Italy*

Correspondence should be addressed to Andrea Zatelli, az@clinicaveterinariapirani.it

Academic Editor: Jiannong Liu

Chitosan and alkalinizing agents can decrease morbidity and mortality in humans with chronic kidney disease (CKD). Whether this holds true in dog is not known. Objective of the study was to determine whether a commercial dietary supplement containing chitosan, phosphate binders, and alkalinizing agents (Renal), compared to placebo, reduces mortality rate due to uremic crises in dogs with spontaneous CKD, fed a renal diet (RD). A masked RCCT was performed including 31 azotemic dogs with spontaneous CKD. Dogs enrolled in the study were randomly allocated to receive RD plus placebo (group A; 15 dogs) or RD plus Renal (group B; 16 dogs). During a first 4-week period, all dogs were fed an RD and then randomized and clinically evaluated up to 44 weeks. The effects of dietary supplements on mortality rate due to uremic crises were assessed. At 44 weeks, compared to group A, dogs in group B had approximately 50% lower mortality rate due to uremic crises ($P = 0.015$). Dietary supplementation with chitosan, phosphate binders, and alkalinizing agents, along with an RD, is beneficial in reducing mortality rate in dogs with spontaneous CKD.

1. Introduction

There is a strong consensus to use dietary modification in dogs affected by chronic kidney disease (CKD) [1–7]. Feeding a renal diet (RD) in dogs with mild and moderate spontaneous CKD had beneficial effects on uremia and mortality rate compared to a maintenance diet [1]. In addition, phosphate retention and renal secondary hyperparathyroidism are common complications of CKD [2–7], and hyperphosphatemia is associated with the development of renal lesions in dogs and cats [2–7]. In humans and cats, oral supplementation with compounds such as chitosan (produced by deacetylation of chitin, which is the structural element in the exoskeleton of crustaceans and cell wall of fungi), calcium carbonate, and potassium citrate has been advocated to control hyperphosphatemia [4–11]. In addition, chitosan is recognized to reduce azotemia during spontaneous CKD in humans and cats [8–10]. However, whether this holds true for dog has not been previously assessed. Aim of the present study was to evaluate the efficacy of a commercial oral supplement rich in chitosan, enteric phosphate binders, and alkalinizing agents (Renal—Istituto Farmaceutico Candioli SpA, Italy), in reducing mortality rate due to uremic crises in dogs affected by spontaneous CKD, in International Renal Interest Society (IRIS) stages 2, 3, and 4 [4, 12], fed an RD.

2. Materials and Methods

2.1. Animals. Dogs affected by CKD, in IRIS stages 2, 3, and 4, were recruited at the Clinica Veterinaria Pirani of Reggio Emilia, Italy. Results of history, physical examination, including body weight (BW) and body condition score (BCS) (1 to 5 scoring system (3 optimal)), CBC, serum biochemical profile, urinalysis, urine protein-to-creatinine (UPC) ratio, venous blood gas analysis, and indirect blood pressure measurement were collected. All dogs underwent abdominal ultrasonographic examination, which was performed by the same operator and with the same instrument (Philips HD11XE or Philips HD7XE, Philips Ultrasound, Bothell, Washington, USA). Dogs of any age were included if presenting inactive urine sediment and stable renal function, as defined by serum creatinine concentrations above 1.4 mg/dL (IRIS stages ≥ 2) that did not increase or decrease by 20% or more within 4 weeks from initial determination [4]. In the first 4-week period, all dogs were started on an RD (Royal Canin Renal Canine, Royal Canin SA, Aimargues, France; Hill's Prescription Diet Canine k/d, Hill's Pet Nutrition Inc, Topeka, Kansas, USA).

Dogs were excluded if clinically affected or suspected to be affected by genitourinary tract inflammation or infection, cardiac disease, neoplasia, and endocrinopathies. As a standard, dogs with arterial pressure (AP) substage 3 of the IRIS staging system [12] were treated with oral amlodipine at 0.1 to 0.5 mg/kg, *q* 24 hr, in order to reduce AP to substage 1 or 0 [6, 7, 13, 14]. Dogs with serum albumin concentration ≤ 2.0 g/dL received oral acetylsalicylic acid at 2.0 mg/kg *q* 24 hr, to prevent thrombosis [6] (Shearer L, Kruth SA, Wood D. Effects of aspirin and clopidogrel on platelet function in healthydogs. J Vet Intern Med 2009; 23(3): 745 (abstract)).

2.2. Study Design. A randomized, blinded, placebo-controlled clinical trial was performed using a software to allocate cases (MedCalc, Version 11.3.0.0). Informed consent to participate in the study was signed by dog owners.

In the first 4 weeks following inclusion all dogs were started on an RD (Royal Canin Renal Canine, Royal Canin SA, Aimargues, France; Hill's Prescription Diet Canine k/d, Hill's Pet Nutrition Inc, Topeka, Kansas, USA). At the end of this first period, all dogs were clinically reevaluated, performing all above-mentioned laboratory and instrumental analyses and assigned to group A (RD plus placebo), or treatment group B (RD plus Renal). Compositions of the dietary supplements are provided in Table 1.

To mask the identity of the two supplements, they were formulated as powders with identical colours and contained in the same package. After assignment to group A and B, dogs were reassessed between week 4 and 8. Thereafter, examinations were scheduled every 4 months and up to 44 weeks of treatment, or earlier if worsening of clinical signs was noted by the owner.

2.3. Blood Sampling and Assay. During each examination, a blood sample was collected in overnight fasted dogs, and serum was obtained within 30 minutes, stored at 4°C and analyzed within 24 hours. Venous blood gas analysis (Rapidpoint 400, Bayer Health Care, Tarrytown (NY), USA) was immediately performed in all cases.

CBC and serum biochemical analysis, including albumin, total protein, glucose, bilirubin, cholesterol, amylase, alanine transferase, alkaline phosphatase, blood urea nitrogen (BUN), creatinine, ionized calcium, sodium, potassium, chloride, and phosphate, were determined by the use of standard methods (Cobas Mira, Roche Diagnostic, Basel, Switzerland). Blood samples were labelled with alphanumeric codes assigned by randomization to ensure that laboratory personals were blinded during processing. All of the above-mentioned biochemical parameters were used for inclusion and exclusion evaluation.

TABLE 1: Composition of placebo and Renal.

Placebo
Maltodextrin
Renal
Maltodextrin
Calcium carbonate (Ca 38%)
Potassium Cytrate (K 36%)
Chitosan

2.4. Urine Sample and Urinalysis. During abdominal ultrasonography, an echo-guided cystocentesis was performed in all dogs, by the use of a 5 mL syringe connected to a 23-gauge needle. All urine samples were put in 10 mL, sterile, evacuated collection tubes labelled with alphanumeric codes based on the previous randomization. All urine samples were analyzed by the same operator. Urines were examined within 60 minutes from collection if samples were stored at room temperature (approx. 20°C), or within 4 hours if samples were stored at 4° to 8°C. Urine sediment was obtained by centrifugation (10 minutes at 900 ×g) of 5 mL of urine, followed by removal of 4.5 mL of supernatant, and by resuspension of the remaining 0.5 mL of urine. A sample of 12 μL of the resuspended urine was microscopically assessed. The supernatant was transferred into separate tubes and stored at −20°C to determine urine protein and creatinine concentration within 7 days. RBCs and WBCs were expressed as mean number of cells/10 hpf (40x magnification). Urine sediment with bacteriuria, and/or >5 RBCs or WBCs/hpf, was considered indicative of active inflammation.

2.5. UPC Ratio. To calculate the UPC ratio, protein concentration (mg/dL) was measured with pyrogallol red, and creatinine (mg/dL) was measured by the use of the Jaffé method in undiluted urine that was thawed before the analysis. Analytes were measured in an automated spectrophotometer (Cobas Mira, Roche Diagnostic, Basel, Switzerland). Dogs were classified as nonproteinuric, borderline proteinuric, or proteinuric according to the IRIS staging system (UPC ratio < 0.2 = nonproteinuric, UPC ratio 0.2 to 0.5 = borderline proteinuric, and UPC ratio > 0.5 = proteinuric) [4, 12].

2.6. Blood Pressure Measurement. Systolic blood pressure measurements were obtained by the use of an ultrasonic Doppler device (DOP 2001, SAMED Elettromedicali srl, Merlino (LO), Italy) in all dogs [13, 14].

2.7. Diagnosis of Uremic Crisis. Diagnosis of uremic crisis was established by clinicians involved in patient management unaware of the supplement being administered. As previously suggested by Jacob and colleagues [1], uremic crisis

Table 2: Mean, median, and 25% and 75% for BW and BCS, hematocrit, serum creatinine, BUN, phosphate, blood pH, bicarbonate, and UPC ratio, for Group A and B at time of randomization. Differences between groups are depicted by P value (statistically significant $P < 0.05$).

	Group A	Group B	P value (A Versus B)
BW (kg)			
mean	*18.2*	*21.0*	
median	14.4	17.8	0.17
25% percentile; 75% percentile	(8.5; 29.0)	(9.7; 29.9)	
BSC (1–5)			
mean	*2.8*	*2.7*	
median	3.0	3.0	1.00
25% percentile; 75% percentile	(3.0; 3.0)	(2.0; 3.0)	
Serum Creatinine (mg/dL)			
mean	*5.7*	*4.9*	
median	3.1	4.1	0.66
25% percentile; 75% percentile	(1.9; 10.5)	(2.1; 7.23)	
BUN (mg/dL)			
mean	*97.1*	*86.2*	
median	69.0	75.1	0.76
25% percentile; 75% percentile	(32.2; 204.0)	(42.9; 150.1)	
Phosphorus (mg/dL)			
mean	*8.9*	*7.1*	
median	7.2	7.2	0.90
25% percentile; 75% percentile	(5.4; 11.0)	(5.0; 9.5)	
Blood pH			
mean	*7.30*	*7.29*	
median	7.30	7.34	0.55
25% percentile; 75% percentile	(7.25; 7.40)	(7.20; 7.39)	
$HCO3^-$ (mEq/L)			
mean	*18.9*	*18.4*	
median	19.1	18.2	0.14
25% percentile; 75% percentile	(16.0; 23.4)	(14.6; 22.7)	
Hct (%)			
mean	*30.7*	*32.1*	
median	34.00	33.0	0.37
25% percentile; 75% percentile	(24.6; 39.0)	(24.5; 41.0)	
UPC ratio			
mean	*2.90*	*0.62*	
median	0.68	0.39	0.41
25% percentile; 75% percentile	(0.24; 1.60)	(0.29; 0.80)	

was defined when the 3 following findings were observed: (i) identification of at least 2 clinical signs consistent with uremia including depression, lethargy, anorexia, vomiting, uremic breath odour; (ii) serum creatinine concentration at least 20% greater than the previously determined value; (iii) no plausible alternative for these clinical signs.

2.8. Establishing Cause of Death. Causes of death were categorized as nonrenal, probably renal or renal, based on results of anamnesis, physical examination, blood and urine tests, and criteria used to define uremic crisis. To avoid bias, only dogs classified in the third category were considered to have died from a renal event (uremic crisis). Necropsies were not performed in any case.

2.9. Statistical Analysis. Dogs characteristics between groups were compared at the time of group assignment, and intragroup during reexamination at 4–8 weeks of treatment, using the Mann-Whitney nonparametric test. We statistically evaluated the following parameters: BCS and BW, hematocrit, serum creatinine, BUN, phosphate, blood pH, bicarbonate, and UPC ratio.

Kaplan-Meier was used to evaluate the survival probability in both groups and the Logrank test was used to compare rates of death due to uremic crisis between groups. In addition, the Kaplan-Meier was used to evaluate the probability of maintaining stable serum creatinine (serum creatinine concentration not increased above 20% compared to randomization time) in both groups, and the Logrank test

Table 3: Mean, median, and 25% and 75% percentile for BW and BCS, hematocrit, serum creatinine, BUN, phosphate, blood pH, bicarbonate, and UPC ratio, for group B at time of randomization (T0) and after 4–8 weeks (T1) of treatment. Differences between values at different examinations are depicted by P value (statistically significant $P < 0.05$).

	T0	T1	P value (T0 Versus T1)
BW (kg)			
mean	*21.0*	*23.9*	
median	17.8	23.0	0.06
25% percentile; 75% percentile	(9.7; 29.9)	(9.5; 33.9)	
BSC (1–5)			
mean	*2.7*	*2.8*	
median	3.0	3.0	1.00
25% percentile; 75% percentile	(2.0; 3.0)	(2.5; 3.0)	
Serum Creatinine (mg/dL)			
mean	*4.9*	*4.4*	
median	4.1	3.4	0.50
25% percentile; 75% percentile	(2.1; 7.23)	(1.7; 6.0)	
BUN (mg/dL)			
mean	*86.2*	*87.6*	
median	75.1	63.3	0.55
25% percentile; 75% percentile	(42.9; 150.1)	(55.0; 77.0)	
Phosphorus (mg/dL)			
mean	*7.1*	*6.9*	
median	7.2	5.4	0.87
25% percentile; 75% percentile	(5.0; 9.5)	(4.2; 10.7)	
Blood pH			
mean	*7.29*	*7.30*	
median	7.34	7.30	0.69
25% percentile; 75% percentile	(7.20; 7.39)	(7.25; 7.40)	
$HCO3^-$ (mEq/L)			
mean	*18.4*	*19.8*	
median	18.2	20.5	0.20
25% percentile; 75% percentile	(14.6; 22.7)	(16.1; 22.6)	
Hct (%)			
mean	*32.1*	*34.2*	
median	33.0	34.0	0.49
25% percentile; 75% percentile	(24.5; 41.0)	(29.6; 40.7)	
UPC ratio			
mean	*0.62*	*0.58*	
median	0.39	0.3	0.39
25% percentile; 75% percentile	(0.29; 0.80)	(0.25; 0.79)	

was used to compare rates of creatinine variation between groups. Statistical analysis was performed with a commerciall software, using the intention-to-treat principle. Significance was defined as $P < 0.05$.

3. Results

3.1. Dogs and Groups. Thirty-one dogs were enrolled in the study. The median age of all dogs was 6 years (range 10 months–13 years). The median age of dogs in group A was 5 years. The median age of dogs in group B was 7 years. Four dogs were intact females, 16 were spayed females, 11 were males. Seven dogs were mixed breed, 2 each Dalmatian, German Shepherd, and Boxer, 1 each Beagle, Boxer, Cavalier King Charles Spaniel, American Pittbull, Dobermann, Golden Retriever, Labrador Retriever, Rottweiler, Border Collie, Bullmastiff, English Bulldog, English Cocker, English Setter, Greyhound, Irish Wolfhound, York-Shire Terrier, and Miniature Poodle.

Fifteen dogs were allocated in group A, and 16 in group B. At the time of allocation, there was no statistical difference between groups with regard to BW and BCS, hematocrit, serum creatinine, BUN, phosphate, blood pH, bicarbonate, and UPC ratio (Table 2).

Four dogs in both groups had arterial pressure (AP) in substage 3 of the IRIS staging system [12] and were treated with oral amlodipine (Norvasc, Pfizer Manufacturing Deutschland GmbH, Illertissen, Germany). Five dogs in

TABLE 4: Mean, median, 25% and 75% percentile for BW and BCS, hematocrit, serum creatinine, BUN, phosphate, blood pH, bicarbonate, and UPC ratio, for group A at time of randomization (T0) and after 4–8 weeks (T1) of treatment. Difference between values at different examinations are depicted by P-value (statistically significant $P < 0.05$).

	T0	T1	P value (T0 Versus T1)
BW (kg)			
mean	*18.2*	*24.4*	0.66
median	14.4	27.9	
25% percentile; 75% percentile	(8.5; 29.0)	(18.1; 31.9)	
BSC (1–5)			
mean	*2.8*	*3.2*	1.00
median	3.0	3.0	
25% percentile; 75% percentile	(3.0; 3.0)	(3.0; 4.0)	
Serum Creatinine (mg/dL)			
mean	*5.7*	*4.2*	0.77
median	3.1	2.0	
25% percentile; 75% percentile	(1.9; 10.5)	(1.5; 5.8)	
BUN (mg/dL)			
mean	*97.1*	*77.0*	
median	69.0	32.8	0.54
25% percentile; 75% percentile	(32.2; 204.0)	(18.9; 121.6)	
Phosphorus (mg/dL)			
mean	*8.9*	*6.6*	
median	7.2	5.5	0.97
25% percentile; 75% percentile	(5.4; 11.0)	(4.7; 7.8)	
Blood pH			
mean	*7.30*	*7.32*	
median	7.30	7.30	0.65
25% percentile; 75% percentile	(7.25; 7.40)	(7.30; 7.35)	
$HCO3^-$ (mEq/L)			
mean	*18.9*	*20.2*	
median	19.1	19.5	0.43
25% percentile; 75% percentile	(16.0; 23.4)	(16.3; 24.4)	
Hct (%)			
mean	*30.7*	*38.7*	
median	34.0	40.0	0.40
25% percentile; 75% percentile	(24.6; 39.0)	(28.8; 45.3)	
UPC ratio			
mean	*2.90*	*1.39*	
median	0.68	0.55	0.54
25% percentile; 75% percentile	(0.24; 1.60)	(0.26; 0.70)	

Group A and 6 dogs in Group B had low serum albumin level (serum albumin concentration ≤ 2.0 g/dL) and received oral acetylsalicylic acid at 2.0 mg/kg *q* 24 hr.

3.2. Followup: BW and BCS, Hematocrit, Serum Creatinine, BUN, Phosphate, Blood pH, Bicarbonate, Potassium, Calcium, and UPC Ratio. When values recorded at 4–8 weeks following supplement administration were compared with those collected at randomization time, in both groups, there was an improvement for mean serum concentrations of creatinine, BUN, phosphate, bicarbonate, and results of venous blood gas analysis, but it was statistically insignificant (Tables 3 and 4). Potassium and calcium remained stable in both groups A and B, and no episodes of hyperkalemia or of hypercalcemia were identified during the study period. There were a significant increase in BW in group B 4–8 weeks following enrolment (Table 3).

3.3. Associations between Dietary Supplements and Serum Creatinine or Death for Uremic Crises. There was a statistically significant difference ($P = 0.0063$; chi-square = 7.44; 95% CI 0.1231 to 0.8615) between groups A and B regarding the probability of maintaining stable level of serum creatinine, with a median period of 16 weeks for group A and 32 weeks for group B (Figure 1(a)). By the end of the study, 9 out of 15 dogs in group A were dead (8 for uremic crises), against 6

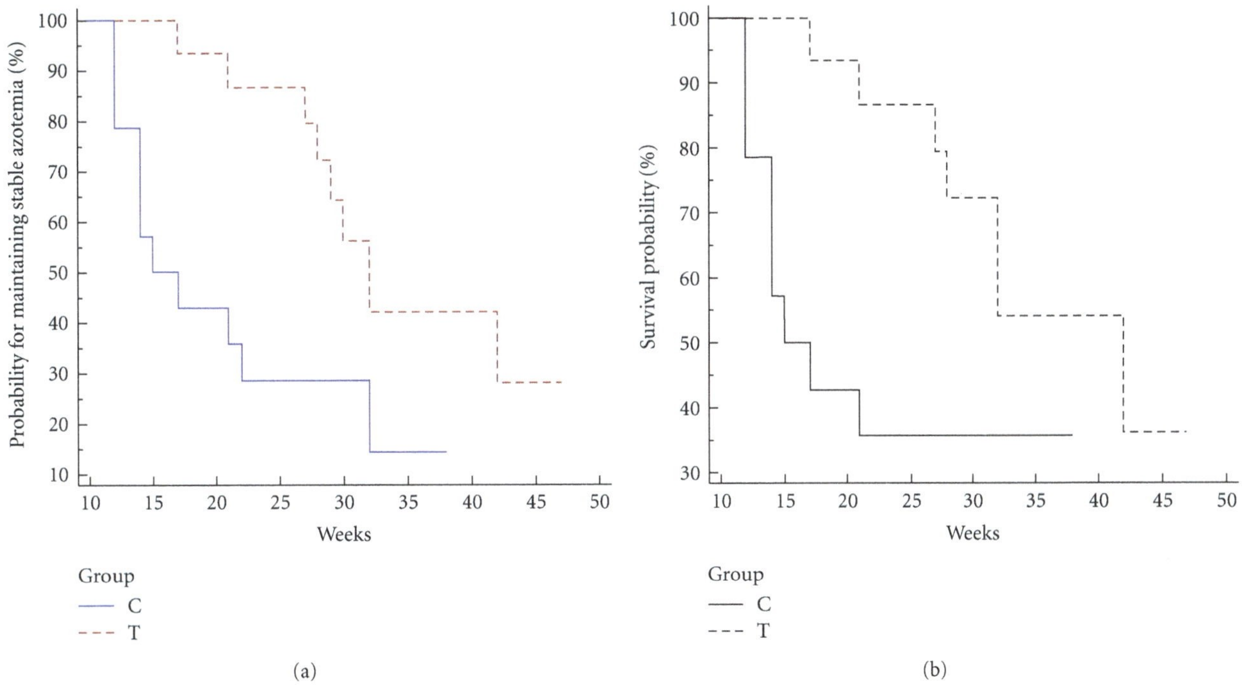

FIGURE 1: (a) Kaplan-Meier evaluating the probability of maintaining stable level of serum creatinine in treatment group B and in placebo group A. Legend: C: placebo control group A; T: treatment group B. (b) Survival curves (death from renal causes) in CKD dogs in IRIS stages 2, 3, and 4 in treatment group B and in placebo control group A. Legend: C: placebo control group A; T: treatment group B.

out of 16 in group B (5 for uremic crises). Median survival of dogs in group B was 42 weeks and was significantly longer than in the control group, with a median survival of 16 weeks ($P = 0.0015$; chi-square = 5.88; 95% CI 0.1093 to 0.9476) (Figure 1(b)). Nonrenal causes of death included one case of aspiration pneumonia in group B, and in group A one dog died because of metastatic hemangiosarcoma. The percentage of deaths due to nonrenal causes did not differ between groups.

4. Discussion

In a previously published study, admission concentration of serum creatinine did not influence survival in dogs with spontaneous CKD if an RD was administered [1]. Indeed, median survival for 21 dogs fed an RD and with a mean serum creatinine concentration of 3.3 mg/dL was 615 days, and median survival for dogs with serum creatinine between 2.0 and 3.1 mg/dL was also 615 days [1]. Differently, among 17 dogs fed a maintenance diet, median survival for dogs with a mean serum creatinine of 3.7 mg/dL was of only 252 days, whereas that of the subpopulation with serum creatinine between 2.0 and 3.1 mg/dL was 461 days [1].

In the present investigation, all dogs were fed an RD, and the mean serum creatinine concentration at the time of randomization was 5.7 mg/dL in group A and 4.9 mg/dL in group B. After 336 days of treatment, 10 out of 16 dogs in group B were alive, compared to 6 out of 15 dogs in group A, with a median survival time of 42 and 16 weeks, respectively ($P = 0.0015$), suggesting that chitosan together with alkalinizing agents are useful in maintaining long-term good clinical conditions in dogs, similar to previous studies performed in humans and cats [8–10]. In addition, the beneficial effect of the dietary supplement was evident on renal function which was stable, based on creatinine concentration, twice as much longer in group B compared to group A ($P = 0.0063$). It is worth mentioning that the improvement of blood analytes observed in the placebo-treated group A after 4–8 weeks of treatment was biased by 3 dogs that died due to severe renal failure and were therefore not included in the analysis. In contrast, none of the dogs in group B had died by 4–8 weeks and was excluded from analysis.

In humans, two possible explanations have been proposed for the reduction of serum concentrations of nitrogen metabolites, including their increased clearance due to compensatory hypertrophy of the remaining nephrons, and their enhanced excretion bound to chitosan in the digestive tract [8, 15]. Furthermore, it has been reported that chitosan can combine with acidic substances suspected to be uremic toxins, resulting in their greater excretion from the body, thus in improved clinical conditions [8, 16]; whether these same effects are exerted in dogs has not been studied but the present results may suggest that one or more of these mechanisms operate also in this species. Furthermore, because the supplement contains different substances, it cannot be excluded that phosphate binders and alkalinizing agents, or their combination, are active against uremic toxins rather than chitosan. In summary, the present study shows the beneficial effect of a commercial dietary supplement including chitosan, enteric phosphate binders, and alkalinizing agents in dogs affected by spontaneous CKD in IRIS stages 2, 3, and 4, fed an RD. The fact that serum creatinine concentration was significantly more stable and for a longer period of time in dogs receiving the supplement (Group B) is consistent with the hypothesis that delay in development of uremic crises and associated mortality rate was related, at least in part, with a reduction in the progression of renal failure.

Abbreviations

CKD:	Chronic kidney disease
RD:	Renal diet
IRIS:	International Renal Interest Society
BW:	Body weight
BCS:	Body condition score
BUN:	Blood urea nitrogen
UPC:	Urine protein–to-creatinine
AP:	Arterial pressure
RR:	Relative risk
95% CI:	95% confidence interval.

Acknowledgment

This study was supported by a grant of Istituto Farmaceutico Candioli, Italy.

References

[1] F. Jacob, D. J. Polzin, C. A. Osborne et al., "Clinical evaluation of dietary modification for treatment of spontaneous chronic renal failure in dogs," *Journal of the American Veterinary Medical Association*, vol. 220, no. 8, pp. 1163–1170, 2002.

[2] D. J. Polzin, C. A. Osborne, F. Jacob et al., "Chronic renal failure," in *Textbook of Veterinary Internal Medicine*, S. J. Ettinger and C. R. Feldman, Eds., pp. 1634–1662, WB Saunders, Philadelphia, Pa, USA, 5th edition, 2000.

[3] S. A. Brown, "Chronic renal failure: recent developments in medical managements," in *Manual of Canine and Feline Nephrology and Urology*, J. Bainbridge and J. Elliott, Eds., pp. 195–208, British Small Animal Veterinary Association, Cheltenham, UK, 1996.

[4] J. Elliott and A. D. J. Watson, "Chronic kidney disease: staging and management," in *Kirk's Current Veterinary Therapy*, J. D. Bonagura and D. C. Twedt, Eds., pp. 883–892, Elsevier Saunders, St. Louis, Mo, USA, 14th edition, 2009.

[5] D. J. Polzin, "Chronic kidney disease," in *Textbook of Veterinary Internal Medicine*, S. J. Ettinger and E. C. Feldman, Eds., pp. 1990–2021, Elsevier Saunders, St. Louis, Mo, USA, 7th edition, 2010.

[6] D. J. Polzin, C. A. Osborne, and S. Ross, "Evidence-based management of CKD," in *Kirk's Current Veterinary Therapy*, J. D. Bonagura and D. C. Twedt, Eds., pp. 872–879, Elsevier Saunders, St. Louis, Mo, USA, 14th edition, 2009.

[7] http://www.iris-kidney.com/pdf/IRIS_2009_Treatment_Recommendations_Summary.pdf.

[8] S.-B. Jing, L. Li, D. Ji, Y. Takiguchi, and T. Yamaguchi, "Effect of chitosan on renal function in patients with chronic renal failure," *Journal of Pharmacy and Pharmacology*, vol. 49, no. 7, pp. 721–723, 1997.

[9] V. Savica, L. A. Calò, P. Monardo et al., "Salivary phosphate-binding chewing gum reduces hyperphosphatemia in dialysis patients," *Journal of the American Society of Nephrology*, vol. 20, no. 3, pp. 639–644, 2009.

[10] E. Wagner, I. Schwendenwein, and J. Zentek, "Effects of a dietary chitosan and calcium supplement on Ca and P metabolism in cats," *Berliner und Munchener Tierarztliche Wochenschrift*, vol. 117, no. 7-8, pp. 310–315, 2004.

[11] S. A. Brown, M. Rickertsen, and S. Sheldon, "Effects of an intestinal phosphate binder on serum phosphate and parathyroid hormone concentration in cats with reduced renal function," *Journal of Applied Research in Veterinary Medicine*, vol. 6, no. 3, pp. 155–160, 2008.

[12] http://www.iris-kidney.com/pdf/IRIS2009_Staging_CKD.pdf.

[13] S. Brown, C. Atkins, R. Bagley et al., "Guidelines for the identification, evaluation, and management of systemic hypertension in dogs and cats," *Journal of Veterinary Internal Medicine*, vol. 21, no. 3, pp. 542–558, 2007.

[14] S. A. Brown, R. A. Henik, and D. R. Finco, "Diagnosis of systemic hypertension in dogs and cats," in *Kirk's Current Veterinary Therapy*, J. D. Bonagura, Ed., pp. 835–838, WB Saunders, Philadelphia, Pa, USA, 13th edition, 2000.

[15] Y. Maezaki, K. Tsuji, Y. Nakagawa et al., "Hypocholesterolemic effect of chitosan in adult males," *Bioscience, Biotechnology, and Biochemistry*, vol. 57, pp. 1439–1446, 1983.

[16] H. Yoshimoto, S. Jing, and T. Yamaguchi, "Application of chitosan for oral sorbents," *Chitin Chitosan Research*, vol. 1, pp. 6–14, 1995.

6

Molecular Characterization of Shiga Toxin-Producing *Escherichia coli* Isolated from Ruminant and Donkey Raw Milk Samples and Traditional Dairy Products in Iran

Hassan Momtaz,[1] Rahil Farzan,[2] Ebrahim Rahimi,[3] Farhad Safarpoor Dehkordi,[2] and Negar Souod[4]

[1] *Department of Microbiology, College of Veterinary Medicine, Islamic Azad University, Shahrekord Branch, Shahrekord 166, Iran*
[2] *Young Researchers Club, Islamic Azad University, Shahrekord Branch, Shahrekord 166, Iran*
[3] *Department of Food Hygiene, College of Veterinary Medicine, Islamic Azad University, Shahrekord Branch, Shahrekord 166, Iran*
[4] *Young Researchers Club, Islamic Azad University, Jahrom Branch, Jahrom 74135-355, Iran*

Correspondence should be addressed to Hassan Momtaz, hamomtaz@iaushk.ac.ir

Academic Editors: Y.-Y. M. Chen, M. Dunn, V. Fedorenko, and J. L. Romalde

The aims of the current study were to detect the virulence factors and antibiotic resistance of Shiga toxin-producing *E. coli*, in animal milk and dairy products in Iran. After *E. coli* dentification with culture method, PCR assay were developed for detection of pathogenic genes, serotypes and antibiotic resistance genes of *E. coli*. Results showed that out of 719 samples, 102 (14.18%) were confirmed to be positive for *E. coli* and out of 102 positive samples, 17.64% were O26 and 13.72% were O157 and 1.96% were O91 and 1.96% were O145 serotypes. Totally, the prevalence of *stx*1 and *papA* genes were the highest while the prevalence of *sfaS* and *fyuA* were the lowest in the positive samples. PCR results showed that *tetA*, *tetB* were the highest (64.70%) and *aac*(3)-*IV* were the lowest (27.45%) antibiotic resistant genes in *E. coli* positive samples. Our study indicated that the isolated *E. coli* trains in these regions had a highest antibiotic resistance to tetracycline (58.82%) and the lowest to nitrofurantoin (3.92%). *tetA* gene and *E. coli* O157 serotype had highest and *aac*(3)-*IV* gene, and *E. coli* O145 serotype had a lowest frequency rates of antibiotics resistance genes, in the region.

1. Introduction

Escherichia coli (*E. coli*) is a gram-negative, rod-shaped, flagellated, nonsporulating, and facultative anaerobic bacterium which belongs to Enterobacteriaceae Family. This bacterium classified into several categories based on its virulence factors such as enterotoxigenic *E. coli* (ETEC), attaching and effacing *E. coli* (AEEC), enteropathogenic *E. coli* (EPEC), enterohemorrhagic *E. coli* (EHEC), and Shiga toxin-producing *E. coli* (STEC or VTEC) [1–5]. On the other hand, pathogenic *E. coli* are classified into groups of strains that cause a common disease using common and remarkable assortments of virulence factors that called pathotypes [6].

The Shiga toxin-producing *E. coli* (STEC) are the causative agents of severe clinical syndromes in humans like HUS. Four of the most important virulence factors of STEC are the two phage-encoded cytotoxins, called Shiga toxin 1 (*stx1*) and Shiga toxin 2 (*stx2*), the protein intimin (*eae*), and the plasmid-encoded enterohaemolysin or enterohaemorrhagic *E. coli* haemolysin (*ehly*) [7]. Gastrointestinal diseases, food poisoning, and even death in some cases make this microorganism an insidious threat to human health and food safety [4, 8]. Trough outbreaks in the European Union [9] and several reports of septicemia in human and animals [10, 11] up to recent studies in England [12], all of them have doubled the importance of addressing the issue.

Studies showed that raw animal milk samples and different dairy products are considered the primary reservoir of STEC [4, 13, 14]. Based on our knowledge, in the majority of cases STEC outbreaks were associated with consumption of raw seafood products, traditional dairy products, unpasteurized milk, contaminated food with pollution sources such as feces, contaminated water, contaminated equipments, infected water, and even infected chief, fast-food, contaminated plants' food, and finally raw or even undercooked foods ([15–18]. There are many *E. coli* serogroups such as O157, O26, O103, O111, O145, O45, O91, O113, O121 and O128 which produce Shiga toxins [16, 17, 19–21].

Reports showed that among the non-O157 STEC, O26 has been the most common serogroup [22]. Other studies indicated that O157, O26, and O111 serogroups have been responsible for many outbreaks of HC and HUS cases [1]. Another researches recommended that *E. coli* O157 is the most commonly implicated in outbreaks while O111, O26, O103, and O145 serotypes have also been associated with HC and HUS [2].

There are different cultural methods for enrichment and detection of STEC [23]; however none of them guarantee the speed, accuracy, sensitivity, specificity, and safety. On the other hand, many studies were advertising the safety, accuracy, sensitivity, and specificity of molecular methods like polymerase chain reaction (PCR) for detection of STEC [4, 18]. To the author's knowledge, in the majority of cases, if the treatment was not sufficient, diseases caused by *E. coli*, in addition to weakening the body immunity and susceptibility to other diseases, it can lead to death. Treatment of diseases caused by this bacterium often requires antimicrobial therapy; however antibiotic-resistant strains of bacteria cause more severe diseases for longer periods of time than their antibiotic-susceptible counterparts. Several studies showed that antibiotic resistance in *E. coli* is increasing in these days [24]. Therefore, identification of resistance genes of bacteria seems to be so essential in reduction of treatment costs.

Therefore, the purpose of the current survey was to study the prevalence of virulence factors and antibiotic resistance properties of Shiga toxin-producing *E. coli* isolate from bovine, ovine, caprine, buffalo, camel, and donkey raw milk samples and traditional dairy products in Iran.

2. Materials and Methods

2.1. Sampling and Detecting E. coli. Overall 424 milk samples were collected: bovine (n = 110), caprine (n = 85), ovine (n = 98), buffalo (n = 52), camel (n = 44), and donkey (n = 35) raw milk samples were collected from farm bulk tanks and milk collection centers from several geographic regions of Iran, from March 2010 to March 2011. Bovine and buffalo milk samples were collected throughout this time period. Because the lactating periods of ewes, donkeys, and goats in Iran is seasonal (from March through May and September to November of the subsequent year), caprine, donkey, and ovine milk samples were only available through these months within the forementioned time frame. At each site, sampling of milk was performed according to the International Dairy Federation Guidelines [34]. Samples (100 mL, in sterile glass containers) were transported to the laboratory at ca. 4°C within a maximum of 6–12 h after sampling.

For dairy products, 106 samples of soft cheese, 99 soft butter, and 90 soft ice-cream made up of raw milk were purchased from Shiraz, Isfahan, and Shahrekord—three big cities of Iran supermarkets. All of these dairy products were made traditionally and after collection were kept under refrigeration in plastic bags; information about dates of production and of assigned shelf-lives was not presented. Dairy product samples were collected over a period of six months between May and November 2010 and were analyzed on the day of acquisition. Samples were transported under refrigeration (4–6°C) in thermal boxes containing ice packs and were tested immediately after collection. A 25 g portion of each sample was blended with 225 mL of nutrient broth (Merck, Germany) for 2 min at normal speed, using a Stomacher lab blender and incubated at 37°C for 24 h. A 1 mL sample of the nutrient broth culture was mixed with 9 mL of MacConkey broth (Merck, Germany) and further incubated at 37°C for 24 h. One loop of each tube was streaked on MacConkey agar (Merck, Germany). Four colonies from each plate with typical *E. coli* morphology were selected and examined by biochemical tests, including hydrogen sulphide, citrate, urease, and indol.

2.2. DNA Isolation. Bacterial strains were overnight grown in trypticase soy agar (TSA—Merck, German) at 37°C. One colony was suspended in 100 μL of sterile distilled water. After boiling the suspension for 13 min, this was followed by freezing and subsequently centrifuged at 14,000 rpm for 15 min to pellet the cell debris [35]. The supernatant was used as a template for amplification reaction.

2.3. Polymerase Chain Reaction. PCR assays for detection of STEC serotypes, virulence factors, and antibiotic resistance genes in *E. coli* isolated from animal milk samples and traditional dairy products were performed in 3 states as follows.

The PCR assays, specific primer sequences and the predicted size of the amplified products for the different pathogenic gene coding regions including, *cnf1, cnf2, stx1, stx2, eaeA, cdtB, papA, sfaS, fyuA, iutA, traT,* and *hlyA* were employed as previously described [36–40]. Strains of *E. coli* O157:K88ac:H19, CAPM 5933 and *E. coli* O159:H20, CAPM 6006 were used as positive controls.

Another PCR was performed for detection of *E. coli* serotypes by application of specific primers shown in Table 1. The PCR reaction was performed in a total volume of 50 μL containing 2.5 μL of DNA template, 1.5 mM $MgCl_2$, 200 μM dNTP (Fermentas), 0.5 μM of each primers (F & R), 1.25 U Taq DNA polymerase (Fermentas), and 5 μL PCR buffer 10X. Reactions were initiated at 1 cycle 95°C for 3 min, followed by 30 cycles of 95°C for 20 s, 58°C for 40 s, 72°C for 30 s, and a final elongation step at 72°C for 8 min, in a DNA thermal cycler for detection of O157, O145, O103, O26, and O111 serotypes and 5 μL PCR buffer 10X, 2 mM $Mgcl_2$, 150 μM dNTP, 0.75 μM of each primers F & R, 1.5 U Taq DNA

Table 1: Primer sequence for detection of STEC serotypes in animals milk and different traditional dairy products.

Primer name	Sequence	Size of product (bp)	Target gene	Reference
O26-F O26-R	CAG AAT GGT TAT GCT ACT GT CTT ACA TTT GTT TTC GGC ATC	423	*wzx*	[25]
O103-F O103-R	TTGGAGCGTTAACTGGACCT GCTCCCGAGCACGTATAAG	321	*wzx*	[25]
O111-F O111-R	TAG AGA AAT TAT CAA GTT AGT TCC ATA GTT ATG AAC ATC TTG TTT AGC	406	*wzx*	[25]
O145-F O145-R	CCATCAACAGATTTAGGAGTG TTTCTACCGCGAATCTATC	609	*wzx*	[25]
O157-F O157-R	CGG ACA TCC ATG TGA TAT GG TTG CCT ATG TAC AGC TAA TCC	259	*wzx*	[25]
O45-F O45-R	CCG GGT TTC GAT TTG TGA AGG TTG CAC AAC AGC CAC TAC TAG GCA GAA	527	*wzx1*	[26]
O91-F O91-R	GCTGACCTTCATGATCTGTTGA TAATTTAACCCGTAGAATCGCTGC	291	*gnd*	[27]
O113-F O113-R	GGGTTAGATGGAGCGCTATTGAGA AGGTCACCCTCTGAATTATGGCAG	771	*wzx*	[19]
O121-F O121-R	TGGCTAGTGGCATTCTGATG TGATACTTTAGCCGCCCTTG	322	*wzx*	[28]
O128-F O128-R	GCTTTCTGCCGATATTTGGC CCGACGGACTGATGCCGGTGATT	289	*galF*	[29]

polymerase, and finally 3 μL DNA template with initiated at 1 cycle 94°C for 6 min, followed by 34 cycles of 95°C for 50 s, 58°C for 70 s, 72°C for 55 s, and a final elongation step at 72°C for 5 min, for detection of O91, O128, O121, O113, and O45 serotypes of *E. coli*.

The presence of genes associated with resistance to streptomycin, tetracycline, trimethoprim, fluoroquinolone, gentamicin, sulfonamide, cephalothin, ampicillin, and chloramphenicol was determined by PCR, and a set of primers was used for each gene showed in Table 2. PCR reactions were performed in a total volume of 25 μL, including 2 mM $MgCl_2$, 50 mM KCl, 10 mM Tris-HCl (pH 9.0), 0.1% Triton X-100, 150 μM dNTPs each, 0.4 μM primers, 1 U of Taq DNA polymerase, and 4 μL (40–260 ng/μL) of DNA. Amplification reactions were carried out using a DNA thermocycler as follows: three min at 95°C, 35 cycles each consisting of 1 min at 94°C, 90 s at ~55°C (show in Table 2), 1 min at 72°C, and a final extension step of 8 min at 72°C.

Finally, a DNA thermocycler (Eppendorf Mastercycler, Eppendorf-Nethel-Hinz GmbH, Hamburg, Germany) was used. The amplified products were visualized by ethidium bromide staining after gel electrophoresis of 10 μL of the final reaction mixture in 1.5% agarose.

2.4. Antimicrobial Susceptibility Testing. Antimicrobial susceptibility tests were performed by the Kirby-Bauer disc diffusion method using Mueller-Hinton agar (HiMedia Laboratories, Mumbai, India, MV1084), according to the Clinical and Laboratory Standards Institute guidelines [41]. After incubating the inoculated plate aerobically at 37°C for 18–24 h in an aerobic atmosphere, the susceptibility of the *E. coli* isolates to each antimicrobial agent was measured, and the results were interpreted in accordance with interpretive criteria provided by CLSI (2006). *E. coli* ATCC 25922 was used as quality control organisms in antimicrobial susceptibility determination.

2.5. Statistical Analysis. Statistical analysis were performed using *SPSS/16.0* software for significant relationship between incidences of virulence factors and antibiotics resistance genes of *E. coli* isolated from various animal milk samples and dairy products. Statistical significance was regarded at a P value < 0.05.

3. Results

In the current study, all *E. coli* colonies were tested by applying PCR method in order to detect 16S rRNA gene of bacterium. According to data, out of 424 animal milk samples, 57 (13.44%) and out of 295 traditional dairy products 45 (15.25%) were positive for presence of *E. coli* (Table 3). Therefore, it was shown that incidences of *E. coli* in different traditional dairy products were higher than animal milk species. Our results showed that bovine (20.9%) and soft cheese (23.58%) had a highest and camel (6.81%) and soft ice cream (10%) had a lowest rate of *E. coli* in raw milk and traditional dairy products, respectively (Table 3). Statistical analysis of data showed significant differences ($P < 0.05$) between bovine, ovine, caprine, and camel samples as well as donkey and camel milk samples for presence of *E. coli*. On the other hand, significant differences ($P < 0.05$) were observed in soft cheese, soft butter, and ice cream in incidence of this bacterium. It was concluded that the total prevalence of *E. coli* in all samples in Iran was 14.18% (102 out of 719).

By applying specific primers for detection of STEC serotypes in various samples, it was indicated that out of 102 positive samples for *E. coli*, 14 (13.72%), 2 (1.96%),

Table 2: *E. coli*-resistant antibiotic genes, primer sequence, and product size.

Antibiotic	Resistant gene	Sequence	Size (bp)	Annealing temperature (°C)	References
Streptomycin	*aadA1*	(F) TATCCAGCTAAGCGCGAACT (R) ATTTGCCGACTACCTTGGTC	447	58	[30]
Tetracycline	*tetA*	(F) GGTTCACTCGAACGACGTCA (R) CTGTCCGACAAGTTGCATGA	577	57	[30]
Tetracycline	*tetB*	(F) CCTCAGCTTCTCAACGCGTG (R) GCACCTTGCTGATGACTCTT	634	56	[30]
Trimethoprim	*dfrA1*	(F) GGAGTGCCAAAGGTGAACAGC (R) GAGGCGAAGTCTTGGGTAAAAAC	367	45	[31]
Fluoroquinolone	*qnr*	(F) GGGTATGGATATTATTGATAAAG (R) CTAATCCGGCAGCACTATTTA	670	50	[32]
Gentamicin	*aac(3)-IV*	(F) CTTCAGGATGGCAAGTTGGT (R) TCATCTCGTTCTCCGCTCAT	286	55	[33]
Sulfonamide	*Sul1*	(F) TTCGGCATTCTGAATCTCAC (R) ATGATCTAACCCTCGGTCTC	822	47	[33]
Cephalothin	*blaSHV*	(F) TCGCCTGTGTATTATCTCCC (R) CGCAGATAAATCACCACAATG	768	52	[33]
Ampicillin	*CITM*	(F) TGGCCAGAACTGACAGGCAAA (R) TTTCTCCTGAACGTGGCTGGC	462	47	[33]
Chloramphenicol	*cat1*	(F) AGTTGCTCAATGTACCTATAACC (R) TTGTAATTCATTAAGCATTCTGCC	547	55	[33]
Chloramphenicol	*cmlA*	(F) CCGCCACGGTGTTGTTGTTATC (R) CACCTTGCCTGCCCATCATTAG	698	55	[33]

4 (3.92%), 3 (2.94%), 3 (2.94%), 10 (9.8%), 6 (5.88%), 2 (1.96%), 6 (5.88%), and 18 (17.64%) samples were positive for incidences of O157, O145, O128, O121, O113, O111, O103, O91, O45, and O26 serotypes, respectively, while 34 (33.33%) samples have been determined as nondetected serotypes. So the prevalence of O26 was the highest and both O91 and O145 were the lowest of STEC serotypes (Table 3). In addition, O157 (19.29%) and O145 (1.75%) were the highest and lowest serotypes of STEC in raw animal milk samples and O26 (28.88%) and O91 (0.0%) were the highest and lowest serotypes of STEC in traditional dairy products, respectively (Table 3). Statistical analysis of data indicated significant differences ($P < 0.05$) between total presence of O26, O91, 113, 121, 128, and 145 also O157, O91, and 145 serotypes in samples.

Another part of our study was specialized to determine *E. coli's* virulence genes. Totally *stx1*, *papA*, *cnf1*, *traT*, *cnf2*, and *eae* were the highest and *sfaS* was the lowest virulence genes of *E. coli* which were isolated from raw animal milk samples and traditional dairy products (Table 4). Statistical analysis showed significant differences ($P < 0.05$) between *stx1*, *papA*, and *sfaS* virulence genes which were isolated from raw animal milk samples and traditional dairy products.

On the other hand, our results revealed that out of 102 *E. coli*-positive samples, 34 (33.33%) were non-STEC and 68 (66.66%) were diagnosed as STEC serotypes (Table 5). Our results showed that raw bovine milk samples and traditional soft cheese had several virulence genes especially *stx1* and *traT*, so were the main sources of pathogenic *E. coli* for human in Iran.

The last part of our study was allotted to antibiotic resistance patterns in *E. coli* that isolated from raw milk samples and traditional dairy products which evaluated by application of PCR for presences of genes associated with resistance to various antibiotics and disc diffusion method. PCR assays were successfully developed for detection of twelve different resistance genes of genomic DNA of *E. coli* isolates from milk and dairy products.

Our result indicated that overall the prevalence of resistance to tetracycline (*tetA* + *tetB*) was 64.70% and both trimethoprim (*dfrA1*) and streptomycin (*aadA1*) were 41.17%, respectively (Table 6).

Therefore totally, the prevalence of antimicrobial resistance especially for tetracycline, streptomycin, sulfonamide, chloramphenicol, and finally cephalothin was so high in this survey.

Besides, statistical analysis revealed a statistical significant association ($P < 0.05$) between *tetA* and *tetB* genes in dairy production, *tetB* with *aac(3)-IV*, *qnr*, *cat1*, and *cmlA* in bovine, ovine, caprine, and buffalo milk samples, *aadA1* with *qnr*, *dfrA1*, *tetB*, *blaSHV*, *CITM*, *cat1*, and *cmlA* in soft cheese, butter, and ice cream. Moreover, our results showed that all STEC serotypes which were isolated from raw animal milk samples and traditional dairy products had resistance to more than one antibiotic. Also, based on our data, out of 102 *E. coli*-positive isolates, all of them were resistant to one or more antimicrobial agent.

Finally, antibiogram tests, beside PCR assays, revealed the highest resistance to tetracycline, penicillin, and enrofloxacin with the frequency rate of 58.82%, 46.07%, and 45.09%,

TABLE 3: Prevalence of STEC serotypes isolated from raw animal milk samples and traditional dairy products in Iran.

Samples	*E. coli* positive (%)	O157 (%)	O145 (%)	O128 (%)	O121 (%)	O113 (%)	O111 (%)	O103 (%)	O91 (%)	O45 (%)	O26 (%)	Not detected (%)
Bovine milk (110)	23 (20.9)	3 (13.04)	1 (4.34)	2 (8.69)	1 (4.34)	1 (4.34)	3 (13.04)	1 (4.34)	1 (4.34)	3 (13.04)	2 (8.69)	5 (21.73)
Ovine milk (98)	9 (9.18)	1 (11.11)	—	—	—	—	—	1 (11.11)	1 (11.11)	1 (11.11)	1 (11.11)	4 (44.44)
Caprine milk (85)	8 (9.41)	1 (12.5)	—	1 (12.5)	—	—	1 (12.5)	—	—	1 (12.5)	1 (12.5)	3 (37.5)
Buffalo milk (52)	8 (15.38)	1 (12.5)	—	—	1 (12.5)	—	1 (12.5)	—	—	—	1 (12.5)	4 (50)
Camel milk (44)	3 (6.81)	1 (33.33)	—	—	—	1 (33.33)	—	—	—	—	—	1 (33.33)
Donkey milk (35)	6 (17.14)	4 (66.66)	—	—	—	—	1 (16.66)	—	—	—	—	1 (16.66)
Total milk (424)	57 (13.44)	11 (19.29)	1 (1.75)	3 (5.26)	2 (3.5)	2 (3.5)	6 (10.52)	2 (3.5)	2 (3.5)	5 (8.77)	5 (8.77)	18 (31.57)
Soft cheese (106)	25 (23.58)	2 (8)	1 (4)	1 (4)	1 (4)	1 (4)	2 (8)	1 (4)	—	1 (4)	8 (32)	7 (28)
Soft butter (99)	11 (11.11)	1 (9.09)	—	—	—	—	1 (9.09)	1 (9.09)	—	—	3 (27.27)	5 (45.45)
Soft ice cream (90)	9 (10)	—	—	—	—	—	1 (11.11)	2 (22.22)	—	—	2 (22.22)	4 (44.44)
Total dairy products (295)	45 (15.25)	3 (6.66)	1 (2.22)	1 (2.22)	1 (2.22)	1 (2.22)	4 (8.88)	4 (8.88)	—	1 (2.22)	13 (28.88)	16 (35.55)
Total (719)	102 (14.18)	14 (13.72)	2 (1.96)	4 (3.92)	3 (2.94)	3 (2.94)	10 (9.8)	6 (5.88)	2 (1.96)	6 (5.88)	18 (17.64)	34 (33.33)

Table 4: Distribution of virulence genes in *E. coli* isolated from raw animal milk samples and traditional dairy products in Iran.

Samples	Virulence genes											
	stx1	*stx2*	*eae*	*ehly*	*cnf1*	*cnf2*	*iutA*	*cdtB*	*papA*	*traT*	*sfaS*	*fyuA*
Bovine milk	9	3	4	1	4	3	2	2	2	3	—	1
Ovine milk	3	1	2	—	2	1	5	—	2	2	—	—
Caprine milk	3	1	1	—	2	1	1	—	5	2	—	—
Buffalo milk	4	2	3	1	2	4	2	1	2	2	—	—
Camel milk	2	1	1	2	1	3	—	2	5	1	—	1
Donkey milk	1	1	1	2	6	1	—	1	1	3	1	2
Total milk	22	9	12	6	17	13	10	6	17	13	1	4
Soft cheese	2	1	2	2	2	1	2	—	2	6	—	—
Soft butter	—	—	2	1	2	1	2	1	2	1	—	—
Soft ice cream	1	1	2	—	1	3	1	1	4	1	—	—
Total dairy products	3	2	6	3	5	5	5	2	8	8	—	—
Total	25	11	18	9	22	18	15	8	25	21	1	4

TABLE 5: Prevalence of virulence genes in Shiga toxin-producing *E. coli* serotypes isolated from raw animal milk samples and traditional dairy products in Iran.

Serotype		Number of positive samples (%)	Virulence gene (%)
Non-STEC		34 (33.33)	—
STEC (68 = 66.66%)	EHEC	14 (20.58)	*stx1, eae, ehly*: 14 (100)
	AEEC	54 (79.41)	*stx1*: 25 (46.29) *stx2*: 11 (20.37) *eae*: 18 (33.33) *stx1, eae*: 12 (22.22) *stx2, eae*: 7 (12.96) *stx1, stx2, eae*: 4 (7.4)

TABLE 6: Distribution of antibiotic resistance genes in various serotypes of *E. coli* isolated from raw animal milk samples and traditional dairy products in Iran.

STEC serotypes	Antibiotic resistance genes										
	aadA1	*tetA*	*tetB*	*dfrA1*	*qnr*	*aac(3)-IV*	*sul1*	*blaSHV*	*CITM*	*cat1*	*cmlA*
O157 (14)	10	7	5	12	14	7	8	7	8	6	4
O26 (18)	13	11	4	5	5	8	11	10	9	3	8
O103 (6)	1	2	1	2	2	1	2	2	2	1	—
O111 (10)	3	3	2	7	12	1	4	6	4	4	1
O145 (2)	—	—	—	—	—	—	1	—	—	—	1
O45 (6)	1	1	—	6	1	—	1	3	5	1	—
O91 (2)	—	—	1	1	—	1	1	—	—	—	—
O113 (3)	—	1	—	1	—	1	1	1	1	—	1
O121 (3)	—	—	1	—	—	—	1	—	1	1	—
O128 (4)	1	2	—	1	—	—	1	1	1	1	1
Not detected (34)	13	10	15	7	26	9	12	13	9	6	8
Total (102)	42 (41.17)	37 (36.27)	29 (28.43)	42 (41.17)	60 (58.82)	28 (27.45)	43 (42.15)	43 (42.15)	40 (39.21)	23 (22.54)	24 (23.52)

respectively, as well as the lowest resistance to nitrofurantoin and ciprofloxacin with the frequency rate of 3.92% and 7.84% (Table 7). On the other hand, in the current situations in Iran, the use of nitrofurantoin and ciprofloxacin due to low antibiotic resistance, can be more effective for treatment of diseases caused by *E. coli*. This survey indicated the highest antimicrobial resistance in O157, O26 and O111 serotypes. Unfortunately, our results showed that nondetected serotypes had a highest incidence of antibiotics resistance. Besides, bovine had highest and camel had lowest rates of resistance to antibiotics. Statistical analysis showed significant differences ($P < 0.05$) between O157, O26, and nondetected serotypes with O103, 145, 91, 113, 121 and 128 serotypes and between resistance to trimethoprim, streptomycin, lincomycin, penicillin, and tetracycline with nitrofurantoin and ciprofloxacin antibiotics. Totally *E. coli* antibiotic resistances against common antibiotics which use in veterinary in Iran were so high. Based on Table 6, between these ten serotypes, *E. coli* O157 and *E. coli* O145 had a highest and lowest prevalence of antibiotic resistance genes. Results showed that in nondetected serotypes, prevalence of antibiotic resistance genes were so high too.

4. Discussion

The present study like the previous studies which introduced ruminants as reservoirs of *E. coli* O157 [42], for the first time, has been introduced donkeys, camels, and buffaloes as the other sources of *E. coli* serotypes especially O157. Despite the highest prevalence of *E. coli* O157 in recent studies [2, 43], our results showed that *E. coli* O26 had a highest frequency rate in traditional dairy products. On the other hand, our study indicated that in spite of raw animal milk samples, pathogenic *E. coli* had a highest prevalence in traditional dairy products. Probably using contaminated water in processing traditional dairy products, infected people who produce dairy products, using contaminated equipments, basic infections of dairy sources which are necessary for producing dairy products, and finally lack of public and individual hygiene, are the factors that can be responsible for the higher prevalence of *E. coli* in traditional dairy products than raw animal milk samples. Only one recent study showed that presence of *E. coli* O157 in foods may be derived from polluted water [44].

There are several studies which have detected *E. coli* species in yogurt [45], soft cheeses [46], cheddar cheese [47],

TABLE 7: Antibiotic resistance properties in STEC serotypes isolated from raw animal milk and traditional dairy products in Iran (disk diffusion method).

STES serotypes	P10 (%)	TE30 (%)	S10 (%)	C30 (%)	SXT (%)	GM10 (%)	NFX5 (%)	L2 (%)	CF30 (%)	CIP5 (%)	TMP5 (%)	F/M300 (%)	AM10 (%)
O157 (14)	12	11	9	9	8	5	12	9	6	1	10	1	6
O26 (18)	4	14	12	9	10	6	3	10	8	1	5	1	8
O103 (6)	—	3	1	—	1	—	1	2	2	—	2	—	2
O111 (10)	8	4	3	4	3	1	9	3	5	2	7	—	3
O145 (2)	—	—	—	—	1	—	—	—	—	—	—	—	—
O45 (6)	4	1	2	1	1	—	1	1	2	—	5	—	1
O91 (2)	—	—	—	—	—	—	—	—	—	—	1	—	—
O113 (3)	—	1	—	—	—	1	—	—	—	—	1	—	1
O121 (3)	1	1	—	—	1	—	—	1	—	—	—	—	1
O128 (4)	1	1	1	1	—	—	—	1	1	—	1	—	1
Not detected (34)	17	24	10	12	7	7	20	15	11	4	9	2	4
Total (102)	47 (46.07)	60 (58.82)	38 (37.25)	36 (35.29)	32 (31.37)	20 (19.6)	46 (45.09)	42 (41.17)	35 (34.31)	8 (7.84)	41 (40.19)	4 (3.92)	27 (26.47)

In this table P10: penicillin (10 u/disk); TE30: tetracycline (30 μg/disk); S10: streptomycin (10 μg/disk); C30: chloramphenicol (30 μg/disk); SXT: sulfamethoxazole (25 μg/disk); GM10: gentamycin (10 μg/disk); NFX5: enrofloxacin (5 μg/disk); L2: lincomycin (2 μg/disk); CF30: cephalothin (30 μg/disk); CIP5: ciprofloxacin (5 μg/disk); TMP5: trimethoprim (5 μg/disk); F/M300: nitrofurantoin (300 μg/disk); AM10: ampicillin (10 u/disk).

and Feta cheese [48]; however in this survey it is for the first time that we observed that this bacterium can be detected in soft cheese, soft butter, and soft ice cream which were produced in traditional conditions too.

According to Meshref in 2010 from Egypt on cooking butter, 31.7% of the samples were contaminated by *E. coli* [49], in which this rate was higher than ours (11.11%). Another study, performed on dairy products, showed that when the assay was applied with 60 market dairy food samples, one sample each of raw milk, paneer, and ice cream was found to be positive for *E. coli* O157:H7 [50] that was lower than our study.

Another study in Iran showed that only *E. coli* O157 subtype was isolated from traditional cheese (4.2%), ice cream (3.33%), and yoghurt (0%) [51] that was more limited than our study. The other study in Pantnagar revealed that out of 135 dairy product samples, 11 samples (8.14%) were positive for *E. coli* [52] that was lower than our study (14.18%). Recent study from Iran indicated that *E. coli* O157:H7 can be detected in high rates from white cheese and probiotic cheese [53]. Besides, a 3-year study of *E. coli* O157:H7 in cattle, camel, sheep, goat, chicken, and beef-minced meat in Iran revealed that 1.7% and 2.1% of samples were positive for *E. coli* O157:H7 and *E. coli* O157:NM, respectively [54]. According to a study in Kerman on raw milk cheese producing, *stx* genes detected in 6.4% of the samples, but STEC strains could be isolated in only five of them (4%) [55]. Another study from Iran showed that about 21.8% of *E. coli* isolates from cattle were positive for *ehxA*, *stx1*, and/or *stx2* genes [56], but our study indicated that *stx1*, *cnf1*, and *eae* with incidences of 24.5%, 21.56%, and 17.64% had a highest frequency rate of virulence genes of *E. coli* isolates from raw bovine milk samples.

Therefore, according to the results, the food contamination with animal fecal origin is so obvious in Iran. Based on the other surveys, the presence of *E. coli* O157 in raw milk and dairy products is proven, however in this investigation we found O26, O111, O103, and even O45 in addition to O157 as a predominant serotypes of *E. coli* in animal's raw milk and dairy products with the frequency of 17.64%, 9.8%, 5.88%, 5.88%, and 13.72%, respectively. So in our study *E. coli* O26 was the predominant serotype, AEEC was the predominant subtype, and *papA* and *stx1* were the predominate genes.

Another study in Swiss in 2006 on 432 cheese samples and in 2007 on 364 cheese samples showed 16 (3.7%) and 23 (6.3%) *E. coli*-positive samples, respectively, so their results were lower than ours in cheese (23.58%) specimens. Further more in this study the investigators found non-O157 STEC strains in 16 samples in which 11 samples based on their O groups typed into 7 categories (O2, O15, O22, O91, O109, O113, O174), whereas 5 strains were nontypeable. They detect *stx1* in only 1 sample and *stx2* in 15 samples of 16 non-O157 STEC specimens. Furthermore this study showed that 3 STEC strains harbored *E-hlyA* as a further putative virulence factor and none of the strains tested positive for *eae* gene [14]. In another study in Irish bovine dairy herds, 85 out of 117 milk filters and 43 out of 120 bulk-tank milk samples were positive for *vt* genes of *E. coli*. Out of *vt*-positive samples, 58, 162, 1, 324, and 26 samples were positive for O26, O103, O111, O145, and O157 serotypes, and 10 of these isolates contained at least one of the four virulence genes of *vt1*, *vt2*, *eaeA*, and *hlyA* [57].

Recent study in United State reported that EHEC subtype of *E. coli* was detected in 23% of strains and *eaeA* gene was found in 4.2%, and one or both Shiga-like toxin genes (*stx1* and *stx2*) were positive in bulk-tank milk too. Based on real-time PCR, they proved that 5 samples were contaminated with O157:H7 [58] while our study showed that out of 102 positive samples for *E. coli*, 13.72% were EHEC, 17.64% had *eaeA* gene, and 35.29% had both Shiga-like toxin genes.

The prevalence of Shiga toxin in our study (66.66%) was obviously higher than Lowa (4.08%) [59]. Another study on lamb food chain showed that all three virulence genes, *eae*, *stx1*, and *stx2*, were the most prevalent genes in slaughterhouses (69%), processing plant (32%), and butcheries (9-10%) [60], but our results indicated that in raw milk and dairy products, *stx1* and *papA* with frequency rate of 24.5% had a highest prevalence of *E. coli*'s virulence genes.

Detection of bacteria in milk samples has some merits like being available and economical. In some geographic places of Iran because of bad climate conditions, bovines, ovine, caprine, and buffaloes are not able to survive, so camels are the main milk supplier for people. So camel's milk hygiene can be essential for human health especially in those especially in that area where the climate is arid and desert. Donkeys' milk samples due to high similarity with human milk and high-sweet components due to high presence of lactose sugar sometimes can be used instead of human milk. Buffaloes' milk hygiene due to high fat and protein contents is very important especially for producing some dairy products.

Studies showed that the antibiotic resistance bacteria which exist in the milk of infected animals can be transmitted to human by the ingestion of unpasteurized milk or dairy products such as cheese, butter, yoghurt, and ice cream. However, the mechanism of spreading antibiotic resistance from food animals to humans remains controversial [61, 62].

Our study showed that *E. coli* O157 was the most prevalent serotype in donkey's milk. Furthermore, this serotype had the highest antibiotic resistance to penicillin and enrofloxacin. To our knowledge, veterinary service-like treatments are very low for donkeys in Iran and unfortunately if a veterinarian wants to apply antibiotical treatments, in most of cases uses penicillin and enrofloxacin for donkeys. Therefore, the high antibiotic resistance in donkeys to these two antibiotics (in our study) may be occurred due to these successive and ectopic treatments, but in bovines the best choices for antibiotic treatment were enrofloxacin, trimethoprim, and tetracycline. So due to the high administration of antibiotics, the prevalence of antibiotic resistance against these antibiotics was so high in bovine's milk samples in the current study. Veterinary interventions and antibiotic administrations are not common in camels in Iran. In most regions of Iran, camel's distribution is so low and reports about the occurrences of diseases in camels usually were low in Iran. Therefore based on our results, it seems logical that the prevalence of antibiotics resistance in camel samples was low.

Our results showed that 58.82% of isolated *E. coli* from raw milk and traditional dairy products were tetracycline resistant. As well as an other study, substantial numbers of human *E. coli* isolates were tetracycline resistant [63]. Recent study indicated that 61% of *E. coli* which isolated from humans, cattle, swine, and food during 1985 to 2000 was susceptible to all 13 antimicrobials tested, while 27% of them were resistant to tetracycline, 26% to sulfamethoxazole, 17% to cephalothin, and 13% to ampicillin [63]. As the present study indicates, there is a high antibiotic resistance in *E. coli* which isolated from raw milk and traditional dairy products.

A report from Scotland revealed that the frequency of antibiotic-resistant *E. coli* was 10.6% in milk samples and suggested that the prevalence of antibiotic-resistant strains in milk was higher in housed bovines than in outdoor bovines. This study showed that out of 1125 *E. coli* isolates tested, 22.2% were antibiotic resistant, and out of these resistant strains, 42.4% were resistant to more than one antibiotic [64]. Another study in Iran indicated that the resistance of the *E. coli* strains isolated from traditional cheese, ice cream, and yoghurt to ampicillin and gentamycin was the most common findings (44.4%), followed by resistance to erythromycin (33.3%), amoxicillin (11.1%), tetracycline (11.1%), and nalidixic acid (11.1%) [51]. Our study showed that two of the most prevalent resistant genes of *E. coli* were *tetA* + *tetB* (64.70%), and this is similar to previous study that was performed on cow's milk [65].

Unfortunately, indiscriminate prescribing of antibiotics in veterinary is so high and in a report from Netherland 300 000 kg of antibiotics are used annually on veterinary prescription in animals [66]. These high amounts of antibiotics can be kept in animals and lead to antibiotics resistance in bacteria. Then resistance genes of bacteria shedding from milk and meat can be used in humans. So these resistance genes will be causing drug resistance in human too. Our results showed that simultaneous application of culture and PCR can easily be effective in diagnosis of pathogens and their resistance factors especially in food for human consumption.

Our results revealed that (i) using raw milk without pasteurization and milking with unsanitary methods and using traditional dairy products that are produced in unsanitary conditions and probably from unpasteurized milk are the main resources for growth, proliferation, and survival of *E. coli* and cause several disorders for human. Therefore, vaccinating dairy animals (if necessary), improving methods of milking, checking milking halls in order to detect *E. coli* especially in the animal feces monthly, fumigating milking halls frequently, observing hygiene during milking, boiling milk, using pasteurized milk for dairy products, keeping dairy products in cool and dry places, away from sunlight, and finally preventing contamination of dairy products with extrinsic factors like insects and dust are the best ways to prevent *E. coli* infections. (ii) Chloramphenicol is a forbidden antibiotic, and the high antibiotic resistance to drug in our study indicated the irregular and unauthorized use of this antibiotic, in veterinary treatment in Iran. Unfortunately, veterinarians in many fields of veterinary such as large animal internal medicine, poultry, and even aquaculture use this antibiotic as a basic one. Therefore, in a very short period of time, antibiotic resistance will appear. (iii) We recommend PCR method as an accurate, safe, and fast diagnostic one for detection of pathogens in milk and dairy products (iv) due to antibiotic resistance especially in *E. coli*, the veterinarians should pay more attention to prescribing the antibiotics. (v) *E. coli* virulence genes especially *stx1*, *stx2*, *eae*, *cnf1*, *cnf2*, *iutA*, *papA*, and finally *traT* are well distributed in milk and dairy products in Iran. (vi) STEC serotypes and especially AEEC are the predominant strains and O157, and O26 serotypes are the predominant serotypes of bacterium in animal raw milk and traditional dairy products in Iran. (vii) Bovine and camel raw milk and soft cheese and ice cream had a highest and lowest frequency rate of pathogenic *E. coli* in raw milk and dairy product samples in Iran, respectively. (viii) In order to prevent antibiotic resistance in bacteria, we should apply antibiotics more cautiously in animals, detect resistance genes, and finally use different antibiotics periodically. Our results recommended the use of PCR for detection of antibiotic resistance genes of bacteria as a safe, rapid, and accurate method in laboratories.

Acknowledgments

The authors would like to thank Dr. E. Tajbakhsh and Mr. M. Momeni at the Biotechnology Research Center of the Islamic Azad University of Shahrekord for their important technical and clinical support. This work was supported by the Islamic Azad University, Shahrekord Branch, Iran, Grant 90/9025.

References

[1] I. Holko, T. Bisova, Z. Holkova, and V. Kmet, "Virulence markers of *Escherichia coli* strains isolated from traditional cheeses made from unpasteurised sheep milk in Slovakia," *Food Control*, vol. 17, no. 5, pp. 393–396, 2006.

[2] H. Karch, P. I. Tarr, and M. Bielaszewska, "Enterohaemorrhagic *Escherichia coli* in human medicine," *International Journal of Medical Microbiology*, vol. 295, no. 6-7, pp. 405–418, 2005.

[3] E. Fröhlicher, G. Krause, C. Zweifel, L. Beutin, and R. Stephan, "Characterization of attaching and effacing *Escherichia coli* (AEEC) isolated from pigs and sheep," *BMC Microbiology*, vol. 8, article 144, 2008.

[4] N. Solomakos, A. Govaris, A. S. Angelidis et al., "Occurrence, virulence genes and antibiotic resistance of *Escherichia coli* O157 isolated from raw bovine, caprine and ovine milk in Greece," *Food Microbiology*, vol. 26, no. 8, pp. 865–871, 2009.

[5] Q. Wang, X. Ruan, D. Wei et al., "Development of a serogroup-specific multiplex PCR assay to detect a set of *Escherichia coli* serogroups based on the identification of their O-antigen gene clusters," *Molecular and Cellular Probes*, vol. 24, no. 5, pp. 286–290, 2010.

[6] J. B. Kaper, J. P. Nataro, and H. L. T. Mobley, "Pathogenic *Escherichia coli*," *Nature Reviews Microbiology*, vol. 2, no. 2, pp. 123–140, 2004.

[7] D. Law, "Virulence factors of *Escherichia coli* O157 and other Shiga toxin- producing *E. coli*," *Journal of Applied Microbiology*, vol. 88, no. 5, pp. 729–745, 2000.

[8] J. Meng, M. P. Doyle, T. Zhao, and S. Zhao, "Enterohemorrhagic *Escherichia coli*," in *Food Microbiology: Fundamentals and Frontiers*, M. P. Doyle and L. R. Beuchat, Eds., ASM Press, Washington, DC, USA, 3rd edition, 2007.

[9] European Food Safety Authority (EFSA), "The community summary report on trends and sources of zoonoses, zoonotic agents, antimicrobial resistance and foodborne outbreaks in the European Union in 2006," *EFSA Journal*, vol. 130, pp. 1–352, 2007.

[10] J. Harel, J. Fairbrother, C. Forget, C. Desautels, and J. Moore, "Virulence factors associated with F165-positive *Escherichia coli* strains isolated from piglets and calves," *Veterinary Microbiology*, vol. 38, no. 1-2, pp. 139–155, 1993.

[11] C. Martin, E. Rousset, and H. De Greve, "Human uropathogenic and bovine septicaemic *Escherichia coli* strains carry an identical F17-related adhesin," *Research in Microbiology*, vol. 148, no. 1, pp. 55–64, 1997.

[12] I. A. Gillespie, S. J. O'Brien, G. K. Adak, T. Cheasty, and G. Willshaw, "Foodborne general outbreaks of Shiga toxin-producing *Escherichia coli* O157 in England and Wales 1992–2002: where are the risks?" *Epidemiology and Infection*, vol. 133, no. 5, pp. 803–808, 2005.

[13] H. S. Hussein and T. Sakuma, "Invited review: prevalence of Shiga toxin-producing *Escherichia coli* in dairy cattle and their products," *Journal of Dairy Science*, vol. 88, no. 2, pp. 450–465, 2005.

[14] R. Stephan, S. Schumacher, S. Corti, G. Krause, J. Danuser, and L. Beutin, "Prevalence and characteristics of Shiga toxin-producing *Escherichia coli* in Swiss raw milk cheeses collected at producer level," *Journal of Dairy Science*, vol. 91, no. 7, pp. 2561–2565, 2008.

[15] H. Sanath Kumar, S. K. Otta, I. Karunasagar, and I. Karunasagar, "Detection of Shiga-toxigenic *Escherichia coli* (STEC) in fresh seafood and meat marketed in Mangalore, India by PCR," *Letters in Applied Microbiology*, vol. 33, no. 5, pp. 334–338, 2001.

[16] L. Heijnen and G. Medema, "Quantitative detection of *E. coli*, *E. coli* O157 and other shiga toxin producing *E. coli* in water samples using a culture method combined with real-time PCR," *Journal of Water and Health*, vol. 4, no. 4, pp. 487–498, 2006.

[17] M. C. Erickson and M. P. Doyle, "Food as a vehicle for transmission of Shiga toxin-producing *Escherichia coli*," *Journal of Food Protection*, vol. 70, no. 10, pp. 2426–2449, 2007.

[18] J. Madic, N. Vingadassalon, C. P. de Garam et al., "Detection of Shiga toxin-producing *Escherichia coli* serotypes O26:H11, O103:H2, O111:H8, O145:H28, and O157:H7 in raw-milk cheeses by using multiplex real-time PCR," *Applied and Environmental Microbiology*, vol. 77, no. 6, pp. 2035–2041, 2011.

[19] C. DebRoy, E. Roberts, J. Kundrat, M. A. Davis, C. E. Briggs, and P. M. Fratamico, "Detection of *Escherichia coli* Serogroups O26 and O113 by PCR Amplification of the *wzx* and *wzy* Genes," *Applied and Environmental Microbiology*, vol. 70, no. 3, pp. 1830–1832, 2004.

[20] C. Jenkins, M. C. Pearce, A. W. Smith et al., "Detection of *Escherichia coli* serogroups O26, O103, O111 and O145 from bovine faeces using immunomagnetic separation and PCR/DNA probe techniques," *Letters in Applied Microbiology*, vol. 37, no. 3, pp. 207–212, 2003.

[21] A. Lin, L. Nguyen, T. Lee et al., "Rapid O serogroup identification of the ten most clinically relevant STECs by Luminex microbead-based suspension array," *Journal of Microbiological Methods*, vol. 87, pp. 105–110, 2011.

[22] Infectious Agents Surveillance Center, National Institute of Infectious Diseases, "The status of enterohemorrhagic *Escherichia coli* Escherichia coli infection, 1998-March 2000," *Infectious Agents Surveillance Reports*, vol. 21, pp. 92–93, 2000.

[23] De Boer E and A. E. Heuvelink, "Methods for the detection and isolation of Shiga toxin-producing *Escherichia coli*.," *Symposium Series Society of Applied Microbiology*, vol. 88, pp. 133S–143S, 2000.

[24] P. Cortés, V. Blanc, A. Mora et al., "Isolation and characterization of potentially pathogenic antimicrobial-resistant *Escherichia coli* strains from chicken and pig farms in spain," *Applied and Environmental Microbiology*, vol. 76, no. 9, pp. 2799–2805, 2010.

[25] B. Possé, L. De Zutter, M. Heyndrickx, and L. Herman, "Metabolic and genetic profiling of clinical O157 and non-O157 Shiga-toxin-producing *Escherichia coli*," *Research in Microbiology*, vol. 158, no. 7, pp. 591–599, 2007.

[26] C. DebRoy, P. M. Fratamico, E. Roberts, M. A. Davis, and Y. Liu, "Development of PCR assays targeting genes in O-antigen gene clusters for detection and identification of *Escherichia coli* O45 and O55 serogroups," *Applied and Environmental Microbiology*, vol. 71, no. 8, pp. 4919–4924, 2005.

[27] S. Perelle, F. Dilasser, J. Grout, and P. Fach, "Identification of the O-antigen biosynthesis genes of *Escherichia coli* O91 and development of a O91 PCR serotyping test," *Journal of Applied Microbiology*, vol. 93, no. 5, pp. 758–764, 2002.

[28] P. M. Fratamico, C. E. Briggs, D. Needle, C. Y. Chen, and C. DebRoy, "Sequence of the *Escherichia coli* O121 O-antigen gene cluster and detection of enterohemorrhagic *E. coli* O121 by PCR amplification of the wzx and wzy genes," *Journal of Clinical Microbiology*, vol. 41, no. 7, pp. 3379–3383, 2003.

[29] J. Shao, M. Li, Q. Jia, Y. Lu, and P. G. Wang, "Sequence of *Escherichia coli* O128 antigen biosynthesis cluster and functional identification of an α-1,2-fucosyltransferase," *FEBS Letters*, vol. 553, no. 1-2, pp. 99–103, 2003.

[30] L. P. Randall, S. W. Cooles, M. K. Osborn, L. J. V. Piddock, and M. J. Woodward, "Antibiotic resistance genes, integrons and multiple antibiotic resistance in thirty-five serotypes of Salmonella enterica isolated from humans and animals in the UK," *Journal of Antimicrobial Chemotherapy*, vol. 53, no. 2, pp. 208–216, 2004.

[31] C. S. Toro, M. Farfán, I. Contreras et al., "Genetic analysis of antibiotic-resistance determinants in multidrug-resistant Shigella strains isolated from Chilean children," *Epidemiology and Infection*, vol. 133, no. 1, pp. 81–86, 2005.

[32] H. Mammeri, M. Van De Loo, L. Poirel, L. Martinez-Martinez, and P. Nordmann, "Emergence of plasmid-mediated quinolone resistance in *Escherichia coli* in Europe," *Antimicrobial Agents and Chemotherapy*, vol. 49, no. 1, pp. 71–76, 2005.

[33] T. T. H. Van, J. Chin, T. Chapman, L. T. Tran, and P. J. Coloe, "Safety of raw meat and shellfish in Vietnam: an analysis of *Escherichia coli* isolations for antibiotic resistance and virulence genes," *International Journal of Food Microbiology*, vol. 124, no. 3, pp. 217–223, 2008.

[34] International Dairy Federation (IDF), *Milk and Milk Products—Guidance on Methods of Sampling*, IDF Standard, Brussels, Belgium, 1995.

[35] U. Reischl, M. T. Youssef, J. Kilwinski et al., "Real-time fluorescence PCR assays for detection and characterization

of Shiga toxin, intimin, and enterohemolysin genes from Shiga toxin-producing *Escherichia coli*," *Journal of Clinical Microbiology*, vol. 40, no. 7, pp. 2555–2565, 2002.

[36] M. J. Brian, M. Frosolono, B. E. Murray et al., "Polymerase chain reaction for diagnosis of enterohemorrhagic *Escherichia coli* infection and hemolytic-uremic syndrome," *Journal of Clinical Microbiology*, vol. 30, no. 7, pp. 1801–1806, 1992.

[37] A. E. Heuvelink, N. C. A. J. Van de Kar, J. F. G. M. Meis, L. A. H. Monnens, and W. J. G. Melchers, "Characterization of verocytotoxin-producing *Escherichia coli* O157 isolates from patients with haemolytic uraemic syndrome in Western Europe," *Epidemiology and Infection*, vol. 115, no. 1, pp. 1–14, 1995.

[38] M. Blanco, J. E. Blanco, J. Blanco et al., "Polymerase chain reaction for detection in *Escherichia coli* strains producing cytotoxic necrotizing factor type 1 and type 2 (CNF1 and CNF2)," *Journal of Microbiological Methods*, vol. 26, no. 1-2, pp. 95–101, 1996.

[39] J. R. Johnson and A. L. Stell, "Extended virulence genotypes of *Escherichia coli* strains from patients with urosepsis in relation to phylogeny and host compromise," *Journal of Infectious Diseases*, vol. 181, no. 1, pp. 261–272, 2000.

[40] M. Idress, U. Mussarat, Y. Badshah, R. Qamar, and H. Bokhari, "Virulence factors profile of drug-resistant *Escherichia coli* isolates from urinary tract infections in Punjab, Pakistan," *European Journal of Clinical Microbiology and Infectious Diseases*, vol. 29, no. 12, pp. 1533–1537, 2010.

[41] Clinical Laboratory Standards Institute (CLSI), *PerFormance Standards for Antimicrobial Disk Susceptibility Tests, Approved Standard-Ninth Edition (M2-A9)*, Clinical and Laboratory Standards Institute, Wayne, Pa, USA, 2006.

[42] B. Oporto, J. I. Esteban, G. Aduriz, R. A. Juste, and A. Hurtado, "*Escherichia coli* O157:H7 and non-O157 Shiga toxin-producing *E. coli* in healthy cattle, sheep and swine herds in Northern Spain," *Zoonoses and Public Health*, vol. 55, no. 2, pp. 73–81, 2008.

[43] I. Caro, V. M. Fernández-Barata, A. Alonso-Llamazares, and M. R. García-Armesto, "Detection, occurrence, and characterization of *Escherichia coli* O157:H7 from raw ewe's milk in Spain," *Journal of Food Protection*, vol. 69, no. 4, pp. 920–924, 2006.

[44] P. Zhu, D. R. Shelton, J. S. Karns et al., "Detection of waterborne *E. coli* O157 using the integrating waveguide biosensor," *Biosensors and Bioelectronics*, vol. 21, no. 4, pp. 678–683, 2005.

[45] A. Govaris, P. Koidis, and K. Papatheodorou, "Behaviour of *Escherichia coli* O157:H7 in sour milk, cows' milk yogurt and ewes' milk yogurt," *Journal of Dairy Research*, vol. 69, no. 4, pp. 655–660, 2002.

[46] C. Vernozy-Rozand, C. Mazuy-Cruchaudet, C. Bavai et al., "Growth and survival of *Escherichia coli* O157:H7 during the manufacture and ripening of raw goat milk lactic cheeses," *International Journal of Food Microbiology*, vol. 105, no. 1, pp. 83–88, 2005.

[47] J. E. Schlesser, R. Gerdes, S. Ravishankar, K. Madsen, J. Mowbray, and A. Y. L. Teo, "Survival of a five-strain cocktail of *Escherichia coli* O157:H7 during the 60-day aging period of Cheddar cheese made from unpasteurized milk," *Journal of Food Protection*, vol. 69, no. 5, pp. 990–998, 2006.

[48] A. Govaris, D. K. Papageorgiou, and K. Papatheodorou, "Behavior of *Escherichia coli* O157:h7 during the manufacture and ripening of Feta and Telemes cheeses," *Journal of Food Protection*, vol. 65, no. 4, pp. 609–615, 2002.

[49] A. M. S. Meshref, "Microbiological quality and safety of cooking butter in Beni-Suef governorate-Egypt," *African Health Sciences*, vol. 10, no. 2, pp. 193–198, 2010.

[50] J. Singh, V. K. Batish, and S. Grover, "A scorpion probe-based real-time PCR assay for detection of *E. coli* O157:H7 in dairy products," *Foodborne Pathogens and Disease*, vol. 6, no. 3, pp. 395–400, 2009.

[51] E. Rahimi, S. Shekarchian Chaleshtori, and P. Parsaei, "Prevalence and antimicrobial resistance of *Escherichia coli* O157 isolated from traditional cheese, ice cream and yoghurt in Iran," *African Journal of Microbiology Research*, vol. 5, pp. 3706–3710, 2011.

[52] R. Kumar and A. Prasad, "Detection of *E. coli* and staphylococcus in milk and milk products in and around pantnagar," *Veterinary World*, vol. 3, pp. 495–496, 2010.

[53] H. K. Darehabi and P. Nikmaram, "Assessment of the growth and survival of *Escherichia coli* O157:H7 during the manufacture and storage of Iranian white cheese and probiotic cheese," *Global Veterinaria*, vol. 6, no. 3, pp. 228–232, 2011.

[54] S. Hajian, E. Rahimi, and H. Mommtaz, "A 3-year study of *Escherichia coli* O157:H7 in cattle, camel, sheep, goat, chicken and beef minced meat," in *Proceedings of the International Conference on Food Engineering and Biotechnology (IPCBEE '11)*, IACSIT Press, Singapoore, 2011.

[55] L. Mansouri-Najand and M. Khalili, "Detection of shiga-like toxigenic *Escherichia coli* from raw milk cheeses produced in Kerman-Iran," *Veterinarski Arhiv*, vol. 77, no. 6, pp. 515–522, 2007.

[56] R, G. Mazhaheri Nejad Fard, T. Behzadian Nezhad, Zahraei Salehi, and N. Atash Parvar, "Evaluation of ehxA, stx1, and stx2 virulence gene prevalence in cattle *Escherichia coli* isolates by multiplex PCR," *Archives of Razi Institute*, vol. 60, pp. 55–66, 2005.

[57] M. J. Lynch, E. M. Fox, L. O'Connor, K. Jordan, and M. Murphy, "Surveillance of verocytotoxigenic *Escherichia coli* in Irish bovine dairy herds," *Zoonoses and Public Health*, vol. 59, no. 4, pp. 264–271, 2012.

[58] J. S. Karns, J. S. Van Kessel, B. J. McClusky, and M. L. Perdue, "Incidence of *Escherichia coli* 0157:H7 and *E. coli* virulence factors in US bulk tank milk as determined by polymerase chain reaction," *Journal of Dairy Science*, vol. 90, no. 7, pp. 3212–3219, 2007.

[59] H. W. Moon, L. J. Hoffman, N. A. Cornick, S. L. Booher, and B. T. Bosworth, "Prevalences of some virulence genes among *Escherichia coli* isolates from swine presented to a diagnostic laboratory in Iowa," *Journal of Veterinary Diagnostic Investigation*, vol. 11, no. 6, pp. 557–560, 1999.

[60] S. M. Osés, K. Rantsiou, L. Cocolin, I. Jaime, and J. Rovira, "Prevalence and quantification of Shiga-toxin producing *Escherichia coli* along the lamb food chain by quantitative PCR," *International Journal of Food Microbiology*, vol. 141, pp. S163–S169, 2010.

[61] O. E. Adeleke, B. A. Adeniyi, and A. A. Akinrinmisi, "Microbiological quality of local soymilk: a public health appraisal," *African Journal of Biomedical Research*, vol. 3, pp. 89–92, 2000.

[62] A. C. Fluit and F. J. Schmitz, "Resistance integrons and super-integrons," *Clinical Microbiology and Infection*, vol. 10, no. 4, pp. 272–288, 2004.

[63] C. M. Schroeder, C. Zhao, C. DebRoy et al., "Antimicrobial resistance of *Escherichia coli* O157 isolated from humans, cattle, swine, and food," *Applied and Environmental Microbiology*, vol. 68, no. 2, pp. 576–581, 2002.

[64] D. W. Johnston, J. Bruce, and J. Hill, "Incidence of antibiotic-resistant *Escherichia coli* in milk produced in the west of

Scotland," *Journal of Applied Bacteriology*, vol. 54, no. 1, pp. 77–83, 1983.

[65] A. Skočková, S. Cupáková, R. Karpíšková, and B. Janštová, "Detection of tetracycline resistance genes in *Escherichia coli* from raw cow's milk," *Journal of Microbiology, Biotechnology and Food Sciences*, vol. 1, pp. 777–784, 2012.

[66] A. E. Van den Bogaard, "Antimicrobial resistance—relation to human and animal exposure to antibiotics," *Journal of Antimicrobial Chemotherapy*, vol. 40, no. 3, pp. 453–454, 1997.

Molecular Characterization of the Porcine Group A Rotavirus NSP2 and NSP5/6 Genes from São Paulo State, Brazil, in 2011/12

Bruna Rocha Passos Barbosa, Nara Thiers Cacciatori Galleti Bernardes, Laila Andreia Rodrigues Beserra, and Fábio Gregori

Department of Preventive Veterinary Medicine and Animal Health, Faculty of Veterinary Medicine, University of São Paulo, Avenida Prof. Dr. Orlando Marques de Paiva 87, Cidade Universitária, 05508-270 São Paulo, SD, Brazil

Correspondence should be addressed to Bruna Rocha Passos Barbosa; bruna888@hotmail.com

Academic Editors: C. DebRoy, D. Endoh, and B. I. Yoon

Rotaviruses are responsible for the acute diarrhea in various mammalian and avian species. The nonstructural proteins NSP2 and NSP5 are involved in the rotavirus replication and the formation of viroplasm, cytoplasmic inclusion bodies within which new viral particles morphogenesis and viral RNA replication occur. There are few studies on the genetic diversity of those proteins; thus this study aims at characterizing the diversity of rotavirus based on NSP2 and NSP5 genes in rotaviruses circulating in Brazilian pig farms. For this purpose, 63 fecal samples from pig farms located in six different cities in the São Paulo State, Brazil, were screened by nested RT-PCR. Seven strains had the partial nucleotide sequencing for NSP2, whereas in six, the total sequencing for NSP5. All were characterized as genotype H1 and N1. The nucleotide identity of NSP2 genes ranged from 100% to 86.4% and the amino acid identity from 100% to 91.5%. For NSP5, the nucleotide identity was from 100% to 95.1% and the amino acid identity from 100% to 97.4%. It is concluded that the genotypes of the strains circulating in the region of study are in agreement with those reported in the literature for swine and that there is the possibility of interaction between human and animal rotaviruses.

1. Introduction

Group A rotaviruses (GARV) are the major causes of viral diarrhea in a variety of animal young species worldwide [1]. In pig farms, they are responsible for economic losses due to death of animals, poor growth performance, and costs of diagnostic and treatment [2, 3]. Porcine GARVs are associated with weaning and postweaning enteritis in piglets and more often detected in piglets between 1 and 8 weeks of age [4, 5].

Rotavirus belongs to the family Reoviridae, subfamily Sedoreovirinae, and its genome consists of 11 segments of double-stranded RNA (dsRNA), which encode six structural proteins (VP1, VP2, VP3, VP4, VP6, and VP7) and six nonstructural proteins (NSP1–NSP6), with all genes being monocistronic except for segment 11 which encodes two proteins, NSP5 and NSP6 [6].

Encoded by segment 8 (1059 bp), NSP2 is a 35 kDa protein which assembles into octamers and is composed of 317 amino acids [7]. NSP2 has a role in packaging and replication, performing activities of nonspecific binding to single-stranded RNA (ssRNA) to start the synthesis of dsRNA, translocation of viral RNA during packaging, and helicase ATP-independent, triphosphatase, and NDP kinase activities [7–10].

NSP5 encoded by segment 11 (667 bp) is a 21 kDa protein that is hyperphosphorylated and O-glycosylated, and it consists of 198 amino acids, with abundance of serine (21%) and threonine (4.5%) [11–13]. NSP5 interacts with NSP2 to form cytoplasmic structures known as viroplasms, inside of which RNA replication and morphogenesis of new viral particles occur [1, 14, 15]. The interaction with NSP2 also enhances the process of NSP5 hyperphosphorylation [9, 16]. The segment 11 also contains the coding sequence of NSP6 in a second ORF, whose function is still unknown, but it preliminarily interacts with NSP5 in dimerization and hyperphosphorylation processes. However, given the low levels of expression of

TABLE 1: Primers designed for amplification and sequencing of the NSP2 and NSP5/6 genes from the samples of this study. bp: base pairs.

Gene	Primer	Primer sequence (5′→3′)	Amplicon (bp)	Reference
NSP2	GEN-NSP2F	GGCTTTTAAAGCGTCTCAG	728	[21]
	NSP2-RW707	GTACCATTTCCAGTGATRTCTC		Developed in this study
	NSP2-FW707	CATGGTAAAGGTCACTAYAGAG	247	Developed in this study
	NSP2-RW975	ACAGTTGACTATCTTTYTACCT		
NSP5	GEN-NSP5F	GGCTTTTAAAGCGCTACAG	667	[21]
	GEN-NSP5R	GGTCACAAAACGGGAGT		

NSP6, this suggests that this protein did not have an essential regulatory role [17–19].

Traditionally, GARVs are classified on the basis of two outer capsid proteins (VP4 and VP7), which induce the formation of neutralizing antibodies, with the VP7 determining the genotype G, whereas VP4 determines P genotype [1, 6]. However, a new classification for rotavirus was recently proposed which takes into account all 11 genomic segments, and the genotype N was determined for NSP2 protein and genotype H for NSP5 [20]. So far, nine genotypes N (N1 to N9) and 11 genotypes H (H1 to H11) have been defined. In humans, genotypes N1, N2, and N3 and H1, H2, and H3 have been described, whereas in pigs, H1 and N1 have been identified [5, 20]. As observed for VP4 and VP7, NSP2 and NSP5 also share genotypes between humans and animals, as previously reported by Martella et al., Matthijnssens et al., Tsugawa and Hoshino, and Khamrin et al. [5, 21–23].

The zoonotic aspect and interspecies transmission of rotavirus have been described by several authors [5, 21, 24, 25], and in this context the swines are considered as a major source of infection and important reservoirs for genetic and antigenic diversity of human rotaviruses [26, 27].

Despite the importance of genetic characterization of rotavirus circulating strains, data on the NSP2/5/6 molecular characterization in pigs in Brazil are scarce. Therefore, the objective of this study was to sequence the NSP2 and NSP5/6 genes of group A porcine rotavirus isolated from different pig herds in the São Paulo State, Brazil, in order to understand the phylogenetic relationships among them, as well as regarding other strains previously isolated from several regions around the world.

2. Materials and Methods

2.1. Samples. A total of 63 fecal samples from 34-day-old piglets with and without symptoms of diarrhea were used to study the NSP2 and NSP5 genes of GARV. The samples were collected in pig farms located in six different cities in the state of São Paulo, Brazil, from 2011 to 2012.

The rotavirus strain NCDV was used as positive control and ultrapure water previously treated with 0.1% diethyl pyrocarbonate (DEPC water) (Invitrogen) as negative control.

2.2. Detection of Rotavirus. For initial screening, the viral RNA was extracted from fecal samples using the TRIzol Reagent method (Invitrogen) according to the manufacturer's instructions, followed by nested RT-PCR technique as described by Salem et al. [28]. The extracted RNA was denatured at 95°C for 5 minutes and then subjected to RT-PCR.

2.3. RT-PCR. The reverse transcription reaction (cDNA synthesis) was performed using the following protocol. Briefly, 7 μL of extracted RNA was added to a mixture containing 1x First Strand Buffer (Invitrogen), dNTP (1 mM each), 10 mM DTT, 1 mM Random Hexamers (50 ng/μL, Invitrogen), 200 U MMLV Reverse Transcriptase (Invitrogen), and ultrapure DEPC-treated water for a final reaction volume of 20 μL. The RT was performed at 37°C for 1 h, followed by incubation at 70°C for 15 min.

The amplification of the NSP2 partial gene (975 bp) was performed using four primers, one of them described by Matthijnssens et al. [21] and others developed in the present study based on alignments of sequences retrieved from GenBank (Table 1). For NSP5/6, the complete segment of 667 bp was amplified using the primers previously described by Matthijnssens et al. [21] (Table 1).

Thus, the PCR reaction consisted of adding 5 μL of cDNA to a mixture containing 1x PCR Buffer (Invitrogen), dNTP (0.2 mM each), 0.2 μM of each primer (Table 1), 2 mM $MgCl_2$, 5 U of Taq DNA Polymerase (Invitrogen), and ultrapure DEPC-treated water for a final reaction volume of 25 μL. The PCR was performed at 94°C/3 min, followed by 40 amplification cycles (94°C/45 s, 45°C/45 s, and 70°C/2,5 min) and a final extension of 70°C for 7 min.

2.4. DNA Sequencing. The amplicons were purified with ExoSAP-IT (Affymetrix) according to the manufacturer's instructions and sequenced in both directions using the BigDye Terminator Cycle Sequencing Kit v. 3.1 (Life Technologies) followed by the application of the BigDye Xterminator kit (Life Technologies) for the removal of unincorporated DNA terminators, also according to the manufacturer's instructions, on an automated DNA sequencer ABI-3500 (Applied Biosystems).

2.5. Phylogenetic Analysis. The sequences obtained were edited using Bioedit v. 7.1.3.0 program [29], and multiple alignments were done using the Clustal W v. 2.1 software [30]. The nucleotide and deduced amino acid sequences of NSP2 and NSP5/6 genes were compared with those of reference strains available at NCBI (National Center for Biotechnology Information) GenBank database using the BLAST (Basic Local Alignment Search Tool) server [31].

Phylogenetic analyses were conducted using MEGA version 5.1 [32], and the phylogenetic tree was built using the neighbor-joining method (1,000 bootstrap trials) with maximum composite likelihood as substitution model.

2.6. Nucleotide Sequence Accession Numbers. The nucleotide sequences of NSP2 and NSP5/6 genes of the rotavirus strains from this study have been deposited in GenBank under the accession numbers KC117140 to KC117146 for NSP2 and KC117147 to KC117152 for NSP5.

3. Results

3.1. Detection of Rotavirus. Seventeen of the 63 fecal samples (17/63 or 27%) tested positive for rotaviruses by nested RT-PCR [28] from five different cities (5/6).

3.2. Analysis of NSP2 Gene Sequences. We sequenced a partial NSP2 fragment (975 bp or 97%) in 7 of the 17 positive strains analyzed (SWRV1 to SWRV7).

Comparing the nucleotide and predicted amino acid sequences of the strains of the present study with others already deposited in GenBank, the data revealed that SWRV 1, 2, 6, and 7 were more closely related to the porcine rotavirus strain, YM, in terms of nucleotides (94.7–95.4%) and to bovine strains, KJ44 and KJ75, in terms of amino acid (98.0–98.3%). With regard to the strains SWRV 3, 4, and 5, they shared maximum identities with the human rotavirus strain, IAL28 (94.0–95.1% in terms of nucleotide and 96.1% for amino acids). The phylogenetic tree revealed that the strains clustered together with the N1 genotype (Figure 1).

The motifs related to the functions of translocation of RNA (75 bases corresponding to the 5′ noncoding region 3′ and the beginning of ORF), to the NTPase (histidine at position 225), and to the cysteine residues 6, 8, 85, and 285, which are involved in the formation of disulfide bridges [10, 33, 34], were conserved between the samples of this study.

There was variability in the RNA-binding domain of NSP2 corresponding to amino acid residues 205–241 (A207S, R215K, I218V and S216F, and I218A) [10, 33].

3.3. Analysis of NSP5/6 Gene Sequences. Complete sequences of these genes and their corresponding proteins were obtained in 6 of the 17 positive strains analyzed (6/17) (SWRV1 to SWRV6).

The comparison among the nucleotide and putative amino acids sequences of the strains of this study with others from human and animal previously deposited in GenBank revealed a high identity among SWRV 1, 2, and 3 and porcine strains Gottfried, RU172 and CMP034 (94.0–95.1% nucleotide and 96.1% amino acid identity). With respect to SWRV 4, 5, and 6, they also shared maximum identities with the porcine rotavirus strains, Gottfried and CMP034 (97.1%, in terms of nucleotide and 99.4% for amino acids). The phylogenetic tree revealed that the strains clustered together with the H1 genotype (Figure 2).

For NSP6, in terms of amino acids, the strains SWRV 1, 2, and 3 shared maximum identities values from 95.6% with human strains 2007744509, 2008747100, and 2007719698, while SWRV 4, 5, and 6 were most closely related to porcine strain, PRG942 (98.9–100%).

The nine phosphorylation sites of NSP5 concerning serine residues at positions 2, 4, 30, 37, 42, 56, 67, 101, 127, and 163 [35] present conserved between the samples of this study, except for the residue at position 37 (S37N).

4. Discussion

Studies carried out about the occurrence of RVA in pigs from different Brazilian regions have shown a relatively wide distribution of this agent in the creations around the country [36–38]. Five of the six cities studied presented samples positive for rotavirus at an overall prevalence of 27% (17/63), very similar to that found by Gregori et al. [36] of 29.9%.

Our study revealed the circulation of genotype N1 of NSP2 in the cities sampled, which, for pigs, is the only N genotype reported so far, but that has also been described in humans, cattle, and cats [5, 20, 39]. Likewise, the genotype H1 detected for NSP5 has been reported in pigs, which also occurs in humans and animals [5, 20]. It should be noted that no genotypic classification was defined for NSP6, since this protein ORF is entirely contained within the NSP5 ORF. Therefore, as suggested by Matthijnssens et al. [39], the phylogenetic analysis of both would be nearly identical.

The NSP2 genes for the strains SWRV 3, 4, and 5 were the closest related to that of the IAL28 strain, a G5 human rotavirus strain isolated in Brazil in 1992 from a child with diarrhea, and that G5 is another genotype commonly described in pigs [40]. Although the highest nucleotide and amino acid identity values for NSP5 had been with porcine rotavirus strains, phylogenetic tree deduced from this gene revealed that the strains SWRV 1, 2, and 3 segregated in a cluster that also included the human strain IAL28 with which those strains showed high nucleotide and amino acid identities ranging from 94.1 to 94.6% and 94.3%, respectively (Figure 2). The findings of genetic relationships of the porcine strains of this study with those of human rotavirus, as well as detection of genotypes common to both species, suggest the occurrence of interspecies transmission, in which the pigs likely act as a source of infection for humans [24, 39].

Several studies corroborated our findings by reporting high degrees of genetic similarity between human and animal strains, as well as the occurrence of N1 and H1 genotypes in human strains (5, 21, 27, 41). Esona et al. showed that in six G8 human African strains, the genes VP7, NSP2, and NSP5 had high identity with animal strains (83–99% and 97–99% nucleotide and amino acid values, resp.) [41]. Additionally, Ghosh et al. determined the nucleotide sequence of the genes encoding VP1, VP2, VP3, and NSP1, NSP2, and NSP3 of the porcine strain, RU172, being that NSP2 clustered in a group predominantly consisting of human rotavirus [42].

It has been shown that NSP2 motif related to the RNA binding consists of the amino acid residues 205–241, while the cysteine residues 6, 8, 85, and 285 are involved in disulfide bridges which ensure the octameric structure of this protein [10, 33]. Furthermore, these studies also reveal an extensive

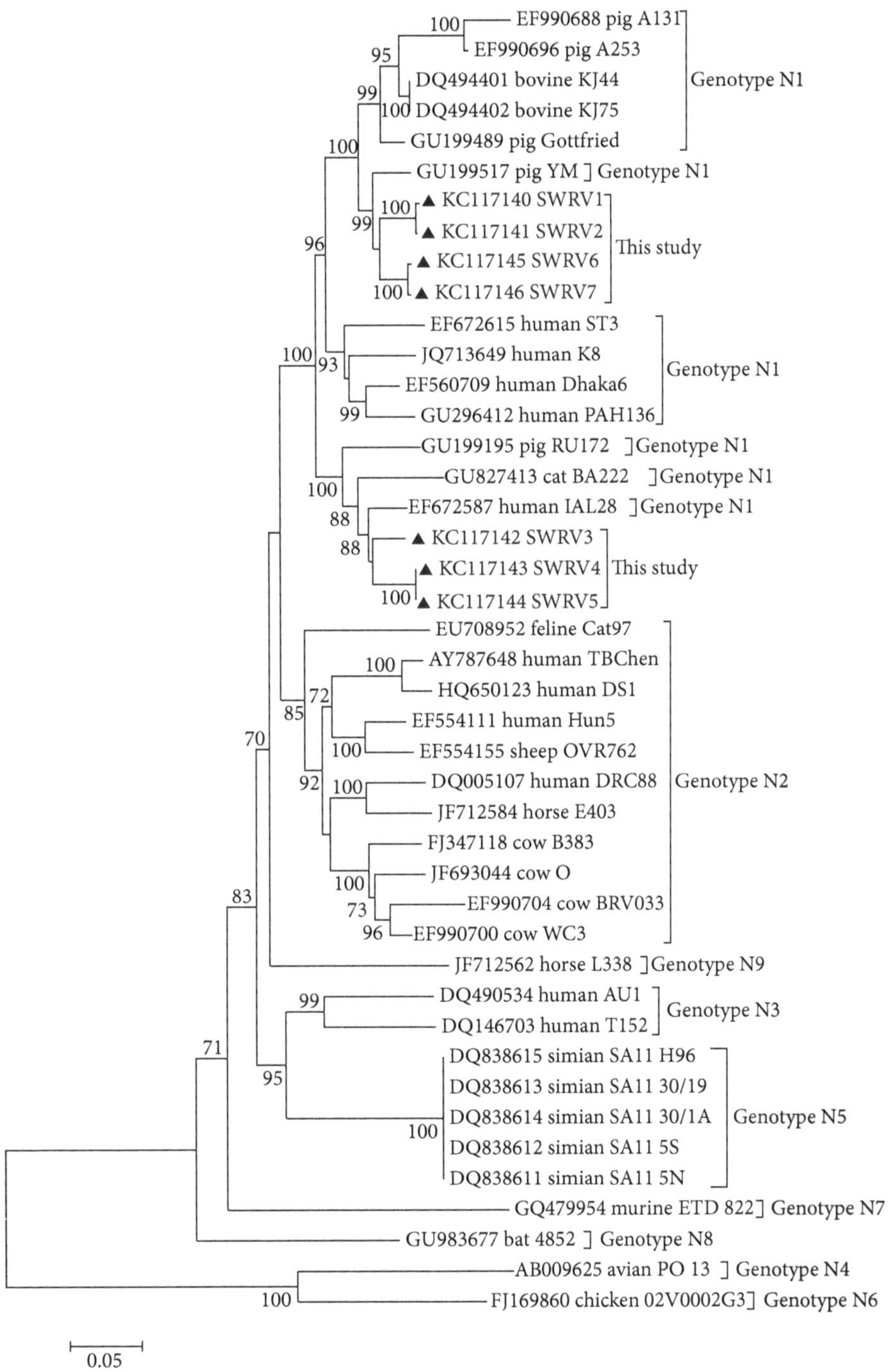

FIGURE 1: Phylogenetic tree constructed with the neighbor-joining method using maximum composite likelihood as substitution model for a partial region (975 bp) of the NSP2 gene of the group A porcine rotavirus of the strains SWRV1 and SWRV7 with others representing human and animal GARVs. The scale represents the number of substitutions per site. Only bootstrap values >70% are shown. Pig strains defined in the present study are preceded by black triangles, and they are identified as accession number/host/strain/NSP2 genotype.

conserved region of 75 bases (b) including 35b in the 5′ noncoding region 3′ and the first 30b of the ORF as a region in which the conformational NSP2 changes occur, leading to translocation of ssRNA. The NTPase activity of NSP2 is related to amino acid histidine at position 225, which acts as a catalyst residue for enzymatic function of this protein, so that the mutation in this residue prevents the synthesis of dsRNA [34]. Thus, mutations in regions concerning the binding domain of NSP2 with the RNA, R215K, S216F, and I218V, found in the strains of the present study in relation to the standard strain Gottfried (Accession number GU199489), have been reported in samples standard OSU, UK, NCDV,

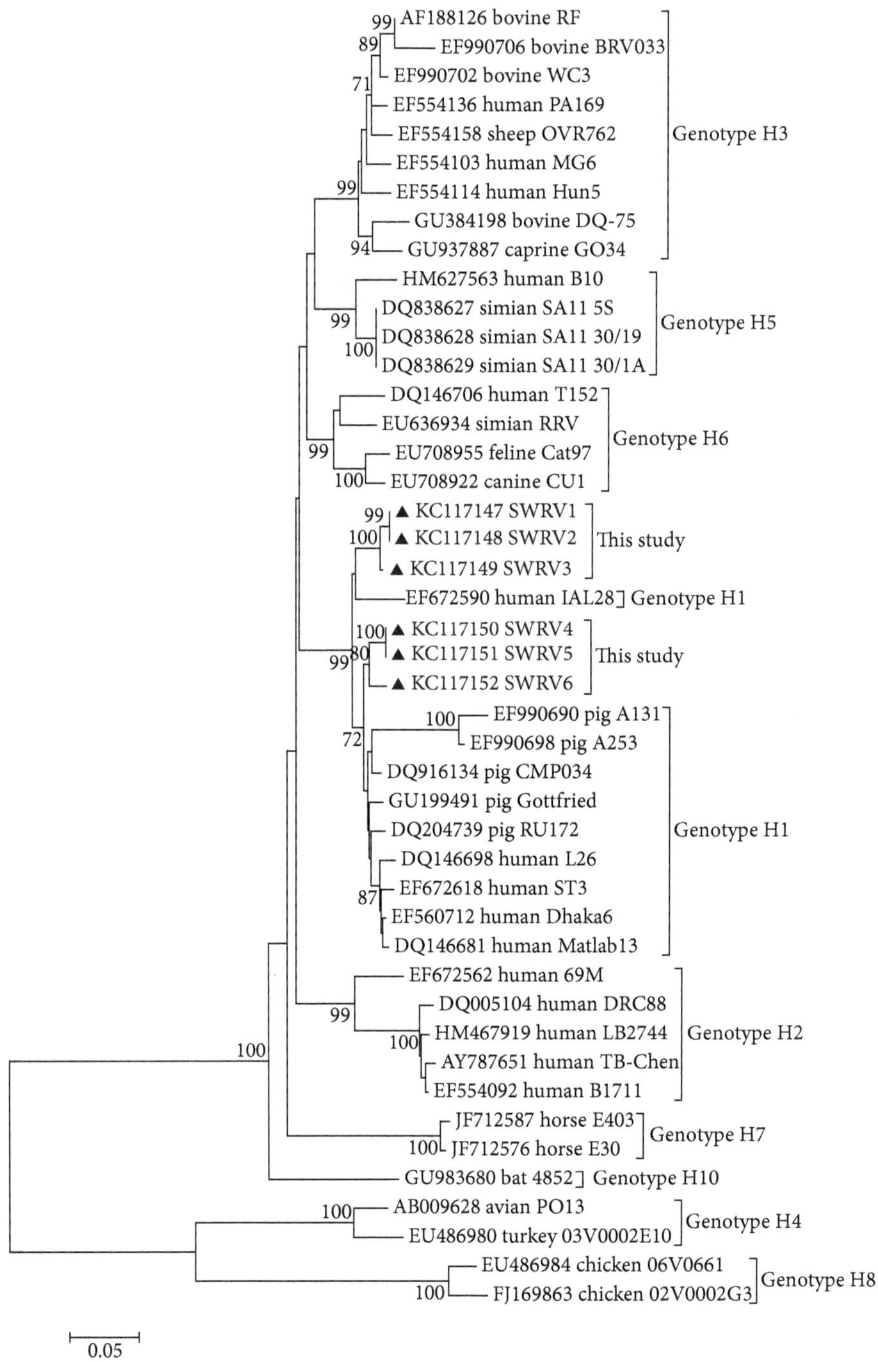

FIGURE 2: Phylogenetic tree constructed with the neighbor-joining method using maximum composite likelihood as substitution model for the NSP5 complete gene of the group A porcine rotavirus of the strains SWRV1 and SWRV6 with others representing human and animal GARVs. The scale represents the number of substitutions per site. Only bootstrap values >70% are shown. Pig strains defined in the present study are preceded by black triangles, and they are identified as accession number/host/strain/NSP5 genotype.

Wa, and SA11 [33, 43, 44]. On the other hand, for mutations at positions I218A and A207S, there are no reports in the literature.

In regard to NSP5, nine phosphorylation sites were identified in this protein concerning serine residues at positions 2, 4, 30, 37, 42, 56, 67, 101, 127, and 163 [35]. Compared to the standard strain Gottfried (Accession number GU199491), the strains of this study showed a mutation from serine to asparagine at position 37 which does not seem to be significant since some isoforms of this protein may not provide the phosphorylation sites at residues 30 and/or 37, and then, serine would be absent at these sites, but without altering the phosphorylation process, as demonstrated by Sotelo et al. [35].

The data showed low rates of genetic variability for NSP2 and NSP5/6 in the strains of the present study. Indeed, these proteins are generally more stable because of structural and functional constraints and lower exposure to immune selection [45].

More genetic characterization studies would be helpful for detection of interspecies transmission [21, 27, 46]; however, only collection and analysis of RV specimens collected in close geographic and temporal proximity in a prospective manner, as shown by Steyer et al. [25], will provide firm evidence. Thus, considering that there are few studies in Brazil aiming at molecular characterization of NSP2 and NSP5 in pigs, it becomes imminent monitoring swine herds and human populations in order to detect and/or prevent such situations of possible cross-infection [25].

5. Conclusion

The molecular analyses performed in this study indicated that most of the samples of rotaviruses circulating in pig herds of the São Paulo State present genotypes consistent with those described in the literature for Brazil and in other countries.

Conflict of Interests

The authors report no conflict of interests, and they have no direct financial relation with the commercial identities mentioned in the paper.

Acknowledgment

The authors would like to thank the FAPESP (São Paulo Research Foundation) for financial support (Process no. 2010/13652-8).

References

[1] M. K. Estes and A. Z. Kapikian, "Rotaviruses," in *Fields Virology*, B. N. Fields, P. M. Knipe, and P. M. Howley, Eds., pp. 1917–1973, Lippincott Williams & Wilkins, Philadelphia, Pa, USA, 5th edition, 2007.

[2] A. A. Alfieri, A. F. Alfieri, and E. A. Beuttemmüller, "Rotavirose suína: tópicos sobre etiologia, infecção e controle," *Semina: Ciências Agrárias*, vol. 20, no. 1, pp. 90–97, 1999.

[3] Paho: Pan American Health Organization, "Rotaviral gastroenteritis," in *Zoonoses and Communicable Diseases Common to Man and Animals: Chlamydioses, Rickettsioses and Viroses*, pp. 286–294, PAHO, Washington, DC, USA, 3rd edition, 2001.

[4] L. J. Saif and B. Jiang, "Nongroup A rotaviruses of humans and animals," *Current Topics in Microbiology and Immunology*, vol. 185, pp. 339–371, 1994.

[5] V. Martella, K. Bányai, J. Matthijnssens, C. Buonavoglia, and M. Ciarlet, "Zoonotic aspects of rotaviruses," *Veterinary Microbiology*, vol. 140, no. 3-4, pp. 246–255, 2010.

[6] A. M. Q. King, M. J. Adams, E. B. Carstens, and E. J. Lefkowitz, Eds., *Virus Taxonomy: Classification and Nomenclature of Viruses*, Elsevier Academic Press, San Diego, Calif, USA, 9th edition, 2012.

[7] P. Schuck, Z. Taraporewala, P. McPhie, and J. T. Patton, "Rotavirus nonstructural protein NSP2 self-assembles into octamers that undergo ligand-induced conformational changes," *The Journal of Biological Chemistry*, vol. 276, no. 13, pp. 9679–9687, 2001.

[8] Z. F. Taraporewala and J. T. Patton, "Identification and characterization of the helix-destabilizing activity of rotavirus nonstructural protein NSP2," *Journal of Virology*, vol. 75, no. 10, pp. 4519–4527, 2001.

[9] T. Bar-Magen, E. Spencer, and J. T. Patton, "An ATPase activity associated with the rotavirus phosphoprotein NSP5," *Virology*, vol. 369, no. 2, pp. 389–399, 2007.

[10] L. Hu, D. C. Chow, J. T. Patton, T. Palzkill, M. K. Estes, and B. V. V. Prasad, "Crystallographic analysis of rotavirus NSP2-RNA complex reveals specific recognition of 5′GG sequence for RTPase activity," *Journal of Virology*, vol. 86, no. 19, pp. 10547–10557, 2012.

[11] I. Afrikanova, E. Fabbretti, M. C. Miozzo, and O. R. Burrone, "Rotavirus NSP5 phosphorylation is up-regulated by interaction with NSP2," *Journal of General Virology*, vol. 79, no. 11, pp. 2679–2686, 1998.

[12] M. Berois, C. Sapin, I. Erk, D. Poncet, and J. Cohen, "Rotavirus nonstructural protein NSP5 interacts with major core protein VP2," *Journal of Virology*, vol. 77, no. 3, pp. 1757–1763, 2003.

[13] C. Eichwald, G. Jacob, B. Muszynski, J. E. Allende, and O. R. Burrone, "Uncoupling substrate and activation functions of rotavirus NSP5: phosphorylation of Ser-67 by casein kinase 1 is essential for hyperphosphorylation," *Proceedings of the National Academy of Sciences of the United States of America*, vol. 101, no. 46, pp. 16304–16309, 2004.

[14] C. Eichwald, J. F. Rodriguez, and O. R. Burrone, "Characterization of rotavirus NSP2/NSP5 interactions and the dynamics of viroplasm formation," *Journal of General Virology*, vol. 85, no. 3, pp. 625–634, 2004.

[15] J. J. Carreño-Torres, M. Gutiérrez, C. F. Arias, S. López, and P. Isa, "Characterization of viroplasm formation during the early stages of rotavirus infection," *Virology Journal*, vol. 7, article 350, 2010.

[16] A. Sen, D. Agresti, and E. R. Mackow, "Hyperphosphorylation of the rotavirus NSP5 protein is independent of serine 67, NSP2, or the intrinsic insolubility of NSP5 and is regulated by cellular phosphatases," *Journal of Virology*, vol. 80, no. 4, pp. 1807–1816, 2006.

[17] M. A. Torres-Vega, R. A. González, M. Duarte, D. Poncet, S. López, and C. F. Arias, "The C-terminal domain of rotavirus NSP5 is essential for its multimerization, hyperphosphorylation and interaction with NSP6," *Journal of General Virology*, vol. 81, no. 3, pp. 821–830, 2000.

[18] M. Samaniego-Hernández, A. León-Rodríguez, R. Aparicio-Fabre, C. Arias-Ortiz, and A. P. Barba de La Rosa, "Expression and purification of rotavirus proteins NSP5 and NSP6 in *Escherichia coli*," *Cell Biochemistry and Biophysics*, vol. 44, no. 3, pp. 336–341, 2006.

[19] E. W. Rainsford and M. A. McCrae, "Characterization of the NSP6 protein product of rotavirus gene 11," *Virus Research*, vol. 130, no. 1-2, pp. 193–201, 2007.

[20] J. Matthijnssens, M. Ciarlet, S. M. Mcdonald et al., "Uniformity of rotavirus strain nomenclature proposed by the Rotavirus Classification Working Group (RCWG)," *Archives of Virology*, vol. 156, no. 8, pp. 1397–1413, 2011.

[21] J. Matthijnssens, M. Rahman, V. Martella et al., "Full genomic analysis of human rotavirus strain B4106 and lapine rotavirus

strain 30/96 provides evidence for interspecies transmission," *Journal of Virology*, vol. 80, no. 8, pp. 3801–3810, 2006.

[22] T. Tsugawa and Y. Hoshino, "Whole genome sequence and phylogenetic analyses reveal human rotavirus G3P[3] strains Ro1845 and HCR3A are examples of direct virion transmission of canine/feline rotaviruses to humans," *Virology*, vol. 380, no. 2, pp. 344–353, 2008.

[23] P. Khamrin, N. Maneekarn, R. Malasao et al., "Genotypic linkages of VP4, VP6, VP7, NSP4, NSP5 genes of rotaviruses circulating among children with acute gastroenteritis in Thailand," *Infection, Genetics and Evolution*, vol. 10, no. 4, pp. 467–472, 2010.

[24] N. Cook, J. Bridger, K. Kendall, M. I. Gomara, L. El-Attar, and J. Gray, "The zoonotic potential of rotavirus," *Journal of Infection*, vol. 48, no. 4, pp. 289–302, 2004.

[25] A. Steyer, M. Poljšak-Prijatelj, D. Barlič-Maganja, and J. Marin, "Human, porcine and bovine rotaviruses in Slovenia: evidence of interspecies transmission and genome reassortment," *Journal of General Virology*, vol. 89, no. 7, pp. 1690–1698, 2008.

[26] V. Martella, M. Ciarlet, R. Baselga et al., "Sequence analysis of the VP7 and VP4 genes identifies a novel VP7 gene allele of porcine rotaviruses, sharing a common evolutionary origin with human G2 rotaviruses," *Virology*, vol. 337, no. 1, pp. 111–123, 2005.

[27] A. Mukherjee, D. Dutta, S. Ghosh et al., "Full genomic analysis of a human group A rotavirus G9P[6] strain from Eastern India provides evidence for porcine-to-human interspecies transmission," *Archives of Virology*, vol. 154, no. 5, pp. 733–746, 2009.

[28] A. N. B. Salem, A. C. Sergei, P. B. Olga, G. A. Olga, A. Mahjoub, and B. P. Larissa, "Multiplex nested RT-PCR for the detection of porcine enteric viruses," *Journal of Virological Methods*, vol. 165, no. 2, pp. 283–293, 2010.

[29] T. A. Hall, "BioEdit: a user-friendly biological sequence alignment editor and analysis program for Windows 95/98/NT," *Nucleic Acids Symposium Series*, vol. 41, pp. 95–98, 1999.

[30] M. A. Larkin, G. Blackshields, N. P. Brown et al., "Clustal W and Clustal X version 2.0," *Bioinformatics*, vol. 23, no. 21, pp. 2947–2948, 2007.

[31] S. F. Altschul, W. Gish, W. Miller, E. W. Myers, and D. J. Lipman, "Basic local alignment search tool," *Journal of Molecular Biology*, vol. 215, no. 3, pp. 403–410, 1990.

[32] K. Tamura, D. Peterson, N. Peterson, G. Stecher, M. Nei, and S. Kumar, "MEGA5: molecular evolutionary genetics analysis using maximum likelihood, evolutionary distance, and maximum parsimony methods," *Molecular Biology and Evolution*, vol. 28, no. 10, pp. 2731–2739, 2011.

[33] J. T. Patton, L. Salter-Cid, A. Kalbach, E. A. Mansell, and M. Kattoura, "Nucleotide and amino acid sequence analysis of the rotavirus nonstructural RNA-binding protein NS35," *Virology*, vol. 192, no. 2, pp. 438–446, 1993.

[34] M. Kumar, H. Jayaram, R. Vasquez-Del Carpio et al., "Crystallographic and biochemical analysis of rotavirus NSP2 with nucleotides reveals a nucleoside diphosphate kinase-like activity," *Journal of Virology*, vol. 81, no. 22, pp. 12272–12284, 2007.

[35] P. H. Sotelo, M. Schümann, E. Krause, and J. Chnaiderman, "Analysis of rotavirus non-structural protein NSP5 by mass spectrometry reveals a complex phosphorylation pattern," *Virus Research*, vol. 149, no. 1, pp. 104–108, 2010.

[36] F. Gregori, C. A. R. Rosales, P. E. Brandão, R. M. Soares, and J. A. Jerez, "Diversidade genotípica de rotavírus suínos no Estado de São Paulo," *Pesquisa Veterinária Brasileira*, vol. 29, pp. 707–712, 2009.

[37] R. C. Linares, A. F. Barry, A. F. Alfieri et al., "Frequency of group A rotavirus in piglet stool samples from non-vaccinated Brazilian pig herds," *Brazilian Archives of Biology and Technology*, vol. 52, pp. 63–68, 2009.

[38] K. C. Médici, A. F. Barry, A. F. Alfieri, and A. A. Alfieri, "Porcine rotavirus groups A, B, and C identified by polymerase chain reaction in a fecal sample collection with inconclusive results by polyacrylamide gel electrophoresis," *Journal of Swine Health and Production*, vol. 19, no. 3, pp. 146–150, 2011.

[39] J. A. Matthijnssens, M. Ciarlet, E. Heiman et al., "Full genome-based classification of rotaviruses reveals a common origin between human Wa-like and porcine rotavirus strains and human DS-1-like and bovine rotavirus strains," *Journal of Virology*, vol. 82, no. 7, pp. 3204–3219, 2008.

[40] E. M. Heiman, S. M. McDonald, M. Barro, Z. F. Taraporewala, T. Bar-Magen, and J. T. Patton, "Group A human rotavirus genomics: evidence that gene constellations are influenced by viral protein interactions," *Journal of Virology*, vol. 82, no. 22, pp. 11106–11116, 2008.

[41] M. D. Esona, A. Geyer, N. Page et al., "Genomic characterization of human rotavirus G8 strains from the African rotavirus network: relationship to animal rotaviruses," *Journal of Medical Virology*, vol. 81, no. 5, pp. 937–951, 2009.

[42] S. Ghosh, N. Kobayashi, S. Nagashima et al., "Full genomic analysis and possible origin of a porcine G12 rotavirus strain RU172," *Virus Genes*, vol. 40, no. 3, pp. 382–388, 2010.

[43] M. L. Dyall-Smith, T. C. Ellemant, P. A. Hoyne, I. H. Holmes, and A. A. Azad, "Cloning and sequence of UK bovine rotavirus gene segment 7: marked sequence homology with simban rotavirus gene segment 8," *Nucleic Acids Research*, vol. 11, no. 10, pp. 3351–3362, 1983.

[44] K. Rushlow, A. Mcnab, K. Olson, F. Maxwell, I. Maxwell, and G. Stiegler, "Nucleotide sequence of porcine rotavirus (OSU strain) gene segments 7, 8, and 9," *Nucleic Acids Research*, vol. 16, no. 1, pp. 367–368, 1988.

[45] K. Taniguchi and S. Urasawa, "Diversity in rotavirus genomes," *Seminars in Virology*, vol. 6, no. 2, pp. 123–131, 1995.

[46] G. I. Parra, G. Vidales, J. A. Gomez, F. M. Fernandez, V. Parreño, and K. Bok, "Phylogenetic analysis of porcine rotavirus in Argentina: increasing diversity of G4 strains and evidence of interspecies transmission," *Veterinary Microbiology*, vol. 126, no. 1–3, pp. 243–250, 2008.

8

Ground Wheat Grain for Midlactation Cows: Challenging a Common Wisdom

A. Nikkhah, F. Amiri, and H. Amanloo

Department of Animal Sciences, Faculty of Agricultural Sciences, University of Zanjan, Zanjan 313-45195, Iran

Correspondence should be addressed to A. Nikkhah, anikkha@yahoo.com

Academic Editor: Antonio Souto

The objective was to determine the effects of ground wheat grain (GW) inclusion rate, grinding extent (GE), and their interaction on lactating cow performance. Eight midlactation cows in 3 × 4 m individual boxes were used in a 4 × 4 replicated Latin square design study with 4 21 d periods. GW was fed at either 10% or 20% of diet dry matter (DM), as either finer or coarser particles. DM intake increased and net energy for lactation (NE_L) intake tended to increase when GW was fed at 10% instead of 20% of diet DM. Milk energy yield, milk solids content and yield, and urine pH were unaffected. Fecal pH tended to increase at 20% versus 10% GW. Total tract apparent NDF, but not DM, digestibility tended to be greater for coarsely than finely GW and tended to be greater at 10% versus 20% GW. GW at 10% versus 20% of diet DM decreased blood BHBA and increased blood concentrations of total proteins and albumin. Data provide novel evidence that both finely and coarsely ground WG can be safely fed up to 20% midlactation cows. Commercial accessibility and cost will determine feeding preference of wheat grain to dairy cows.

1. Introduction

Wheat grain (WG: *Triticum spp.*) is an invaluable energy and amino acids source for livestock. Due to its usually fast and extensive rumen degradation, popular consumption by humans, and climatic, agronomical and economical constraints, WG has less commonly been fed to ruminants compared to corn and barley grains. Subsequent to oats, ground WG (GW) possesses the highest starch and protein degradation extent and rate among cereals [1, 2]. If not managed properly, increased dietary GW levels are, thus, more likely to cause subacute rumen acidosis (SARA), milk fat depression, and laminitis, when compared to corn and barley grains [3, 4]. However, such a SARA risk would exist rather shortly after feeding (44% versus 60% of total starch degraded after 4-h for barley and wheat grains, resp; [5]) because wheat and barley grains have almost similar degradation patterns after few hours after feeding [1, 6]. The traditional belief that feeding GW threatens rumen and ruminant health and production is prone to challenges. As such, in vitro and in vivo digestion and metabolic properties of feeding wheat cultivars to ruminants continue to receive research interests [7–9].

As WG becomes more accessible and cheaper, its dietary inclusion for lactating cows may be more feasible. However, such reports for feeding GW of different particle sizes are lacking. For adequate ruminal and small intestinal utilization, WG should be physically processed. Processing can improve DM digestion of WG in the whole gastrointestinal tract from 16–32% to 87–100% [14, 15]. Crushing, grinding and rolling are the common processing methods. Steam-processing may reduce ruminal degradation rate of rapidly fermentable grains (e.g., WG) via increased particle size, and likely by developing starch-protein and starch-lipids bonds in the endosperm [16]. However, steam-rolling equipment is very expensive to be established and be maintaind, particularly for medium and small size farms. Thus, in vivo data are required to determine if and to what extent differently ground WG, produced by hammer mills, can be fed to lactating cows. Uncovering optimum dietary inclusion rates of differently ground WG without other major investments in chemical and physical processing is of practical importance. Ground GW fed prepartum has recently been shown to increase blood glucose and calcium and improve milk production of periparturient cows and heifers [8, 17]. Nevertheless, GW inclusion rate in lactation diets in relation to processing methods and particle size has not been studied. Doepel et al. [7] found that steam-rolled WG may replace steam-rolled barley grain at 20% of diet DM for second-calf midlactation cows without compromising rumen conditions and nutrient digestibility. Feeding 20% of steam-rolled WG has been found feasible without any sodium bicarbonate in midlactation diets [18]. Whilst grinding is an easy-to-access and widely accessible technique to process WG, in vivo data are lacking on feeding lactating cows different levels of differently ground WG. In light of the higher rumen degradation rate of starch and protein in wheat grain than in barley grain, feeding GW at controlled levels was hypothesized to maintain feed intake and milk production. The primary objective was to determine effects of feeding a higher (20%) versus a lower (10%) level of coarsely versus finely GW in chopped alfalfa- hay- and wheat- straw- based mixed rations on feed intake, peripheral blood metabolites, and milk production of midlactation Holstein cows.

2. Materials and Methods

2.1. Cows, Diets, and Management. Eight midlactation Holstein dairy cows (176 ± 8 d in milk; 554 ± 13 kg body weight (BW), 3.12 ± 0.14 body condition score (BCS); mean ± SE) were randomly assigned to one of four treatments in a 4 × 4 replicated Latin square design with 4 21-day periods. Each period had 14 days of adaptation. Since dietary forage type and level were similar among diets, and treatments involved readily degradable grains, the 14-d was considered sufficiently optimal for rumen microbial adjustment to changes in GW level and particle size [19]. In addition, 14-d was set to avoid period by treatment interactions that are likely to occur with longer periods [20]. Treatments included 4 total mixed rations (TMRs) containing either (1) a higher (20%) or (2) a lower (10%) level of either (1) coarsely or (2) finely ground wheat grain (GW). Thus, GW level and grinding extent (GE) effects were determined in a 2 × 2 factorial arrangement. Ground wheat grain replaced ground barley grain when going from 10% to 20% GW (Table 1). Chopped alfalfa-hay-and wheat-straw-based TMRs with forage to concentrate ratio of 47.5 : 52.5 were fed to individual cows in equal portions 3 times daily at 0900, 1600, and 2300 h to permit about 5–10% daily orts, calculated based on the previous day's intake. Diets were formulated using NRC [13] for Holstein midlactation cows with 560 kg BW, 20 kg DMI, and 30 kg daily milk yield with 3.5% fat (Table 1). Cows were housed indoor in individual 3 × 4 m boxes equipped with concrete feed bunkers and metal water troughs. Cows were allowed 1 h of daily exercise 3 times daily prior to each milking. The experiment was conducted at the Dairy Facilities of the University of Zanjan Research Farm (Zanjan, Iran) according to the guidelines of the Iranian Council of Animal Care [21].

2.2. Grain and Forage Properties and Processing. Wheat (*Triticum spp.*) and barley (*Hordeum spp.*) grains were obtained from bulked sources representing grains fed in broad regions of Iran. Wheat grain DM contained 75% starch, 13% CP, 11% NDF, 3.2% ADF, and 2.3% ether extract. The respective values were 58%, 11%, 20%, 7%, and 2.2% for barley grain. Whole barley and wheat grains densities were 500 and 550 g/L, respectively. Rumen degradation rates of potentially degradable DM of corn, barley and wheat grains were 6%, 10%, and 12%/h, respectively. To produce the coarser and finer particle size treatments, WG was ground by passing through larger and smaller mesh size screens within a commercial hammer mill (model 5543 GEN, Isfahan Dasht, Isfahan, Iran), widely used by dairy farmers in Iran [8, 22]. Ground WG particle size distributions were determined using an electrical laboratory particle size separator-shaker with 7 round screens of decreasing mesh size on a bottom pan. The percentages of particles retained on the bottom pan and 0.8-mm, 1.2-mm, 1.6-mm, 3.0-mm, 5.0 mm and 8-mm screens were, respectively, 6.8%, 26%, 38%, 9.6%, 11%,

Table 1: Dry matter based dietary ingredients at higher and lower inclusion rates of ground wheat grain in midlactation diets.

Ingredients and nutrients (DM based)	Dietary ground wheat grain	
	Lower (10%)	Higher (20%)
Alfalfa hay	42.8	42.8
Wheat straw	4.8	4.8
Ground barley grain	10.5	1.1
Ground wheat grain	9.7	19.1
Ground corn grain	5.8	5.8
Soybean meal	12.0	12.0
Whole cottonseed	6.8	6.8
Fish meal	3.6	3.6
Fatty acids-calcium soaps (powder)[1]	0.8	0.8
NaCl	0.42	0.42
Calcium carbonate	1.05	1.05
Sodium bicarbonate	1.05	1.05
Minerals and vitamins supplement[2]	0.63	0.63
DM %	92.5	93.5
CP %	18.5	18.6
Starch %	18.1	19.5
NDF %	39.5	40.5
$peNDF_{>8}$[3]	18.4	18.0
$peNDF_{>1.18}$[3]	37.3	34.8
NE_L[4], Mcal/kg	1.60	1.62
Calcium %	1.0	1.0
Phosphorous %	0.5	0.5

[1]Berg + Schmidt (GmbH & Co.) KG, Hamburg, Germany.
[2]Contained 250000 IU/kg vitamin A, 50000 IU/kg vitamin D, 1500 IU/kg vitamin E, 2.25 g/kg manganese, 120 g/kg calcium, 7.7 g/kg zinc, 20 g/kg phosphorus, 20.5 g/kg magnesium, 186 g/kg sodium, 1.25 g/kg iron, 3 g/kg sulfur, 1.25 g/kg copper, 14 mg/kg cobalt, 56 mg/kg iodine, and 10mg/kg selenium.
[3]NDF content of TMR or forage multiplied by their physical effective factor (pef) or the proportion of particles retained on the 19-mm, 8-mm, and 1.18-mm sieves of the PSPS [10, 11]. NDF content of TMR or forage multiplied by its pef or the proportion of particles retained on the 19-mm and 8-mm sieves of the PSPS [12].
[4]Estimated from NRC [13].

4.7%, and 3.3% for the coarser GW and 12%, 6.4%, 22%, 21%, 27%, 8.2%, and 3.2% for the finer GW. Alfalfa hay DM contained 13.1% CP and 41.6% NDF, and was chopped using an on-farm chopper machine (Agricultural Machinery Co., Tabriz, Iran) for an average theoretical chop length of 4 cm before mixing with concentrate. Forage and concentrate for individual cows were weighed daily and divided into 3 portions for 3 times daily feed delivery. At each feeding, forage and concentrate were mixed in the individual cow bunks.

2.3. DMI, Feed Analysis, and Total Tract Nutrient Digestibility. The amount of TMR offered and orts were measured daily from d 15–21 of each period to calculate DMI for individual cows. Samples of TMR were taken daily for individual cows during the 7 sampling d of each period. Feed and ort samples were pooled per cow per period and were oven-dried at 100°C for 24-h, ground to pass through 1-mm screen using a Wiley mill (Arthur H. Thomas Co., Philadelphia), and stored at −20°C until analyzed for nutrients. Feed samples were analyzed for CP (method 984.13; [23]), NDF (using heat-stable α-amylase and sodium sulfite), and ADF (method 973.18; [23]). Organic matter was determined by ashing the dried feed and feces for 8 h at 550°C (method 942.05; [23]). The acid insoluble ash (AIA; [22]) was used as an internal marker to determine total tract apparent DM and NDF digestibility. Particle size distribution of TMR samples was measured using Penn State Particle Separator (PSPS) [12]. For the PSPS analysis, the daily samples were composited to obtain 2 TMR and 2 forage samples per period. Physically effective NDF was estimated by multiplying dietary NDF% by (1) the proportion of DM retained on the 19.0-mm and 8.0-mm sieves of the PSPS ($peNDF_{>8}$, [12]) and (2) the proportion of DM retained on the 19.0-mm, 8.0-mm, and 1.18-mm sieves of the PSPS ($peNDF_{>1.18}$; [11]). After sieving, materials from each sieve were removed and dried at 55°C to determine DM content.

2.4. Milk Production and Composition. Cows were milked 3 times daily at 0800, 1500, and 2200 h in a milking parlor. Milk weights for individual cows were recorded daily during the entire experiment. Before milking, cows were monitored for udder inflammation and presence of milk clots to ensure that they were not infected by mastitis. Milk samples were collected during 2 consecutive days from 6 milkings into plastic vials containing potassium dichromate. Samples in plastic vials were analyzed separately for protein, fat, solid nonfats, and lactose using Milk-O-Scan (134 BN Foss Electric, Hillerod, Denmark). Milk components yield and content were calculated as a weighted mean for only the days that milk was sampled.

2.5. Blood Sampling and Analysis. Blood samples from individual cows were taken from tail veins at 0 and 2 h relative to feeding on the last day of each period. Blood was collected into anticoagulant-containing tubes and centrifuged at 1000 g for 15 min to harvest plasma for storage at −20°C until analyzed for β-hydroxybutyric acid (BHBA) (Ultraviolet method; Randox Kits, Cat. # RB1007 Antrim, UK), albumin (Bromocresol Green method), globulin (CHOD-PAR enzymatic method), and glucose (GOD-PAR enzymatic method) concentrations using commercial kits (Pars Azmun Laboratory, Tehran, Iran). The absorbance was read using spectrophotometer (Perkin- Elmer, Coleman Instruments Division, Oak Brook, IL, USA).

2.6. Fecal and Urine Parameters. For pH analysis, urine and fecal samples were collected twice daily at 1100 and 1800 h for the last 4 days of each period. Urine was collected by manual stimulation of the lower vulva. Urine samples in plastic vials were stirred and analyzed for pH immediately after sampling using a portable pH meter (HI 8314 membrane pH meter, Hanna Instruments, Villafranca, Italy). Daily fecal samples were taken from rectum at 1100 h and 1800 h for the entire 7-d sampling and stored at −20°C for digestibility measurements [22]. To determine fecal pH, a portion of it was mixed with an equal portion of distilled water and stirred for sufficient uniformity and thus for a representative pH value.

2.7. BW, BCS, and Back Fat Thickness (BFT). Cow BCS was assessed by skilled individuals at the commencement of the first period and the end of all periods. A 5-point scoring scale, with 1 being an emaciated or extremely thin cow, and 5 being an obese or extremely fat cow, was used [24]. Ultrasound examination of BFT was made on the last d of each period to quantify subcutaneous fat deposition in the back area, as affected by treatments.

2.8. Statistical Analysis. Data were analyzed using MIXED procedures of SAS program [25]. The REML method was used to estimate least squares means, and Kenward-Roger method was used to calculate denominator degrees of freedom. Treatments effects on production variables were subjected to following linear model:

$$Y_{cijps} = \mu + GL_i + GE_j + (GL \times GE)_{ij} + PD_p + Sq_s + Cow(Sq)_{c(s)} + e_{cijps}, \quad (1)$$

where, Y is response variable, GL is ground wheat grain level, GE is grinding extent, PD is period, Sq is square, and e is residuals. The "cow within square" was the main error term for testing the fixed square effect. For blood metabolites, the following linear model was computed:

$$Y_{cijpst} = \mu + GL_i + GE_j + (GL \times GE)_{ij} + Time_t + (GL \times Time)_{it} + (GE \times Time)_{jt} + (GL \times GE \times Time)_{ijt} + PD_p + Sq_s + Cow(Sq)_{c(s)} + e_{cijpst} \quad (2)$$

where, Y is response variable, GL is ground wheat grain level, GE is grinding extent, PD is period, Sq is square, Time

TABLE 2: Treatment effects on DMI and milk parameters of cows fed either finely or coarsely ground wheat grain (GW) at higher and lower inclusion rates.

GW level (GL) %	Grinding extent (GE)							
	Coarser		Finer				*P* value	
	10%	20%	10%	20%	SE	GE	GL	GE × GL
DMI, kg/d	19.7	19.4	20.1	19.4	0.22	0.22	<0.01	0.25
NE_L intake, Mcal/d	31.6	31.4	32.2	31.4	0.35	0.22	0.07	0.26
Milk yield, kg/d	25.4	25.1	25.1	25.5	0.44	0.83	0.99	0.28
Milk energy density[1], Mcal/kg	0.700	0.695	0.696	0.699	0.01	0.97	0.88	0.58
Milk energy yield[1], Mcal/d	17.69	17.30	17.50	17.68	0.42	0.75	0.72	0.34
Milk energy yield: DMI	0.90	0.90	0.87	0.92	0.02	0.72	0.20	0.12
Milk fat, %	3.42	3.37	3.52	3.39	0.11	0.39	0.26	0.60
Fat yield, kg/d	0.86	0.83	0.87	0.86	0.03	0.37	0.20	0.78
Milk protein, %	3.07	3.06	3.16	3.07	0.08	0.43	0.37	0.45
Protein yield, kg/d	0.78	0.77	0.79	0.78	0.02	0.35	0.41	0.98
Milk lactose, %	5.54	5.56	5.51	5.58	0.08	0.87	0.50	0.63
Lactose yield, kg/d	1.40	1.39	1.39	1.42	0.04	0.80	0.81	0.50
Milk SNF, %	9.77	9.71	9.66	9.75	0.10	0.56	0.83	0.30
SNF yield, kg/d	2.48	2.43	2.44	2.48	0.05	0.89	0.90	0.25
Total solids, %	13.39	13.02	13.27	13.33	0.24	0.57	0.36	0.21
TS yield, kg/d	3.39	3.24	3.34	3.37	0.09	0.47	0.38	0.14
Milk fat %: protein %	1.11	1.10	1.11	1.11	0.02	0.81	0.41	0.77

[1]Calculated based on milk components [13]: NE_L (Mcal/kg) = (0.0929 × fat %) + (0.0547 × crude protein %) + (0.0395 × lactose %).

is blood sampling time, and e = residuals. Normality of distribution and homogeneity of variance for residuals were tested and ensured using PROC UNIVARIATE [25]. The *P*-values <0.05 were declared as significant, and *P* values ≤0.10 were declared as trends for significance. The standard errors of differences presented are those for pair-wise comparisons within the GL × GE interactions.

3. Results

3.1. Feed Intake and Milk Properties. Ground wheat grain (GW) inclusion rate affected DMI ($P < 0.01$) and tended to affect NE_L intake ($P = 0.07$), so that cows fed 10% GW had greater DMI and a tendency for greater NE_L intake than cows fed 20% GW (Table 2, $P < 0.01$). However, grinding extent (GE) and its interaction with GW inclusion rate did not affect DMI. Treatments did not affect milk production and composition including milk solids yield, milk energy density and yield, and milk fat to protein ratio (Table 2).

3.2. BW, BCS, and Back Fat Thickness (BFT). Treatments did not affect BW and BCS changes (Table 3, $P > 0.10$). The BCS changes were not statistically different from zero ($P > 0.10$). However, an interaction of GW level and GE existed on BCS, so that GW at 10% instead of 20% of diet DM increased BCS when GW particles were coarser and decreased BCS when GW particles were finer. A tendency for a similar interaction ($P < 0.10$) of GW inclusion rate and GE was found on BFT examined by ultrasound (Table 3).

3.3. Total Tract Apparent Nutrient Digestibility and Fecal and Urine pH. Cows fed coarser versus finer GW tended to have greater total tract NDF digestibility ($P = 0.09$), as did cows on 10% versus 20% dietary GW ($P = 0.07$; Table 4). Total tract DM digestibility was similar among treatments. Whilst urine pH was unaffected by treatments, fecal pH tended to be higher at 20% versus 10% GW ($P = 0.10$, Table 4).

3.4. Blood Metabolites. Blood concentrations of albumin ($P = 0.04$) and total protein ($P = 0.03$) were greater in cows fed 10% GW than in cows fed 20% GW (Table 4). Blood BHBA concentrations increased with increasing dietary GW from 10% to 20% of DM ($P = 0.01$). Neither GW level, nor GE, nor their interaction affected other blood metabolites (Table 4).

4. Discussion

The present study provides novel practical in vivo insights into feeding lactating cows higher and lower dietary levels of finely and coarsely ground wheat grains (GW) in mixed rations with chopped alfalfa hay, wheat straw, and corn grain. Ground wheat has long been overlooked in dairy cattle nutrition [13, 26]. For its rapid degradation, GW has traditionally and not most reasonably been considered a risk to feed intake, rumen fermentation, and milk production. Another main reason for limited GW feeding to dairy cows is the GW popular consumption by humans and non-ruminant industries [1, 13]. Rapidly fermentable starch and proteins could predispose cows to subacute rumen acidosis (SARA), proinflammatory responses, milk fat depression, and laminitis [4, 27]. However, recent studies [7, 18] suggest that major but controlled dietary inclusion rates of steam-rolled WG (e.g., 20% of diet DM) are feasible for midlactaion

TABLE 3: Treatment effects on body weigh (BW), body condition score (BCS), and back-fat thickness in cows fed either finely or coarsely ground wheat grain (GW) at higher and lower inclusion rates.

GW level (GL) %	Grinding extent (GE) Coarser		Finer		SE	P value GE	GL	GE × GL
	10%	20%	10%	20%				
BW, kg	588.1	595.6	591.4	595.9	6.30	0.68	0.19	0.74
BW changes, kg/d	0.50	0.73	0.61	1.06	0.38	0.42	0.22	0.70
BCS	3.34	3.19	3.03	3.25	0.08	0.05	0.61	0.01
Unit BCS changes	0.12	0.00	−0.19	−0.01	0.13	0.11	0.75	0.12
Back fat thickness, mm	21.6	20.4	21.4	23.0	1.00	0.10	0.82	0.07

TABLE 4: Treatment effects on blood metabolites, fecal and urine pH, and total tract apparent DM and NDF digestibility in cows fed either finely or coarsely ground wheat grain (GW) at higher and lower inclusion rates.

GW level (GL) %	Grinding extent (GE) Coarser		Finer		SE	P value GE	GL	GE × GL
	10%	20%	10%	20%				
NDF digestibility, %	34.8	32.0	32.1	31.9	1.10	0.09	0.07	0.11
DM digestibility, %	62.1	60.7	61.0	60.4	1.04	0.34	0.27	0.56
Glucose, mg/dL	51.1	51.6	50.8	51.1	1.70	0.84	0.81	0.96
Total protein, g/dL	8.5	8.2	8.6	8.4	0.08	0.38	0.03	0.42
Albumin, g/dL	3.84	3.75	3.83	3.68	0.07	0.42	0.04	0.56
Globulin, g/dL	4.62	4.46	4.64	4.67	0.14	0.23	0.50	0.32
BHBA, mol/L	0.53	0.64	0.55	0.64	0.07	0.74	0.01	0.71
Fecal pH	6.73	6.77	6.71	6.77	0.03	0.74	0.10	0.66
Urine pH	8.11	8.08	8.09	8.03	0.04	0.45	0.33	0.70

cows. In addition, to maintain milk fat and functional rumen and cow metabolism, no sodium bicarbonate was required at 20% dietary steam-rolled GW [18]. Ground WG has also been feasibly fed to periparturient cows to improve DMI and Ca and energy balances [8]. The current data demonstrate that GW, regardless of its particle size, can feasibly be included in alfalfa hay based midlactation dairy diets at up to 20% of diet DM without compromising nutrient intake and milk properties. It should be considered that ground wheat grain replaced ground barley grain when going from 10% to 20% wheat grain. The greater DMI and NE_L intake of cows on 10% GW than that of cows on 20% GW could suggest that a combination of ground wheat (10.5%), barley (9.7%), and corn (5.8%) grains was more palatable than a blend of ground wheat (19.1%) and corn (5.8%) grains. In addition, the combined ground wheat, barley, and corn grains may have affected satiety signals differently than the blended ground wheat and corn grains. Moreover, the slightly greater dietary starch for the higher versus lower GW diet (19.5% versus 18.1%) could have contributed to decreased DMI of the higher GW diet. Furthermore, possible differences in portal dynamics of glucose might also contribute to the DMI differences via hepatic signals effects on feed intake regulation, despite the similar peripheral glucose concentrations among treatments. Due to the relatively lower NE_L density of the 10% GW diet than that of the 20% GW diet (1.60 versus 1.62 Mcal/kg), cows on 10% GW showed only a tendency for increased NE_L intake, compared to cows on 20% GW. The increased NE_L intake was consistent with the higher blood albumin and total protein at 10% instead of 20% GW, suggesting greater hepatic substrate supply and use for protein synthesis at 10% GW. Liver synthesizes albumin and other proteins for peripheral nutrient transport and optimum immune functioning. Doepel et al. [7] found no effects on DMI of feeding 20% steam-rolled WG to dairy cows in barley silage-based rations. Feed intake and blood metabolite data should be interpreted in light of the midlactation stage and dietary NDF levels of the current study. Midlactation scenarios would be expected to be more resistant to SARA and immune challenges than early and peak lactation cows.

The present study found no interactive and independent effects of GW inclusion rate and GE on milk production and composition of lactating cows. This finding along with DMI data suggest that GW, at 10% of diet DM, did not reduce diet palatability, a traditional concern that has restricted GW feeding to ruminants [26, 28]. Diets with 20% and 10% GW provided 19% and 17.4% cereal starch, respectively. These amounts are within the recommended maximum ranges of 20–25% to minimize health issues. Cows on 20% GW had similar milk energy output as cows on 10% GW while tending to consume less energy. Ground WG replacing barley grain was recently shown to favor prepartal DMI in cows and heifers [8, 17]. Consistent with the current data, rolled WG at lower (17.5%) and medium (19.7%) levels, respectively, corresponding to 24% and 31% dietary starch maintained milk fat and solids production, when compared to slowly degradable potato peelings [29]. In that study, at the low dietary starch level, WG also improved milk true protein content. These data support the hypothesis that feeding GW at major-controlled dietary levels would not compromise rumen and cow metabolism.

Adequately high milk fat and solids percentages and normal milk fat to protein ratios suggest no compromise of rumen conditions and function [10]. Most recent data [16, 30] demonstrated that steam rolling was not superior in DMI and milk production to fine grinding of barley grain at up to 30% barley grain. The numerical decrease in fecal pH of cows fed 10% versus 20% GW might in part be due to increased DMI at 10% GW. This could have increased postrumen flow of partially digested DM, thereby tending to increase hindgut fermentation and reduce fecal pH. Similar urine pH suggests no or little impact of treatments on extracellular fluids anion-cation balance and acidity [22]. The finding that GE did not affect DMI and milk production suggests that at up to 20% GW, its GE has little impact on cow performance. The midlactation stage and dietary NDF levels of the current study require important considerations because cows in midlactation would normally be less sensitive to rumen abnormalities and immune challenges than early lactation cows.

Since the cows were in midlactation and in positive energy balance, the tendency for increased blood BHBA by increasing GW from 10% to 20% has most likely an alimentary origin [31]. Increased peripheral blood BHBA concentrations could indicate a more extensive gastrointestinal epithelial metabolism of organic acids and output of BHBA [32]. Accordingly, gut epithelial BHBA supply may have tended to increase likely due to an increase in rumen degradation of cows fed 20% versus 10% GW. Total tract NDF digestibility was greater at 10% versus 20% GW when wheat particles were coarser, suggesting more favorable rumen conditions for fiber digestion in cows fed a blend of ground barley and wheat versus only 20% GW. The similar total tract DM digestibility among treatments was not unexpected, since differences in rumen digestibility of nonfiber diet components could disappear by the more extensive postrumen digestion processes including hindgut fermentation. Altogether, findings question any significant effects of feeding level and grinding extent of wheat grain on productivity of midlactation dairy cows fed an alfalfa-hay based diet.

5. Conclusions

Dietary inclusion rate (10% versus 20%) and grinding extent (coarser versus finer) of wheat grain and their interactions in chopped alfalfa-hay and wheat-straw-based mixed rations did not affect milk production and composition of midlactation cows. Ground wheat at 10% versus 20% GW increased DMI, and blood concentrations of total protein and albumin, while decreasing blood BHBA concentrations. Coarsely, and not finely, GW at 10% versus 20% of diet DM improved total tract apparent NDF digestibility. Data suggest that feeding midlactation cows finely and coarsely GW at 10% and 20% of diet DM with chopped alfalfa hay and ground corn is feasible. It should be considered that GW replaced ground barley grain when dietary GW was increased from 10% to 20%. Results imply the adequacy of the inexpensive grinding as an effective technique to process WG. These conclusions are made for midlactation cows on chopped alfalfa hay (42.8%) and wheat-straw-(4.8%) based mixed rations.

Acknowledgment

Nature for its inspirations deserves the highest acknowledgement.

References

[1] R. E. Herrera-Saldana, J. T. Huber, and M. H. Poore, "Dry Matter, crude protein, and starch degradability of five cereal grains," *Journal of Dairy Science*, vol. 73, pp. 386–393, 1990.

[2] G. B. Huntington, "Starch Utilization by Ruminants: From Basics to the Bunk," *Journal of Animal Science*, vol. 75, no. 3, pp. 852–867, 1997.

[3] A. L. Slater, M. L. Eastridge, J. L. Firkins, and L. J. Bidinger, "Effects of starch source and level of forage neutral detergent fiber on performance by dairy cows," *Journal of Dairy Science*, vol. 83, no. 2, pp. 313–321, 2000.

[4] W. C. Stone, "Nutritional approaches to minimize subacute ruminal acidosis and laminitis in dairy cattle," *Journal of Dairy Science*, vol. 87, no. 1, pp. E13–E26, 2004.

[5] O. Tománková and P. Homolka, "In vitro ruminal degradability of cereal grain starch," *Czech Journal of Animal Science*, vol. 49, no. 4, pp. 151–155, 2004.

[6] A. Nikkhah and G. R. Ghorbani, "Effects of dry and steam processing on in situ ruminal digestion kinetics of barley grain," *Journal of Animal Science* , vol. 81, p. 338, 2003.

[7] L. Doepel, A. Cox, and A. Hayirli, "Effects of increasing amounts of dietary wheat on performance and ruminal fermentation of Holstein cows," *Journal of Dairy Science*, vol. 92, no. 8, pp. 3825–3832, 2009.

[8] A. Nikkhah, F. Ehsanbakhsh, D. Zahmatkesh, and H. Amanlou, "Prepartal wheat grain feeding improves energy and calcium status of periparturient Holstein heifers," *Animal*, vol. 5, no. 4, pp. 522–527, 2011.

[9] J. Pozdíšek and K. Vaculová, "Study of wheat (*Triticum aestivum* L.) quality for feeding ruminants using in vitro and in vivo methods," *Czech Journal of Animal Science*, vol. 53, no. 6, pp. 253–264, 2008.

[10] D. R. Mertens, "Creating a system for meeting the fiber requirements of dairy cows," *Journal of Dairy Science*, vol. 80, no. 7, pp. 1463–1481, 1997.

[11] P. J. Kononoff, A. J. Heinrichs, and D. R. Buckmaster, "Modification of the Penn State Forage and total mixed ration particle separator and the effects of moisture content on its measurements," *Journal of Dairy Science*, vol. 86, no. 5, pp. 1858–1863, 2003.

[12] B. P. Lammers, D. R. Buckmaster, and A. J. Heinrichs, "A simple method for the analysis of particle sizes of forage and total mixed rations," *Journal of Dairy Science*, vol. 79, no. 5, pp. 922–928, 1996.

[13] National Research Council, *Nutrient Requirements of Dairy Cattle*, National Academy Press, Washington, DC, USA, 7th edition, 2001.

[14] M. A. Faldet, T. Nalsen, L. J. Bush, and G. D. Adams, "Utilization of wheat in complete rations for lactating cows," *Journal of dairy science*, vol. 72, no. 5, pp. 1243–1251, 1989.

[15] W. J. Falkerson and P. J. Michell, "Production response to feeding wheat grain to milking cows," *Australian Journal of Experimental Agriculture*, vol. 25, pp. 253–256, 1985.

[16] A. Nikkhah, "Optimizing barley grain use by dairy cows: a betterment of current perceptions," in *Progress in Food Science and Technology*, Nova Science Publishers, 2011.

[17] H. Amanlou, D. Zahmatkesh, and A. Nikkhah, "Wheat grain as a prepartal cereal choice to ease metabolic transition from gestation into lactation in Holstein cows," *Journal of Animal Physiology and Animal Nutrition*, vol. 92, no. 5, pp. 605–613, 2008.

[18] L. Doepel and A. Hayirli, "Exclusion of dietary sodium bicarbonate from a wheat-based diet: effects on milk production and ruminal fermentation," *Journal of Dairy Science*, vol. 94, no. 1, pp. 370–375, 2011.

[19] W. Z. Yang, K. A. Beauchemin, and L. M. Rode, "Effects of Barley grain processing on extent of digestion and milk production of lactating cows," *Journal of Dairy Science*, vol. 83, no. 3, pp. 554–568, 2000.

[20] P. H. Robinson, J. Wiseman, P. Udén, and G. Mateos, "Some experimental design and statistical criteria for analysis of studies in manuscripts submitted for consideration for publication," *Animal Feed Science and Technology*, vol. 129, no. 1-2, pp. 1–11, 2006.

[21] Iranian Council of Animal Care, *Guide to the Care and Use of Experimental Animals*, vol. 1, Isfahan University of Technology, Isfahan, Iran, 1995.

[22] A. Nikkhah, M. Alikhani, and H. Amanlou, "Effects of feeding ground or steam-flaked broom sorghum and ground barley on performance of dairy cows in midlactation," *Journal of Dairy Science*, vol. 87, no. 1, pp. 122–130, 2004.

[23] AOAC, *Official Methods of Analysis*, Assoc. Offic. Anal. Chem., Arlington, Va, USA, 15th edition, 1990.

[24] E. E. Wildman, G. M. Jones, P. E. Wagner, R. L. Boman, H. F. Troutt, and T. N. Lesch, "A dairy cow body condition scoring system and its relationship to selected production characteristics," *Journal of Dairy Science*, vol. 65, pp. 495–501, 1982.

[25] *SAS User's Guide*, SAS Institute, Cary, NC, USA, Version 9.1 edition, 2003.

[26] F. B. Morrison, "Chapter 4: factors affecting the value of feeds," in *Feeds and Feeding*, pp. 59–71, The Morrison Publishing Co., Ithaca, NY, USA, 1935.

[27] D. G. V. Emmanuel, S. M. Dunn, and B. N. Ametaj, "Feeding high proportions of barley grain stimulates an inflammatory response in dairy cows," *Journal of Dairy Science*, vol. 91, no. 2, pp. 606–614, 2008.

[28] G. W. Mathison, "Effects of processing on the utilization of grain by cattle," *Animal Feed Science and Technology*, vol. 58, no. 1-2, pp. 113–125, 1996.

[29] S. Jurjanz, O. Colin-Schoellen, J. N. Gardeur, and F. Laurent, "Alteration of milk fat by variation in the source and amount of starch in a total mixed diet fed to dairy cows," *Journal of Dairy Science*, vol. 81, no. 11, pp. 2924–2933, 1998.

[30] A. Soltani, G. R. Ghorbani, M. Alikhani, A. Samie, and A. Nikkhah, "Ground versus steam-rolled barley grain for lactating cows: a clarification into conventional beliefs," *Journal of Dairy Science*, vol. 92, no. 7, pp. 3299–3305, 2009.

[31] C. K. Reynolds, "Economics of visceral energy metabolism in ruminants: Toll keeping or internal revenue service?" *Journal of Animal Science*, vol. 80, pp. E74–E84, 2002.

[32] A. Nikkhah, C. Furedi, A. Kennedy, G. Crow, and J. Plaizier, "Effects of feed delivery time on feed intake, rumen fermentation, blood metabolites and productivity of lactating cows," *Journal of Dairy Science*, vol. 91, pp. 1–12, 2008.

Morphology of the Myoepithelial Cell: Immunohistochemical Characterization from Resting to Motile Phase

Germana Beha,[1] Giuseppe Sarli,[1] Barbara Brunetti,[1] Francesco Sassi,[2] Domenico Ferrara,[1] and Cinzia Benazzi[1]

[1] *Department of Veterinary Medical Science, University of Bologna, 40064 Ozzano Emilia, Italy*
[2] *Institute for Cancer Research and Treatment (IRCC), Fourth Floor, 10060 Candiolo, Italy*

Correspondence should be addressed to Cinzia Benazzi, cinzia.benazzi@unibo.it

Academic Editors: C. DebRoy and B. I. Yoon

Myoepithelium is present in canine mammary tumors as resting and proliferative suprabasal and spindle and stellate interstitial cells. The aim of this paper was to evaluate a panel of markers for the identification of four different myoepithelial cell morphological types in the normal and neoplastic mammary gland and to investigate immunohistochemical changes from an epithelial to a mesenchymal phenotype. Cytokeratin 19 (CK19), cytokeratin 5/6 (CK5/6), cytokeratin 14 (CK14), estrogen receptor (ER), p63 protein, vimentin (VIM), and α-smooth muscle actin (Alpha-SMA) antibodies were used on 29 neoplasms (3 benign and 3 malignant myoepithelial tumors, 7 carcinomas in benign-mixed tumors and 16 complex carcinomas) and on normal tissue of mammary glands. All these antibodies were also tested on 3 mammary tissues from animals with no mammary pathology. The myoepithelial markers were well expressed in the suprabasal cells and gradually lost in the motile types, with the stellate cells maintaining only VIM expression typical of mesenchyma. ER labeled some resting and motile myoepithelial cells. On the basis of our results, we propose a transition from myoepithelial immotile cells into migratory fibroblast-like cells. This transition and the characterization of an immunohistochemical panel for resting and motile myoepithelial cells shed more light on the biological behavior of myoepithelial cells.

1. Introduction

Mammary gland tumors of dogs are formed by both epithelial (epithelium and myoepithelium) and mesenchymal components. The origin of the mesenchymal cells is still debated. The elevated frequency of tumors showing myoepithelial or basal cell proliferation is a unique feature of canine mammary tumors [1].

In the normal mammary gland, the lumina are delimitated by an inner layer of polarized epithelial cells resting on two outer or basal layers of epithelial and myoepithelial cells [2]. Both basal and myoepithelial cells synthesize the basement membrane of ducts and alveoli and form a structural barrier between the luminal epithelial cells and the surrounding stroma [3]. In ducts, myoepithelial cells form a nearly continuous layer of cells oriented parallel to the long axis of the ducts. This layer surrounds the luminal epithelial cells and separates them from the basement membrane and the stroma. In alveoli, the myoepithelial cells are discontinuous, forming a basket-like network around the alveoli, allowing some luminal epithelial cells to contact the basement membrane directly [3–5]. Therefore, the myoepithelium is not only located in an ideal position to communicate between these two compartments, but it is also positioned to provide important regulatory signals for the maintenance of normal cell structure [5].

Based on immunohistochemistry, the three layers of cells of the normal mammary gland display different markers: the luminal epithelium is labeled by CK19, and the basal cells and myoepithelial cells are stained by CK5/6 [6] and CK14 [2] and p63, Alpha-SMA, and VIM [2]. Myoepithelial cells are contractile elements exhibiting a combined epithelial and smooth muscle immunoprofile. The markers mentioned above are expressed in the cytoplasm, except for p63 which is a nuclear marker [1]. The myoepithelial cell layer is the sole source of tumor suppressor p63, which is significantly inhibited on proliferation and invasion of associated tumor cells [7]. In addition, basal myoepithelial cells in the normal mammary gland are occasionally labeled by ER antibody [8], which is used for the molecular-based classification of canine mammary tumors [9, 10].

Distinct myoepithelial cell morphologies can be recognized in canine complex and mixed tumors: resting and proliferative suprabasal myoepithelial cells and spindle and stellate motile interstitial myoepithelial cells. Suprabasal cells are located between the basement membrane and the luminal epithelium and exhibit flattened spindle (resting cells) or polygonal morphologies (proliferative cells). Interstitial cells are frequently arranged in solid nests apposed to epithelial elements or isolated in the interstitium [1, 11]. Spindle and stellate myoepithelial cells differentiate toward a more general contractile phenotype [12].

Interstitial myoepithelial cells may eventually become fibroblast-like cells, showing only VIM immunoreactivity [11]. The myoepithelial differentiation may culminate in the formation of various mesenchymal tissues, including cartilage and bone in canine mammary mixed tumor.

The acquisition of typical features of mesenchymal cells is likely to originate through epithelial-mesenchymal transition (EMT). EMT is a biological phenomenon that allows a polarized epithelial cell, which normally interacts with the basement membrane via its basal surface, to undergo multiple biochemical changes enabling it to assume the traits and functions of mesenchymal cells [13].

This paper will focus on various aspects of myoepithelial cells and mammary tumors in dogs, specifically (1) characterization of the four different myoepithelial cell morphological types in the normal and neoplastic mammary gland using a panel of antibodies and (2) the immunohistochemical changes in myoepithelial cells from an epithelial to a mesenchymal phenotype.

2. Materials and Methods

2.1. Samples. Mammary gland specimens of 29 female dogs were retrieved from the database of the Anatomopathological Service of the Faculty of Veterinary Medicine of Bologna. The subjects belonged to different breeds: mongrel (n = 13), German shepherd (n = 3), Poodle (n = ·3), Yorkshire Terrier (n = 3), Dachshund (n = 2), Setter (n = 1), Pointer (n = 1), Cocker spaniel (n = 1), Schnauzer (n = 1), and Siberian Husky (n = 1); they were all females, with an average age of 9.20 ± 2.28 years (mean ± SD). The tumors consisted of: 3 benign myoepithelial tumors, 3 malignant myoepithelial tumors, 7 carcinomas in benign mixed tumors, and 16 complex carcinomas (the last two groups were differentiated by the presence of cartilage and/or bone in the mixed tumors). In addition, 29 specimens from normal mammary glands of the same tumor line and 3 mammary samples from 3 healthy nonmammary tumor-bearing female dogs were evaluated.

Tumors were classified according to Misdorp et al. [14] and Goldschmidt et al. [15] into benign myoepithelial tumors: a rare neoplasm composed of myoepithelial cells arranged in short bundles admixed with an extracellular fibrillar basophilic material; malignant myoepithelial tumors: different from the benign variant with more polymorphic myoepithelial cells; complex carcinoma: a carcinoma composed of both luminal epithelial and myoepithelial components; carcinoma in benign tumor: a tumor with foci of malignant-appearing epithelial cells or distinct nodules of such cells occurring together with mesenchymal cells that have produced cartilage and/or bone possibly in combination with fibrous tissue.

2.2. Immunohistochemistry. Four μm thick sections were cut from formalin-fixed paraffin-embedded blocks containing representative tumor samples. Immunohistochemistry for the following markers was done on these tissues: CK19, ER, CK5/6, CK14, VIM, Alpha-SMA, p63.

Sections were dewaxed in toluene and rehydrated. Endogenous peroxidase was blocked by immersion in 0.3% hydrogen peroxide for 20 min. Sections were then rinsed in Tris buffer. Antigen retrieval was performed with citrate buffer (2.1 g citric acid monohydrate/liter distilled water), pH 6.0 (except for CK5/6 and ER, which used EDTA, pH 8.0), and heating for two 5 min periods in a microwave oven at 750 W, followed by cooling at room temperature for 20 min. The primary antibodies are summarized in Table 1. All primary antibodies were incubated overnight at 4°C, followed by a commercial streptavidin-biotin-peroxidase technique (LSAB Kit, Dako, Amsterdam, The Netherlands). Diaminobenzidine (0.05% for 10 min at room temperature) was used as chromogen. Slides were counterstained with Papanicolaou's hematoxylin.

As a negative control, the primary antibody was replaced with an irrelevant, isotype-matched antibody to control for nonspecific binding of the secondary antibody. Positive tissue controls using the same IHC protocols included canine normal mammary gland (anti-CK19, -ER, -CK14, -VIM, Alpha-SMA, -p63 antibodies) and canine skin (anti-CK5/6).

The number of positive cells by each marker was calculated semiquantitatively: − = no stained cells, ± = less than 5% positive cells, + = 5–50% positive cells, ++ = more than 50% positive cells. Cases were considered positive for ER when nuclear staining was observed in at least 5% tumor cells [16].

3. Results

Four types of myoepithelial cells were recognized on the basis of their morphology. The resting subtype exhibited the elongated features of spindle cells in close contact with luminal epithelial cells as well as proliferating suprabasal cells that instead showed a polygonal shape (Figure 1(a)). The interstitial motile cells were observed both forming nests (the spindle type lined nests and the stellate cells constituted the nest core) and isolated in the interstitium (Figure 2(a)).

3.1. Normal Mammary Gland. In the 3 control cases, all resting and proliferative suprabasal myoepithelial cells were labeled by p63, CK14, Alpha-SMA, and VIM. Resting and

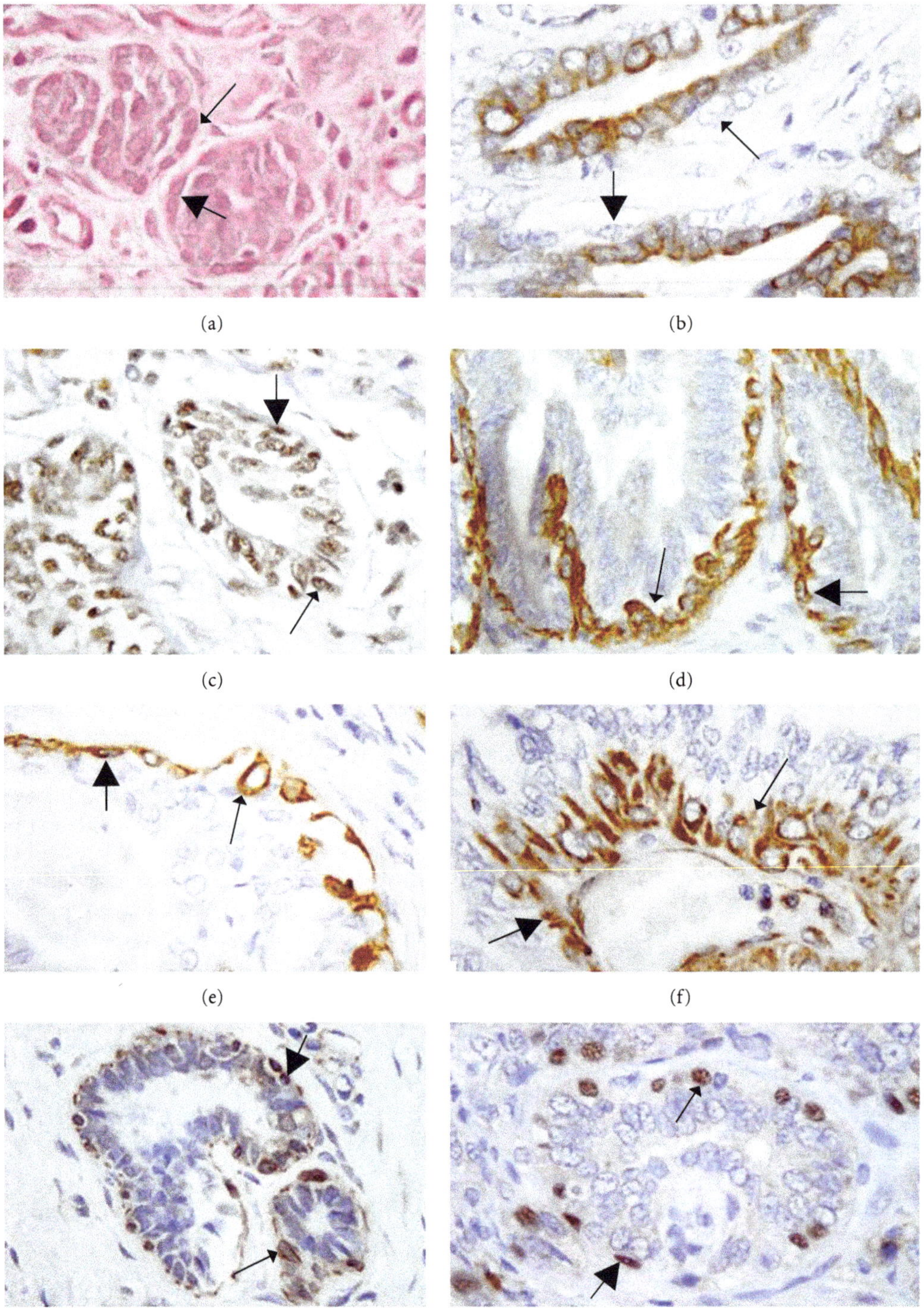

(a) (b) (c) (d) (e) (f) (g) (h)

Figure 1: Suprabasal myoepithelial cells: resting (thin arrows) and proliferative (thick arrows) cells. Immunohistochemical expression of a panel of antibodies applied by IHC, 63x (a) Hematoxylin-eosin; (b) anti-CK19 antibodies labeling the cytoplasm; (c) anti-ER antibodies labeling the nuclei; (d) anti-CK 5/6 antibodies labeling the cytoplasm; (e) anti-CK14 antibodies labeling the cytoplasm; (f) anti-VIM antibodies labeling the cytoplasm; (g) anti-Alpha-SMA antibodies labeling the cytoplasmic membrane; (h) anti-p63 antibodies labeling the nuclei.

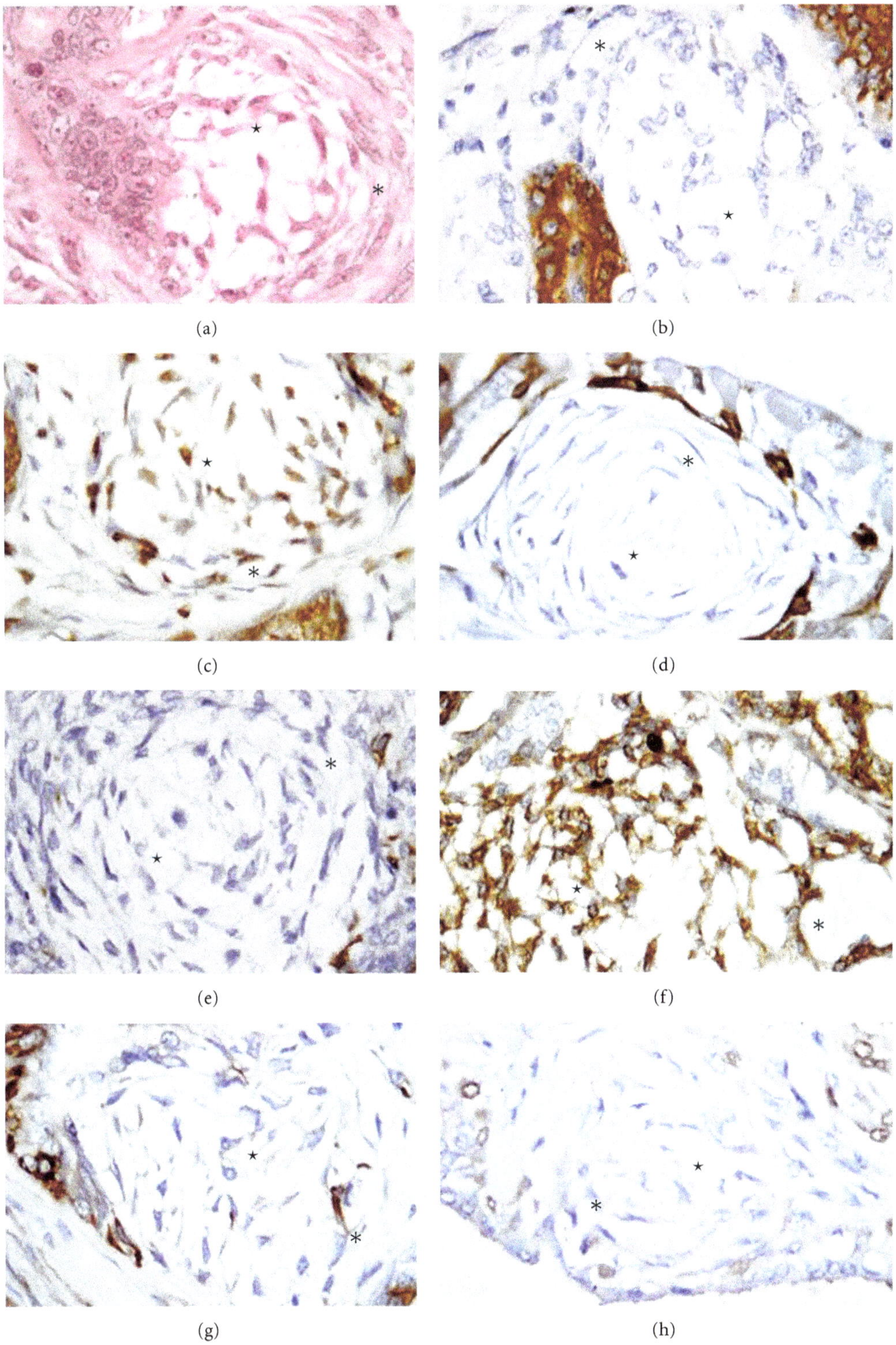

FIGURE 2: Motile myoepithelial cells: spindle (asterisks) and stellate (stars) cells. Immunohistochemical expression of a panel of antibodies applied by IHC. 63x (a) Hematoxylin-eosin; (b) anti-CK19 antibodies labeling the cytoplasm; (c) anti-ER antibodies labeling the nuclei; (d) anti-CK 5/6 antibodies labeling the cytoplasm; (e) anti-CK14 antibodies labeling the cytoplasm; (f) anti-VIM antibodies labeling the cytoplasm; (g) anti-Alpha-SMA antibodies labeling the cytoplasmic membrane; (h) anti-p63 antibodies labeling the nuclei.

Table 1: Primary antibodies, resources, and dilutions used in immunohistochemistry.

Antibody (anti-)	Clone	Manufacturer	Dilution
P63	4A4	Dako (Glostrup, Denmark)	1 : 50
Alpha-SMA	1A4	Dako (Glostrup, Denmark)	1 : 100
Cytokeratin 19	BA17	Dako (Glostrup, Denmark)	1 : 50
Cytokeratin 14	Ab-1 (LL002)	NeoMarkers (Fremont, CA, USA)	1 : 300
Cytokeratins 5/6	D5/16B4	Zymed (South San Francisco, CA, USA)	1 : 100
VIM	V9	Dako (Glostrup, Denmark)	1 : 100
ER	1D5	Dako (Glostrup, Denmark)	1 : 25

Table 2: Immunohistochemical results for suprabasal and motile myoepithelial cells.

Type of lesion	Cell morphology		Antibodies for*						
			p63	CK14	CK5/6	CK19	Alpha-SMA	VIM	ER
Normal mammary gland ($n = 3$)°	Suprabasal	resting	++	++	+	−	++	++	+
		proliferative	++	+	+	−	++	++	+
Mammary tissue in the same tumor line ($n = 29$)°	Suprabasal	resting	++	++	++	−	++	++	+(12/29)
		proliferative	++	+	+	−	++	++	+(12/29)
Benign myoepithelioma ($n = 3$)§	Motile	spindle	−	±(2/3)	−	−	−	++	−
		stellate	−	−	−	−	−	++	−
Malignant myoepithelioma ($n = 3$)§	Motile	spindle	−	±	−	−	−	++	−
		stellate	−	−	−	−	−	++	−
Carcinoma in benign-mixed tumor ($n = 7$)	Suprabasal	resting	++	++	+(5/7)	−	++	++	+(4/7)
		proliferative	++	+/±(2/7)	+(3/7)	−	++	++	+(4/7)
	Motile	spindle	−	±(2/7)	+(3/7)	−	±(5/7)	++	+(3/7)
		stellate	−	−	−	−	−	++	+(3/7)
Complex carcinoma ($n = 16$)	Suprabasal	resting	++	++ (15/16)	+(11/16)	−	++	++	+(7/16)
		proliferative	++	+(15/16)	+(7/16)	−	++	++	+(7/16)
	Motile	spindle	−	±(2/16)	+(7/16)	−	±(5/16)	++	+(6/16)
		stellate	−	−	−	−	±(2/16)	++	+(6/16)

* −: no stained cells; ±: less than 5% positive cells; +: 5–50% positive cells; ++: more than 50% positive cells.
°: the motile phonotype is not updated because not present.
§: the suprabasal phonotype is not updated because not detectable around luminal cells.

proliferative suprabasal myoepithelial cells did not express CK19 in any of the cases.

3.2. Mammary Tissue from the Same Line of the Mammary Tumor. In the 29 normal tissues in the same line as the tumors, all resting and proliferative suprabasal myoepithelial cells were labeled by p63, CK14, Alpha-SMA, and VIM. CK5/6 was positive in all but four cases and ER was detected in 12 cases. CK19 expression was only observed in the luminal epithelium. Myoepithelial motile interstitial cells were not observed. All the results are summarized in Table 2.

3.3. Mammary Tumors. Immunohistochemical results for suprabasal (Figure 1) and motile cells (Figure 2) using p63, CK14, CK5/6, CK19, Alpha-SMA, VIM, and ER are summarized in Table 2. CK5/6 labeled: suprabasal resting cells in 16 of the 29 cases (5 carcinomas in benign mixed tumors and

11 complex carcinomas). CK 5/6 also labeled proliferative suprabasal and spindle motile cells in 10 cases (3 carcinomas in benign mixed tumors and 7 complex carcinomas). Stellate motile cells were present in 25 cases (1 benign myoepithelial tumor, 3 malignant myoepithelial tumors, 5 carcinomas in benign mixed tumors and 15 complex carcinomas) but were negative for CK5/6. Cartilage in mammary mixed tumors was always negative.

CK14 showed positivity in 23 cases in resting cells (with the exception of 1 complex carcinoma and benign and malignant myoepithelial tumors), in 22 cases in proliferative cells (6 carcinomas in benign mixed tumors and 15 complex carcinomas) with a trend to lose the expression when these cells had acquired the more motile phenotype of spindle cells (positive in 2 benign and 3 malignant myoepithelial tumors, 2 carcinomas in benign mixed tumors and 2 complex carcinomas). Chondrocytes of mixed tumors were negative.

VIM was positive in suprabasal cells in the 23 cases of carcinoma in benign tumor and complex carcinoma and in motile myoepithelial cells in all 29 cases. Stromal cells were positive in all cases. Cartilage was VIM positive in all 7 carcinomas in benign-mixed tumors.

Alpha-SMA labeled resting and proliferative suprabasal myoepithelial cells in 23 carcinomas in benign-mixed tumors and complex carcinomas. The spindle cells in 10 cases (5 carcinomas in benign mixed tumor and 5 complex carcinomas) showed positivity for Alpha-SMA. In each case, except for two complex carcinomas, stellate cells were negative. Stroma showed positivity in only 6 cases (1 carcinoma in benign-mixed tumor and 5 complex carcinomas).

P63 was detected in resting and proliferative suprabasal myoepithelial cells of the 23 cases of carcinoma in benign-mixed tumor and complex carcinoma. All spindle and stellate motile cells were negative. Stromal cells and cartilage were negative.

ER expression was present in 11 suprabasal myoepithelial cells (4 carcinomas in benign-mixed tumors and 7 complex carcinomas); spindle and stellate motile cells were positive in 9 cases (3 carcinomas in benign-mixed tumors and 6 complex carcinomas). Cartilage of mixed tumors was negative.

Resting and proliferative suprabasal and spindle/stellate motile myoepithelial cells did not express CK19 in any of the tumors examined. Cartilage of mixed tumors was also negative for CK19.

4. Discussion

Based on the findings of Gama et al. [1] and Tateyama et al. [11], four morphological types of myoepithelial cells are present in the mammary gland: resting and proliferative suprabasal myoepithelial cells lining alveoli and ducts and spindle and stellate interstitial motile cells, which lie in the interstitial space where they may be arranged in nests. Myoepithelial markers, such as p63, CK5/6, CK14, Alpha-SMA, and VIM, proved to be valuable diagnostic adjuncts to facilitate the evaluation of complex and mixed proliferations. CK19 is considered the gold standard marker for luminal epithelium and was used to avoid any misdiagnosis with myoepithelial cells. Because of cross-reactivity patterns and the fact that lesional foci are typically minute, none of the myoepithelial markers enjoyed 100% sensitivity and specificity for myoepithelial cells. As such, at least 2 markers should be used to evaluate any given focus [17].

Based on our results, the best marker for suprabasal cells was p63 especially in association with CK14, which was limited to mature (basal) myoepithelial cells and, to a lesser extent followed by CK5/6, Alpha-SMA and VIM (Figure 1). However, CK5/6 also marked luminal epithelial cells making it difficult to distinguish them from proliferative suprabasal myoepithelial cells [2]. Morphologically, both epithelial and myoepithelial cells may have a polygonal shape. A characteristic of both CK14 and CK5/6, but not of p63, Alpha-SMA, and VIM, was their reduced expression in myoepithelial cells in the suprabasal proliferative state. CK14, CK5/6, and p63 expression was gradually lost in cells in the spindle and stellate motile state.

Alpha-SMA and VIM were present in spindle motile myoepithelial cells with different degrees of intensity. Only VIM proved to be a consistent marker for stellate motile myoepithelial cells. In this study, the stellate motile myoepithelium was arranged in nests and lined by resting cells presumably of alveolar origin. This feature may support the idea that the nests of stellate motile myoepithelial cells, which have lost expression of the main myoepithelial suprabasal markers, but retained affinity for VIM, are the precursors of cartilage, indicating that these cells have completed their transformation into mesenchymal elements. In benign and malignant myoepithelial tumors, VIM labeling in all cases, loss of all other suprabasal myoepithelial markers, and the scant positivity to CK14 in spindle cells were indicative of a prevailing expression of the myoepithelium motile state and a possible passage from simple myoepithelial cells to mesenchymal fibroblasts.

In our study, evidence of the myoepithelial cells shifting to a mesenchymal phenotype, shown by the loss of CK14, CK5/6, and p63 expression, was reinforced by the discontinuous labeling of spindle cells for Alpha-SMA, a marker of both myoepithelial cells and myofibroblasts, which was completely lost in stellate motile cells that have supposedly become fibroblasts.

Further confirmation studies by Tsuda et al. [18] reported the occurrence of myofibroblasts with remnants of CK14 expression (described as "converted myoepithelial cells"). In the cases examined in the present study, CK14 progressively faded, therefore indicating a loss of the (myo-)epithelial phenotype. These results support the EMT hypothesis involving a myoepithelial-like state [19], which undergoes a myoepithelial mesenchymal transition (MMT). This hypothesis was confirmed in the dog by Gärtner et al. [20] who stated that in mammary tumors one of the steps in the evolution of mesenchymal cells involves the expression of typical myoepithelial traits.

An interesting result of the present study was the positivity to ER found in 12/29 suprabasal myoepithelial cells and 9/29 stellate cells of carcinoma in benign-mixed tumors and complex carcinomas. Two isoforms of ER receptors have been described, namely, ER-α and ER-β, the latter being the only form expressed in the nuclei of isolated basal-myoepithelial cells [8]. The antibody used in the present investigation was inclusive of both isoforms: both luminal and basal/stellate cells were labeled, presumably luminal cells by ER-α and basal/stellate cells by ER-β.

In conclusion, the suprabasal myoepithelial cells were well characterized by p63 and CK14 and to a lesser extent by the other marker used. The motile myoepithelial cells are instead characterized by Alpha-SMA and VIM and loss of CK14, CK5/6, and p63 (Figure 2). The present study also demonstrated ER in both luminal epithelial and suprabasal/stellate myoepithelial cells (the latter in about half of the cases) and that ER expression is not influenced by the resting/motile phase. Therefore, in serial or multistained sections, immunohistochemistry to ER in combination with p63 and CK14 may serve to avoid erroneous identification of luminal or myoepithelial cells in canine mammary tumors. The trend of preserved Alpha-SMA and VIM expression in spindle cells, and only VIM positivity in stellate motile cells as well as the decreased p63 expression in both motile types, supports the hypothesis of the EMT involving a myoepithelial-like state [19] in MMT. The spindle motile cell could be considered an earlier transformation than the stellate cell towards a mesenchymal phenotype.

Authors' Contribution

These authors contributed equally to this work.

Conflict of Interests

The authors declare they have no competing interests.

Acknowledgment

The authors thank Ms. Anne Collins for editing the English text.

References

[1] A. Gama, A. Alves, F. Gartner, and F. Schmitt, "p63: a novel myoepithelial cell marker in canine mammary tissues," *Veterinary Pathology*, vol. 40, no. 4, pp. 412–420, 2003.

[2] L. N. Z. Ramalho, A. Ribeiro-Silva, G. D. Cassali, and S. Zucoloto, "The expression of p63 and cytokeratin 5 in mixed tumors of the canine mammary gland provides new insights into the histogenesis of these neoplasms," *Veterinary Pathology*, vol. 43, no. 4, pp. 424–429, 2006.

[3] K. Polyak and M. Hu, "Do myoepithelial cells hold the key for breast tumor progression?" *Journal of Mammary Gland Biology and Neoplasia*, vol. 10, no. 3, pp. 231–247, 2005.

[4] K. U. Sorenmo, R. Rasotto, V. Zappulli, and M. H. Goldschmidt, "Development, anatomy, histology, lymphatic drainage, clinical features, and cell differentiation markers of canine mammary gland neoplasms," *Veterinary Pathology*, vol. 48, no. 1, pp. 85–97, 2011.

[5] T. Gudjonsson, M. C. Adriance, M. D. Sternlicht, O. W. Petersen, and M. J. Bissell, "Myoepithelial cells: their origin and function in breast morphogenesis and neoplasia," *Journal of Mammary Gland Biology and Neoplasia*, vol. 10, no. 3, pp. 261–272, 2005.

[6] T. O. Nielsen, F. D. Hsu, K. Jensen et al., "Immunohistochemical and clinical characterization of the basal-like subtype of invasive breast carcinoma," *Clinical Cancer Research*, vol. 10, no. 16, pp. 5367–5374, 2004.

[7] Y. H. Hsiao, H. D. Tsai, M. C. Chou, and Y. G. Man, "The myoepithelial cell layer may serve as a potential trigger factor for different outcomes of stage-matched invasive lobular and ductal breast cancers," *International Journal of Biological Sciences*, vol. 7, no. 2, pp. 147–153, 2011.

[8] J. Martín De Las Mulas, J. Ordás, M. Y. Millán et al., "Immunohistochemical expression of estrogen receptor β in normal and tumoral canine mammary glands," *Veterinary Pathology*, vol. 41, no. 3, pp. 269–272, 2004.

[9] A. Gama, A. Alves, and F. Schmitt, "Identification of molecular phenotypes in canine mammary carcinomas with clinical implications: application of the human classification," *Virchows Archiv*, vol. 453, no. 2, pp. 123–132, 2008.

[10] F. Sassi, C. Benazzi, G. Castellani, and G. Sarli, "Molecular-based tumour subtypes of canine mammary carcinomas assessed by immunohistochemistry," *BMC Veterinary Research*, vol. 6, article 5, 2010.

[11] S. Tateyama, K. Uchida, T. Hidaka, M. Hirao, and R. Yamaguchi, "Expression of bone morphogenetic protein-6 (BMP-6) in myoepithelial cells in canine mammary gland tumors," *Veterinary Pathology*, vol. 38, no. 6, pp. 703–709, 2001.

[12] L. Rønnov-Jessen and O. W. Petersen, "A function for filamentous α-smooth muscle actin: retardation of motility in fibroblasts," *Journal of Cell Biology*, vol. 134, no. 1, pp. 67–80, 1996.

[13] R. Kalluri and R. A. Weinberg, "The basics of epithelial-mesenchymal transition," *Journal of Clinical Investigation*, vol. 119, no. 6, pp. 1420–1428, 2009.

[14] W. Misdorp, R. W. Esle, E. Hellmén, and T. P. Lipscomb, *Histological Classification of Mammary Tumors of the Dog and Cat*, Armed Forces Institute of Pathology in cooperation with the American Registry of Pathology and the World Health Organization Collaborating Centre for Worldwide Aderence on Comparative Oncology, Washington, DC, USA, 1999.

[15] M. H. Goldschmidt, L. Peña, R. Rasotto, and V. Zappulli, "Classification and grading of canine mammary tumors," *Veterinary Pathology*, vol. 48, no. 1, pp. 117–131, 2011.

[16] F. Millanta, M. Calandrella, G. Bari, M. Niccolini, I. Vannozzi, and A. Poli, "Comparison of steroid receptor expression in normal, dysplastic, and neoplastic canine and feline mammary tissues," *Research in Veterinary Science*, vol. 79, no. 3, pp. 225–232, 2005.

[17] R. Dewar, O. Fadare, H. Gilmore, and A. M. Gown, "Best practices in diagnostic immunohistochemistry: myoepithelial markers in breast pathology," *Archives of Pathology and Laboratory Medicine*, vol. 135, no. 4, pp. 422–429, 2011.

[18] H. Tsuda, T. Takarabe, F. Hasegawa, T. Fukutomi, and S. Hirohashi, "Large, central acellular zones indicating myoepithelial tumor differentiation in high-grade invasive ductal carcinomas as markers of predisposition to lung and brain metastases," *American Journal of Surgical Pathology*, vol. 24, no. 2, pp. 197–202, 2000.

[19] O. W. Petersen, H. L. Nielsen, T. Gudjonsson, R. Villadsen, L. Rønnov-Jessen, and M. J. Bissell, "The plasticity of human breast carcinoma cells is more than epithelial to mesenchymal conversion," *Breast Cancer Research*, vol. 3, no. 4, pp. 213–217, 2001.

[20] F. Gärtner, M. Geraldes, G. Cassali, A. Rema, and F. Schmitt, "DNA measurement and immunohistochemical characterization of epithelial and mesenchymal cells in canine mixed mammary tumours: putative evidence for a common histogenesis," *Veterinary Journal*, vol. 158, no. 1, pp. 39–47, 1999.

10

Transcriptome and Proteome Research in Veterinary Science: What Is Possible and What Questions Can Be Asked?

Robert Klopfleisch and Achim D. Gruber

Institut für Tierpathologie, Universität Berlin, Robert-von-Ostertag-Strasse 15, 14163 Berlin, Germany

Correspondence should be addressed to Robert Klopfleisch, robert.klopfleisch@fu-berlin.de

Academic Editor: Kenneth D. Clinkenbeard

In recent years several technologies for the complete analysis of the transcriptome and proteome have reached a technological level which allows their routine application as scientific tools. The principle of these methods is the identification and quantification of up to ten thousands of RNA and proteins species in a tissue, in contrast to the sequential analysis of conventional methods such as PCR and Western blotting. Due to their technical progress transcriptome and proteome analyses are becoming increasingly relevant in all fields of biological research. They are mainly used for the explorative identification of disease associated complex gene expression patterns and thereby set the stage for hypothesis-driven studies. This review gives an overview on the methods currently available for transcriptome analysis, that is, microarrays, Ref-Seq, quantitative PCR arrays and discusses their potentials and limitations. Second, the most powerful current approaches to proteome analysis are introduced, that is, 2D-gel electrophoresis, shotgun proteomics, MudPIT and the diverse technological concepts are reviewed. Finally, experimental strategies for biomarker discovery, experimental settings for the identification of prognostic gene sets and explorative versus hypothesis driven approaches for the elucidation of diseases associated genes and molecular pathways are described and their potential for studies in veterinary research is highlighted.

1. Background

The molecular aetiology and mechanisms of the many neoplastic, inflammatory, and degenerative veterinary diseases are largely unknown. This information deficit is caused by several constraining factors such as the lack of the complete genomic information or the unavailability of molecular tools, for instance, species-specific antibodies.

Due to this lack of a critical mass of knowledge on the disease mechanisms in veterinary medicine, hypotheses on the pathogenesis of veterinary diseases are often based on the knowledge on homologous human diseases. This approach doubtlessly helped to elucidate the aetiology of several veterinary diseases, such as the impact of mutations in the c-kit receptor for some canine mast cell tumours [1]. However, in at least the same number of studies, this approach failed to identify identical mechanism in human and animal diseases, most probably due to interspecies differences or plainly because of the absence of comparable human diseases.

An alternative approach to develop and test hypotheses is to study known cellular molecular mechanisms or genes whose dysfunction may theoretically cause the clinical symptoms and morphologic lesions. This includes the analysis of the mutational DNA status and the RNA and protein expression levels of these specific genes to elucidate their role in the disease. However, due to the redundancy of gene functions and the complexity of molecular pathways, the chances are rather low to identify "the" disease-associated genes or molecular pathways by this approach. Furthermore, it becomes more and more evident that most diseases and notably the carcinogenesis of veterinary tumours are only rarely caused by a mutation in a single gene but are rather caused by dysfunction of a wider array of multiple genes [2].

In case the above-mentioned hypothesis-driven approaches fail, non-hypothesis-driven, explorative studies are feasible alternatives. This approach, however, needs technologies which facilitate the concurrent analysis of a large

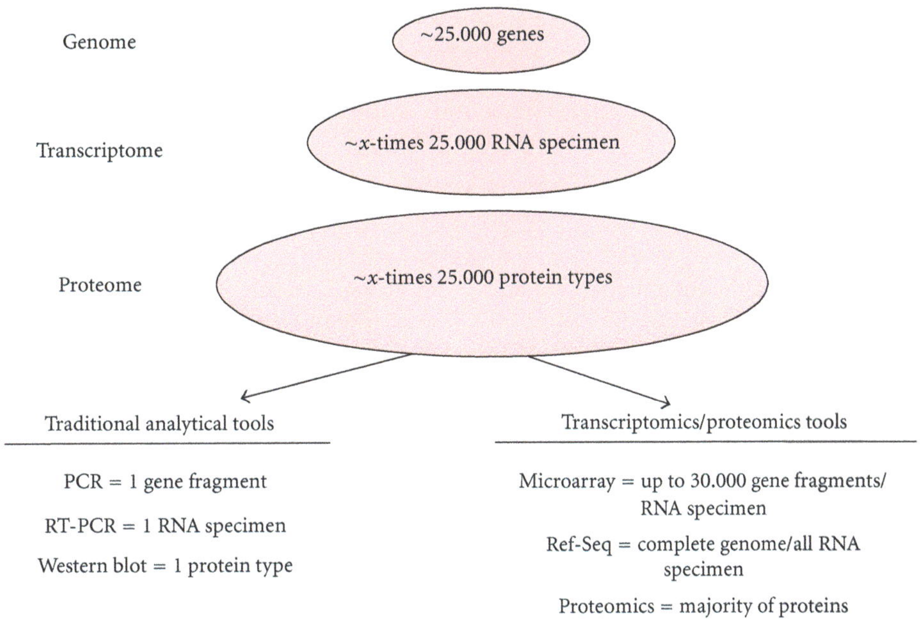

FIGURE 1: Traditional analytical tools for quantification of DNA, RNA, or proteins are restricted to the sequential analysis of one biomolecule specimen at a time. Research based on these tools is therefore strictly hypothesis driven. In contrast, transcriptomics tools permit the parallel quantification of thousands of biomolecules and therefore allowing for explorative, non-hypothesis-driven studies.

scale of the genome, the transcriptome, or the proteome in diseased versus nondiseased tissues (Figure 1).

The so-called "-omics" technologies, which made much headway in the last ten years, enable such an approach to answer hitherto inaccessible scientific questions. The transcriptome [3] which constitutes the complete set of RNA specimen within a tissue, and the proteome [4] the complete set of proteins in a tissue, have been named in analogy to the genome, the complete set of genes of an organism. In addition to these three dominating fields, several other groups of biochemical elements have been coined in analogy to the genome, such as the metabolome [5], the complete set of metabolic intermediates, or the glycome [6], the complete set of cellular sugars, free or in more complex molecules.

This review aims to summarize the current state of the art of technologies in transcriptome and proteome research. Furthermore, the strengths and weaknesses of the technologies will be described, and potential applications in veterinary science will be depicted.

2. Methods in Transcriptomics

The term transcriptome embraces all types of complementary RNA synthesized during transcription of the genome at a given time point [3]. Of these, microRNA (miRNA) and messenger RNA (mRNA) momentarily are the RNA types of greatest interest in transcriptome research. The mRNA expression levels directly reflect the gene activity of a cell, while differences in miRNA expression levels, a major post-transcriptional regulator of gene activity, are thought to be associated with several cellular functions and diseases [7]. Three common methods for the multiplex detection and quantification of miRNA and mRNA at a large scale are momentarily used: microarrays, deep sequencing (RNA-Seq), and quantitative reverse transcription (RT) PCR arrays (Table 1).

2.1. Microarrays. A microarray is a multiplex, high-throughput screening method which uses a two-dimensional arrangement of nucleotide probes on a glass slide or a thin silicon chip [8]. One array can contain ten thousands of nucleotide sequences or hypothetically the complete transcriptome, which is covalently bound to the chip's surface or fixed in parallel rows in microfluidic channels [8, 9]. Depending on the scientific questions asked, these nucleotide sequences may represent short fragments (probes) with exon sequences to analyse the presence and the quantity of specific mRNA or miRNA in expression profiling experiments. Alternatively, genomic DNA sequences with allelic variants, known mutations, or single nucleotide polymorphism (SNP) is spotted on the chips to identify the mutational status of a tissue in comparative genomic analysis or SNP assays [10]. Independent from the spotted sequences, pairwise hybridization of the given sequences on the chip with complementary DNA or cDNA sequences (targets) in a tissue lysate under high-stringency conditions is the general principle of all microarray-based experiments [11]. Successful hybridization is visualized by labelling of bound target oligonucleotides with fluorescent dyes. Fluorescence intensity of the respective spot on the chips is subsequently used to determine the presence or absence of a mutation or SNP or the level of mRNA or miRNA expression in a tissue, respectively [11].

The resulting large data sets on the expression level of up to ten thousands of genes represent a challenge to the commonly used statistic methods. These challenges include the subtraction of background noise, the normalization of data

Table 1: Advantages and limitations of transcriptomics technologies.

	qPCR arrays	Microarrays	Ref-Seq
Advantage	Highest sensitivity/specificity	Costume-made assays available less expensive than Ref-Seq	Combination of quantitative and sequence information
Limitation	Only few hundreds of targets measurable in parallel	Less sensitive and specific than qPCR	Less sensitive and specific than qPCR Expansive

to allow for the comparison of different microarrays and microarray experiments with each other, and the identification of statistically significant changes in large data sets [12]. For the latter, the common statistical test, *t*-test, ANOVA, and Mann-Whitney test have been adjusted to consider the multiple comparisons and permit cluster analysis [13, 14]. However, in most instances, the number of variables is larger than the observational units. Principal component analysis and partial least squares have been used for dimension reduction and to visualize microarray data sets [15]. Furthermore, clustering methods like hierarchical and fuzzy clustering are used to identify differences in gene expression profiles associated with different disease states or treatment response [16].

Ready-to-use whole genome cDNA microarrays are commercially available for several species including human, mouse, and rat (Affymetrix, Illumina, Agilent) but also for canine, bovine, porcine, sheep, equine, chicken, rhesus macaque, salmon, and zebrafish (Affymetrix, Agilent). However, costume-made microarrays with any given DNA of interest are provided by several local and international suppliers. These arrays can be adjusted to each experiment in terms of gene number or type of interest and may therefore represent a low-cost alternative to expensive full-genome microarrays.

Similar to other analytic tools, microarray experiments require technical and biological replicates. In addition, several initiatives are launched to standardize microarray experiments, whose outcome is strongly influenced by tissue and RNA handling, the assay protocols and the microarray platform on the resulting data. For instance, the "minimum information about a microarray experiment (MIAME)" and the "microarray quality control (MAQC) project" are becoming the gold standard of how detailed information on an experiment should be included in a publication [17, 18].

In summary, microarrays are well established and valuable tools to get a first impression on the genetic activity or the genomic composition of a specific tissue under physiologic and pathologic conditions. Despite the high quality of prefabricated microarrays, one has to keep in mind that cross-hybridization and low sensitivity when compared to quantitative PCR are intrinsic problems of this valuable method and may lead to false positive or negative results [19]. Microarray data can therefore in most circumstances not be considered as final and conclusive information but have to be confirmed by other methods such as quantitative PCR or, optimally, on the protein level or by functional cell assays [17, 18].

2.2. Deep Sequencing (RNA-Seq). RNA-Seq is a new approach to obtain complete information on the RNA expression levels in a tissue sample [20]. This approach utilizes the tremendous progress in the development of next generation sequencing technologies, which allow to sequence millions of base pairs in a relatively short time [21]. Initially, these methods were used for whole-genome sequencing of organisms [22] or tumours [23]. Within the past 2-3 years, second-generation sequencing has been applied to cDNA sequencing to obtain information on the full set of all transcribed RNA sequences within a given tissue, that is, the complete transcriptome in so-called RNA-Seq experiments [24, 25].

RNA-Seq uses a cDNA library, which is reverse transcribed from the total RNA in a single tissue or cell culture [20]. Small fragments from each of these cDNA molecules are then sequenced using the different technology platforms Illumina IG [24], Applied Biosystems SOLiD [26], Roche 454 Life Science [27], or Helicos Biosciences tSMS [28].

Although subsumed under the name "next generation" or "deep" sequencing, the three main technologies are based on different principles. Pyrosequencing, which has been developed by 454 Life Sciences, is based on the emulsion amplification of a single DNA sequence attached to a primer-coated bead, on which a clonal DNA colony is formed in a picotitre well [29]. The sequencing procedure employs luciferase to generate light for indication of the addition of one of the four consecutively added dNTP types to the newly synthesised DNA in each well [29].

In contrast, the reversible dye-terminator-based technology of Ilumina employs amplification of DNA fragments to clonal DNA colonies on a glass slide. During each sequencing step, one of the four types of dNTP is added, and the addition of the fluorescently labelled nucleotides is detected by a camera at the respective spot [30]. After each step, the dye is chemically removed, and the next cycle is started.

The SOLiD technology of Applied Biosystems is based on sequencing by ligation. Similar to pyrosequencing, DNA is amplified by emulsion PCR, and the resulting bead with a clonal DNA colony is positioned on a glass slide [31, 32]. The mismatch sensitivity of the DNA ligase is then used to identify the nucleotide present at a given position in a DNA sequence.

The sequences retrieved from any of these technologies are aligned to the reference genome, and the resulting information can be used to analyze both genomic and posttranscriptional mutations and the mRNA expression level of each gene. RNA-Seq therefore extends the information obtained with microarrays by a second dimension, the sequence of the mRNA transcripts [20]. This may permit the identification of disease-associated mutations or SNP in the actively transcribed genes [26].

Another advantage of RNA-Seq is potential analysis of genomes from organisms without complete genomic sequence information, although further data analysis in these cases is often hampered by the lack of gene annotation or the lack of a sequenced genome [33]. This is in strict contrast to the microarray approach that requires knowledge on the sequences to be detected [34]. Finally, RNA-Seq also has a large dynamic range of quantification levels which allows the quantification of very low and high quantities in contrast to the low sensitivity and reduced dynamic range of microarrays [35].

A major disadvantage of this technology is the relatively high costs for a high coverage analysis of a complex mammalian genome [36]. Still, the price per nucleotide is significantly lower than for classic sequence; a reasonable RNA-Seq run requires the analysis of several million bases, making it still an expansive technology for most scientific questions.

2.3. Quantitative Real-Time PCR Arrays. Quantitative real-time PCR (qPCR) arrays are, although less complex, still a very valuable method for the quantification of the gene expression of up to 600 genes [37]. At the moment, qPCR arrays are a commonly used method for the quantification of the "miRNA transcriptome" [37]. This is mainly based on two facts. First, the number of miRNA types per species can be considered at level of hundreds and is therefore much lower than the number of mRNA types (see http://www.mirbase.org/, [38–40]). Second, the high similarity between the different miRNA types makes the development of microarrays difficult due to the high risk of cross-hybridization [41]. In contrast, Taq-Man- or SYBR-Green-based qPCR assays permit a specific and sensitive quantification of miRNA and are a commonly used method in veterinary sciences for the detection of mRNA and miRNA [42–46]. Arranged in an array, qPCR assays are therefore an efficient and highly reproducible method to quantify the miRNA transcriptome.

3. Methods in Proteomics

Transcriptome analysis gives useful information on the transcriptional activity of a cell. However, due to posttranscriptional gene regulation and the different stabilities and biological half-lives of RNA and protein specimens including miRNA, the correlation between mRNA levels and the corresponding protein is often poor [47]. Transcriptome analysis therefore requires confirmation of the results on the protein level for most scientific questions. The analysis of the cellular proteome is, however, a much greater challenge than the transcriptome due to the high chemical diversity of the cellular proteins [48]. Despite these difficulties, proteome analysis has become an important tool for explorative analysis of molecular mechanisms in physiology and pathology [49]. There is a great variety of approaches applied in proteome research that can be grouped into two broader categories: gel-based assays and shotgun proteomics (Table 2).

3.1. Gel-Based Proteomics. One of the major problems of proteome analysis is the complexity of proteins in tissues and cell lysates. Two-dimensional gel electrophoresis (2D-GE) which combines two dimensions of physical protein separation is a common method to separate proteins by their chemical properties [50, 51]. In the first dimension, the proteins are separated by their isoelectric point (IP), that is, they are arranged on a linear gel with an immobilized pH-gradient according to their content of basic or acidic amino acids [51, 52]. In the second dimension, IP-separated proteins are separated by their molecular size similar to a conventional SDS-Page [51, 53]. The orthogonal combination of both techniques results in a two-dimensional arrangement of proteins with a high resolution of single protein types (Figure 2).

TABLE 2: Advantages and limitations of the two major proteomics approaches.

	2D-DIGE	Shotgun Proteomics (MudPit)
Advantage	Moderate costs for necessary equipment (separation phase) Good protein separation	Industrialized work processes Almost all protein types analyzable
Limitation	Gel-based variability Hydrophobic (membrane) proteins difficult to measure	Difficult quantification of low abundance proteins in complex protein mixes High costs for equipment

The separated proteins can be visualized on the gel by different staining methods, for instance, Compassion brilliant blue [54], silver (Figure 2) [55], or fluorescent stainings [56]. Each of the detected spots on the acrylamide gel theoretically consists of one protein species, and each cell or condition of a cell is theoretically associated with a specific pattern of these spots on the gel. Changes in this spot pattern should therefore reflect changes of the cellular proteome, for example, its metabolism and gene activity under diseased or healthy condition [51].

Two approaches have been developed to compare spot presence and intensity in 2D-GE gels. In the original single channel approach, all gels containing one protein sample, are stained with same stain and scanned independently [57]. This approach is, however, prone to the technical intergel variability and has difficulties to normalize spot intensity. The multiplex approach of two-dimensional differential gel electrophoresis (2D-DIGE) uses gels which contain up to three protein samples stained with three different fluorescent dyes to reduce the gel number [58]. One of the three samples on each gel usually represents an internal standard, which allows for normalization of spot intensity between different gels [58].

Detection of the differences in spot intensity even between only two gels usually overstrains the human eyes capacity independent from the method used. Comparison or quantification of spot intensity and presence therefore requires automated digital image analysis [59]. Despite the high efficiency of the available software, comparison of protein expression pattern on polyacrylamide gels is still the major challenge and weakness of gel-based proteome analysis.

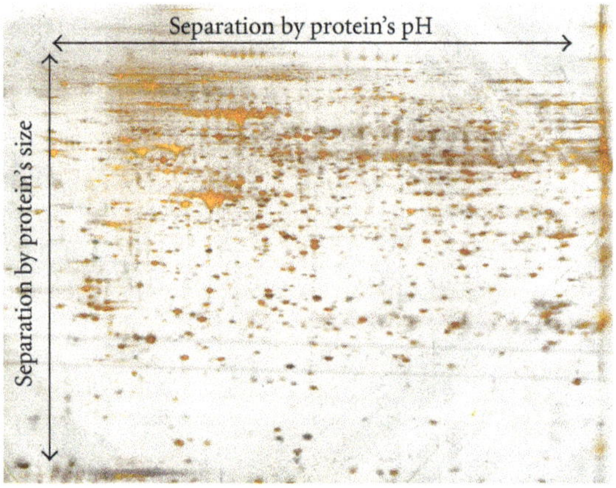

Figure 2: Gel-based proteomics reduces the complexity, of protein lysates by two-dimensional separation of proteins, that is, separation by size and pH. This leads to a high resolution of single protein which facilitates the quantification of their spot size and the extraction of single proteins for subsequent mass spectrometry-based identification of the protein identity.

Even with highest accuracy and long experience of the experimenter, preparation of 2D-GE gels without technical artefacts is not assured mostly due to random polymerization artefacts in nonmanufactured gels. Commercially available, machine-made gels are an interesting but costly alternative that reduces most of these gel-based artefacts [60].

Once protein spots with a significant difference in intensity between the two disease states are identified, the protein type has to be identified using mass spectrometry. To this end, the spots with the respective protein are picked and eluted from the gel and fragmented for mass spectrometry by trypsin-digestion [61]. The molecular weight of the trypsin digested protein fragments is then determined using, for instance, Matrix-assisted Laser Desorption/Ionization (MALDI) [62]. This approach uses trypsin fragment pattern, the so-called "peptide fingerprint" (PF), to identify the regulated protein in open source protein databases [63]. With this PF, protein data bases are searched to determine the peptide/protein with the highest accordance according to statistical calculations. However, PFs for animal proteomes are far from being complete, and PFs obtained from proteome studies in animals are in most cases compared with peptide masses of human protein in the versatile human data bases. This may lead to low sequence coverage [64], and peptide sequencing is required for Mascot MS/MS Ions Search (C. Weise, Freie Universität, personal communication).

In summary, gel-based proteomics is still an acceptable and commonly used approach to analyze the cellular proteome. Its main advantage is the relatively low costs for equipment when compared to non-gel-based approaches. Disadvantages are the restriction on hydrophilic proteins with a pH between 3 and 10, difficult standardization of the gel preparation, the limited dynamic range, and the limited sensitivity [65–69].

3.2. Shotgun Proteomics (MudPIT). The term shotgun proteomics is applied due to its similarities with DNA shotgun sequencing, which sequences multiple short DNA fragments in complex mixtures and recombines them in silico [48]. Similarly, shotgun proteomics analyses trypsin-digested protein fragments in complex mixtures by mass spectrometry after separation by liquid chromatography. This so-called multidimensional protein identification technology (MudPIT) combines at least two chromatography separation steps with tandem mass spectrometry (Figure 3) [70, 71]. The combination of two chromatographic methods allows for the separation of digested peptide fragments by at least two features, for example, charge and hydrophobicity, to reduce the overall protein complexity [72]. The selection of two coupled, thus two-dimensional chromatography methods depends on the scientific question asked and the experience of the experimentator. Microcapillaries packed with strong cation exchange material, reverse phase material, or other affinity-based chromatographic material are most commonly used. In addition, separation before mass spectrometry may also include isoelectric focussing and capillary electrophoresis which enables a high resolution and narrow analyte bands [73].

The different peptide fractions are eluted from the chromatography columns by alternating salt pulses or organic mobile gradients. They are subsequently stored or, more commonly, directly applied to the mass spectrometer [71, 74]. MudPIT approaches commonly use electrospray ionization (ESI) mass spectrometers since the chromatography eluate can be directly "online" analyzed with a connected ESI mass spectrometer [75].

Most proteome experiments do not exclusively aim at identifying the general protein composition in the tissue lysates but require comparative protein quantification. Isotopic labelling or label-free methods have been developed and successfully applied in MudPIT experiments [74]. A simple method for label-free quantification is the spectral counting [76]. It uses the observation that the total number of spectra from a peptide correlates well with the original abundance of the protein in lysates [77]. However, relative quantification by spectral counting is limited to prefractionated, less complex samples [76], while analysis of complex, unfractionated samples and low abundant proteins may result in reduced accuracy [78].

Stable isotope labelling is an alternative strategy to quantify proteins in MudPIT experiments. Stable isotope labelling with amino acids in cell culture (SILAC) is a metabolic labelling strategy that has been applied to both cell cultures and small mammals [79, 80]. It relies on metabolic incorporation of "light", native amino acids in one experimental group or "heavy" amino acids with substituted isotopic deuterium ^{13}C in the other group [80]. A typical experimental design therefore includes a cell line which is grown in cell culture medium with light or heavy amino acids but under otherwise identical conditions. This leads to the complete replacement of the native amino acids in the "heavy" isotope group after a decent incubation period [81], marking the proteome of this cell unequivocal. After the intended experiment, this labelling facilitates the mixture of equal amounts of protein lysates from both experimental groups and parallel analysis by mass spectrometry, thus reducing technical artefacts

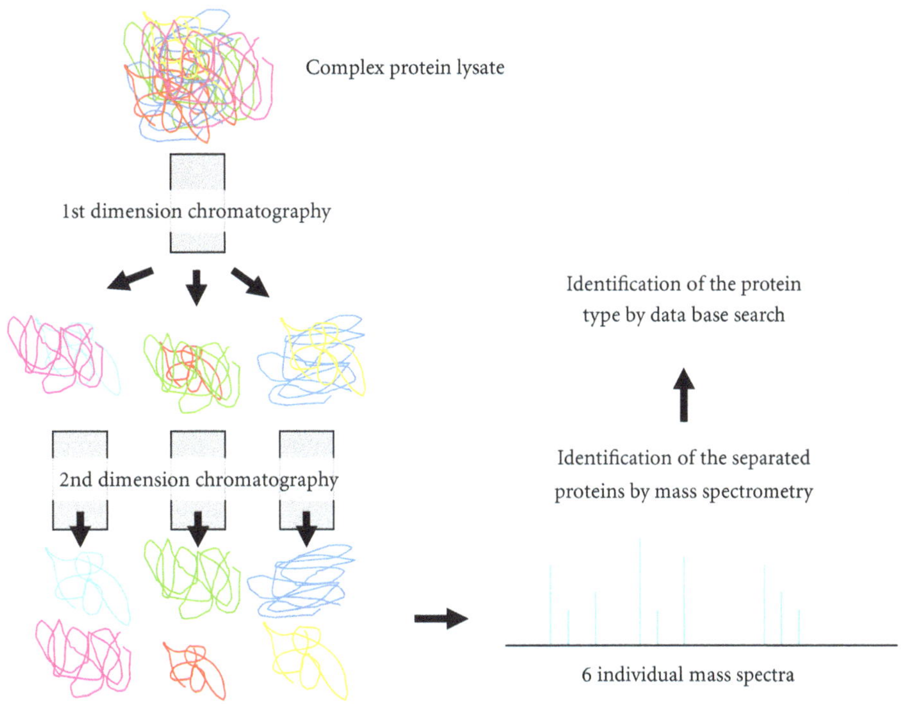

FIGURE 3: Shotgun proteomics or MudPIT uses multidimensional chromatographic separation to reduce complexity of protein lysates. The selection of the type of chromatographic columns depends on the question asked and the technical equipment. The different protein lysate fractions obtained by chromatographic separation ideally contain only one protein type which is subsequently identified by mass spectrometric analysis and data base search.

during the spectrometric quantification. The different isotope mass in the amino acids of the two groups leads to twin peaks which can be quantified relatively according to their intensity ratios [81].

Isotope-coded affinity tags (ICAT) and isobaric tag for relative and absolute quantisation (iTRAQ) rely on the chemical labelling of protein samples after the experiment but before mass spectrometry [82, 83]. ICAT and iTRAQ assays label proteins with reactive groups which contain either heavy or light isotopes, which allows the direct quantification of proteins by mass spectrometry similar to SILAC [82, 83]. In contrast to ICAT and SILAC, the isobaric labelling by iTRAQ does not increase the complexity of the protein lysates and labelling of all peptides in a mixture after the biological experiment [74]. ICAT and iTRAQ therefore enable the proteome quantification in tissue samples of larger mammals which cannot be fed with substituted amino acids only.

In summary, shotgun proteomics analyses the proteome of complex protein lysates in an industrialized manner without gel-based artefacts. It permits the analysis of a wider range of proteins including hydrophobic membrane proteins and strongly acidic and basic proteins. Limitations are the restriction of this method to specialized and appropriately equipped laboratories and the relatively high costs (Table 2).

4. Questions to Be Asked in Transcriptomics and Proteomics

The "-omics" technologies enable the parallel analysis of several thousands of biomolecules in a sample instead of the traditional sequential approach. The comprehensive parallel approach naturally interferes with the sensitivity and specificity of detection and quantification. However, these technologies are now on a technological level that facilitates their application for explorative, descriptive pilot studies on biological phenomena when the present knowledge is not sufficient to establish a substantiated hypothesis on its molecular basis. Furthermore, they may also be applied to overcome deadlocked views and paradigms and to approach well-known diseases unbiased again.

In the following, three major research fields are introduced where "-omics" technologies are successfully applied: biomarker discovery, identification of complex, prognostic gene expression patterns, explorative and hypothesis-driven proteome, and transcriptome analysis (Figure 4).

4.1. Biomarker Discovery. A biomarker can be DNA, mRNA, miRNA, proteins, or any other biomolecule associated with a specific state of the cell or tissue [84]. These markers are synthesized by the diseased tissue itself or by nondiseased cells in response to the neoplastic or inflammatory disease. Biomarkers are further subdivided in diagnostic marker which enable the detection of the disease, prognostic markers which in turn allow for a prediction of the disease course when the initial diagnosis has been established, and stratification markers which predict a response to a specific treatment (reviewed in [84]).

The ideal biomarker therefore permits the diagnosis and classification of a disease with a cheap, sensitive, and specific

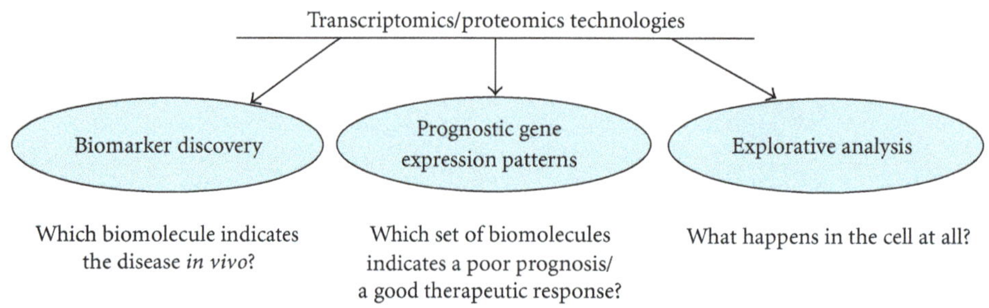

FIGURE 4: The three main fields for the application of transcriptomics and proteomics technologies and the basic questions behind these applications.

assay in a tissue sample which is obtained by a microinvasive intervention such as serum samples or small tissue biopsies.

Several, well-established biomarkers are used in clinical biochemistry in daily diagnostic routine. For instance, enzymatic activity of alkaline phosphatase (ALP) and other enzymes in serum samples are used for the evaluation of the hepatic function or thyroxin, and sex steroid levels are used to identify endocrine diseases. Tumor (bio-) markers are a field of specific interest in the search for biomarkers, and several of them have been introduced in human routine diagnostic, for instance, alpha-fetoprotein and carcinoembryonic antigen [85, 86]. In contrast, several, mostly immunohistochemical but also serum tumor markers have been suggested in veterinary medicine but are in most cases not routinely used in the prediction of disease outcome mostly due to low specificity and sensitivity (reviewed in [87]).

The complete sequencing of the canine, feline, bovine, equine, and chicken genome, the availability of manufactured genome microarrays, and the reduction in costs of transcriptomics and proteomics technology will however accelerate the search biomarker in veterinary sciences, and progress in this filed can be expected in the near future [88–92]. However, biomarker identification is, despite the technological progress, still difficult and requires structured and expansive analysis and comprehensive evaluation of the results.

The first and in most cases a tremendous hurdle for biomarker studies in veterinary medicine is the need for well-preserved, clinical samples with comprehensive clinical data on disease outcome. The appropriate number of samples from a well-defined study population taken with a standard protocol usually requires multicentred efforts to gain the critical mass. Once a sufficient and statistically relevant number of clinical samples are available, biomarker discovery is usually based on a simple comparison of tissue samples from patients with and without the disease (diagnostic biomarkers), certain disease outcomes (prognostic biomarkers), or different responses to therapy (stratification biomarkers). Most biomarker studies are therefore based on the assumption that specific proteins are present in the blood of a patient with a particular disease, disease outcome, or reaction to a drug. However, knowledge on the composition and the biodynamics of the blood proteome or specific proteins in healthy individuals is still far incomplete, and unless these gaps of knowledge are filled, important biomarkers may be possibly missed [93].

Whether proteins, DNA, miRNA, mRNA, or other biomolecules are searched as candidates for biomarkers in these samples depends on the available samples the concurrent knowledge on disease mechanisms, and the general requirements of the intended final assay. Nonetheless, there is a clear trend towards proteomic approaches on easily accessible body fluids like serum to identify biomarkers for clinical routine diagnostics. This is supported by the growing content of the public protein data bases (SwissProt, UniProt, RCSB) for human, murine but also other farm and companion species which facilitates the first biomarker discovery studies in veterinary science.

The work plan for biomarker discovery projects is long and complicated (reviewed in [93]). Briefly, the early detection research network (EDRN) has proposed a five-phase process for the development and testing of disease biomarkers [94].

Explorative preclinical, proteome or transcriptome studies are proposed as initial first phase steps in biomarker discovery. Which of the "-omics" strategies is utilized is in most circumstances determined by the available equipment and the amount of preexisting knowledge of molecular disease mechanisms (reviewed in [84]). Nevertheless, mass-spectrometry-based profiling by MudPIT proteomics of low molecular weight proteins (peptidome) in the clinical serum samples has been given special attention due to the easy and microinvasive obtainment of such samples in a clinical environment [95]. In contrast, the cancer biomarker-family approach is based on the hypotheses that "if a member of protein family is a biomarker, other members of that family might also be good biomarkers" [84]. Finally, the secreted-protein-based approach hypothesizes that a good serological biomarker should be a secreted protein, and biological fluids with contact to the tumor site may help in primary identification of these markers [84, 93].

The initial preclinical, explorative phase of the biomarker discovery which includes proteome or transcriptome profiling of the complete set of proteins has to be followed by the development of clinical assays for the identified few candidates. The assays are tested retrospective longitudinally and prospectively to evaluate their sensitivity and specificity for disease detection in phases two to four [94]. Finally, in phase five, the established assays have to be evaluated in a large patient population to ensure their clinical efficiency and impact, another phase which requires multicenter collaboration to obtain sufficient patient numbers [84, 93]. All of these stages are influenced by several variables that have been carefully planed or standardized by standard operating procedures but are beyond the scope of this review (reviewed in [93]).

Costs are another critical factor of biomarker discovery at each of the discovery phases. In the initial exploratory phase, the high costs of modern instrumentations and reagents for proteome and transcriptome analysis are a limiting. Costs for commercial proteome analysis are dropping. In the proceeding phases, costs are mainly driven by the development and validation of marker-specific assays, for example, ELISA. The cost for the development of the assays varies but numbers of 100,000 up to 1,000,000$ have been suggested [96]. In addition, experience shows that only a small fraction of the total candidates successfully make good clinical biomarkers [96]. The high developmental costs for specific biomarker detection assays and only to a minor extent the costs for explorative "-omics" technologies are therefore considered as the current bottleneck in biomarker discovery [97, 98].

4.2. Detection of Prognostic Gene Expression Patterns by Supervised Gene Expression Profiling. Especially in tumor biology, it becomes more and more evident that for most cancer types a malignant phenotype is associated with specific, complex changes in gene expression levels and not based on the expression levels of single genes [99, 100]. This perception has changed the search for prognostic factors in oncology. In recent years, expression profiling has been used to identify complex, prognostic gene expression patterns [100–102]. Ideally, gene expression profiling focuses on protein expression levels, since mRNA or miRNA expression levels do not fully reflect the protein expression pattern and the biologic activity of a cell. However, the technological head start of mRNA assays like microarrays and next generation sequencer makes these methods superior to proteome analysis for the identification of prognostic gene sets. In addition, prognostic gene expression patterns do not have to reflect the true biologic state of the cell. Their only function is to diagnose a disease or predict a disease outcome even if they are based on biologically irrelevant, phenotypic mRNA patterns.

Two major approaches for gene identification are commonly used, supervised and unsupervised classification (Figure 5) [103]. The principle of supervised gene expression profiling studies is rather simple [99]. According to the diagnostic questions, the complete mRNA of tissue samples from "training" groups of patients with and without the disease or the intended or not intended therapy outcome are analyzed to identify genes whose expression level is significantly associated with the respective group [99]. Thus, the tissue samples are first divided by their disease status, and the data analysis aims at identifying the differences in the gene expression profile behind these clinically observed differences [99]. In contrast, the unsupervised method differentiates tissue samples according to their gene expression profile without preceding information on their diseases status. This approach aims at identifying molecular phenotypes within a by then phenotypically homogeneous disease which may be of interest for treatment and prognosis. Another method is to apply experimentally obtained information on gene expression profiles associated with the activation of certain molecular pathways to classify tumour samples. This hypothesis-driven gene expression profiling approach aims at differentiating tumours that depend on these molecular pathways and may be treated accordingly [99].

The diagnostic value of the gene sets identified with supervised clustering has to be tested in a second, independent "test" group to confirm its usefulness. This group again consists of a large population of patients with and without the disease or the different therapeutic outcomes. In an unsupervised approach, the prognostic gene set is now used to assign tissue samples to one of the groups. According to the ability to attribute clinical samples to the respective group, that is, false negative and false positive results, the specificity and sensitivity of the gene set are determined.

In 2002, van't Veer et al. published one of the first studies that identified a prognostic set of 70 genes for human breast cancer [100]. In a supervised classification approach, they compared lymph-node-negative breast cancer samples with short intervals to distant metastases with samples with long intervals to distant metastasis. By this approach, the authors identified a prognostic set of 70 genes that predicts distant metastases and allows a patient-tailored therapy strategy to identify patients which benefit from the application of adjuvant therapy from [100]. Of interest, first gene expression profiling studies on canine mammary tumours show that similar prognostic gene set may exist for malignant canine mammary tumours although their prognostic relevance has not been tested in larger patient populations yet (Figure 6) [101, 102, 104–107]. It can however be assumed that similar prognostic gene sets will be identified for veterinary diseases in the near future, given that affordable molecular tools like microarrays are now available for the most relevant species in veterinary science.

Unsupervised cluster analysis and hypothesis-driven gene expression profiling are less successful and promising strategies to identify prognostic gene expression profiles but may help to understand disease-associated molecular mechanisms in explorative and hypothesis-driven transcriptome and proteome studies.

4.3. Explorative and Hypothesis-Driven Transcriptome and Proteome Analysis. Ideally, scientific progress is a continuous hypothesis-driven process by which new ideas are based on and refine recent findings. However, occasionally the preexisting knowledge is insufficient to establish a substantial hypothesis. In these cases, transcriptome and proteome analyses are a promising, explorative approach to obtain first exploitable information on potential molecular disease mechanisms. Both supervised and unsupervised gene expression clustering using microarray technology and comparative proteome analysis have been used in veterinary science to explore the molecular basis of various, mostly neoplastic diseases [64, 104, 105, 108–110]. All these studies compared diseased and nondiseased tissues in a supervised approach to identify genes or molecular pathways with significant disease

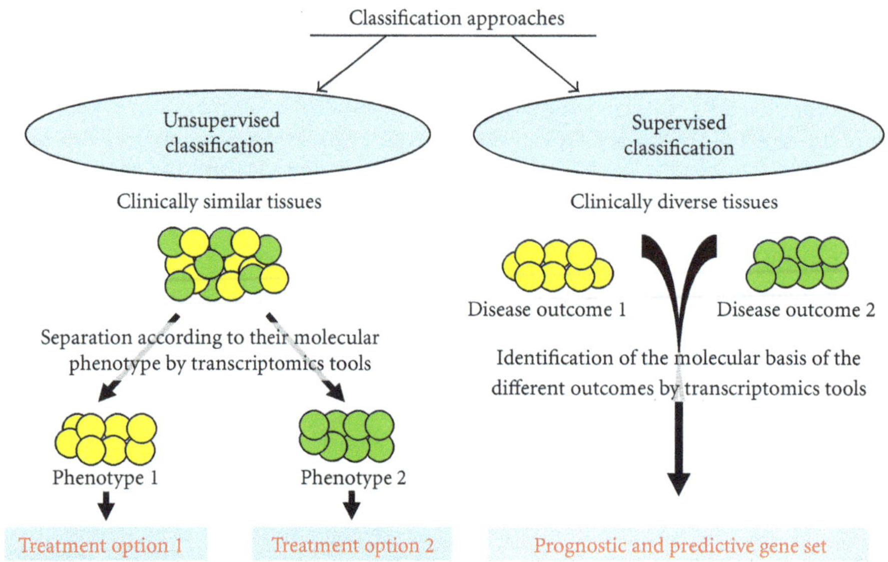

Figure 5: Two major approaches for the identification of disease-relevant gene expression profiles are supervised and unsupervised classification. Unsupervised classification is used to identify different molecular mechanisms in tissues from patients with clinically similar disease phenotypes. Clustering of these tissues according to their molecular phenotype may lead to the identification of different molecular phenotypes behind the identical clinical behaviour. This knowledge may finally lead to diverse therapy protocols of these molecular subtypes. In contrast, during supervised clustering, molecular mechanisms behind different disease outcome or phenotypes are analyzed. Two tissue groups with clinical differences are therefore compared, and the differences in gene expression are thought to be relevant for the distinct clinical behaviour. The resulting set of genes may also serve prognostic markers for the prospective classification tissue samples.

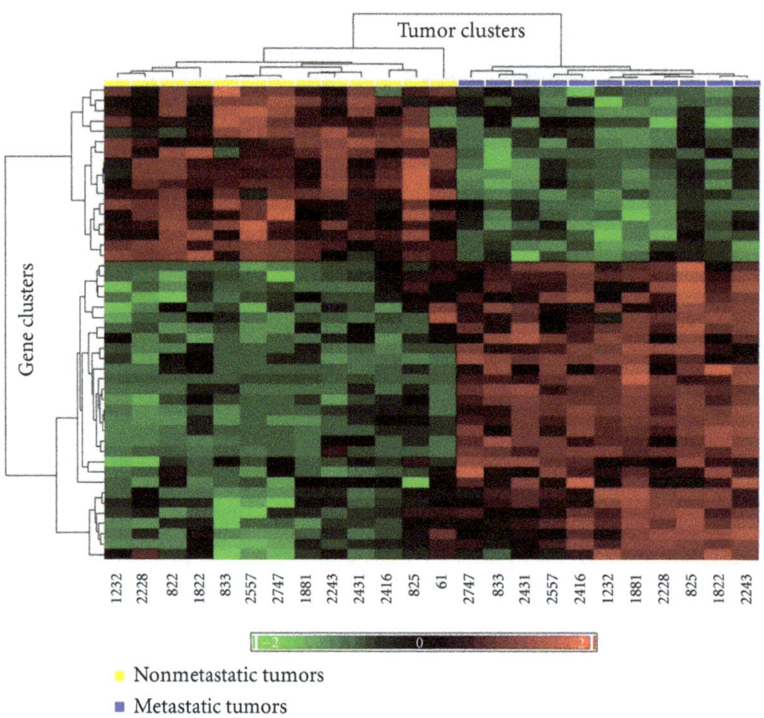

Figure 6: First studies in canine mammary tumours show that clinically different but histologically similar tumours can be clustered in a supervised approach into clinically relevant groups by a prognostically relevant gene sets (modified from [102]).

association. These disease-associated proteins are now to be tested in further hypothesis-driven experiments to prove their relevance as primary disease causes or to identify them as pure phenotypic and secondary effects.

Unsupervised clustering of microarrays data has been used in human oncology to subclassify histologically identical cancer samples by their molecular phenotype. This strategy is based on the general hypothesis that a clinically and morphologically uniform disease may be caused by different molecular mechanisms, that is, that different molecular mechanisms can lead to the same disease or clinical picture. In one of the first studies using this strategy, Perou et al. investigated the gene expression patterns in breast cancer by unsupervised hierarchical cluster analysis [111]. They were able to divide malignant high-grade breast cancer tissue samples into four diverse subgroups with differential gene expression profiles. In several ensuing studies, these subgroups were refined, and their prognostic and therapeutic relevance has been confirmed [112]. Similar studies with impact on the classification of veterinary tumours are lacking but hopefully will be available in the near future.

Hypothesis-driven gene expression profiling is the complete opposite strategy to unsupervised, explorative gene expression profiling. This strategy uses gene expression signatures which either have been identified during in vitro or in vivo experiments using models of the disease of interest or theoretically by comparison with other diseases, species, or consideration of known gene functions [99]. The relevant set of genes or rather "functional" gene expression profiles are applied on preexisting microarray data to subcategorize the tissues according to the activity of the relevant genes. For instance, it has been hypothesized that carcinogenesis is a chronic inflammatory process, and a tumor can therefore be considered as nonhealing wound [99, 113, 114]. Based on this idea, the gene expression profiles of serum-activated fibroblasts were applied to the gene expression profiles of different tumours [113]. It has been shown that signature was an independent prognostic factor and showed a strong prediction of metastasis and overall survival and may therefore represent a hypothesis-based prognostic gene set [115].

Hypothesis-driven gene expression profiling studies on veterinary diseases are not available momentarily, most probably to the delayed accumulation of necessary gene expression data in experimental models. However, due to the successful application of this approach on human diseases, it can be expected that similar studies will be available in the near future.

5. Summary

Transcriptome and proteome analyses have been introduced as a research tool in most fields of biomedical research. They permit the identification of prognostically relevant biomarkers, gene expression profiles, and the understanding of complex molecular mechanisms in cell physiology and pathology.

Methods to analyze the transcriptome have made the greatest advancement so far. cDNA microarrays have been and are widely used to analyse disease mechanisms and to identify prognostic gene sets. With the availability of species-specific, commercially available and affordable microarrays, it is expectable that its use is becoming even more relevant in veterinary science in the next years. However, due to the intrinsic cross-hybridization and sensitivity issues of the microarray technology, there are tendencies towards Ref-Seq or deep sequencing technologies, respectively, as an alternative method for the analysis of the transcriptome. Ref-Seq expands transcriptome analysis by the parallel information on the mutational status of the quantified mRNA types and is less dependent on the full genome coverage of a species in a database. Especially, the latter fact indicates that Ref-Seq will be helpful in areas of veterinary science with deal with rather rare species, where microarrays are commercially not available. A major but most probably temporary disadvantage of Ref-Seq is the relatively high costs and the need of computational power and biostatistical expertise required to appraise the resulting data masses. The questionable relevance of mRNA expression levels on the biology of a tissue is, however, a general problem of transcriptome analyses, independent from the applied technology.

Proteome analysis is therefore considered the ultimate method for the analysis of disease-associated mechanisms. Momentarily, the two competing methodical approaches are 2D-gel electrophoresis-based proteomics and shotgun proteomics. While 2D-gel electrophoresis allows protein separation with less expansive equipment and experience, chromatography-based proteomics seems to be of greater development potential in terms of mechanisation and standardization. General hurdles of proteome analyses itself that still need further development are problems to standardize the analysis of chemically and biochemically highly diverse proteins when in tissue lysates, that is, to cover the full proteome in each case. Furthermore, there are still sensitivity issues in mixtures of high-and low-abundance proteins and the general instability of proteins in tissue samples.

Biomarker discovery is a constantly growing scientific field which attracted high investments and efforts in the recent years. Although it can be based on all kinds of biologic elements, that is, RNA, metabolites, it is commonly based on proteome analysis of tissue samples or body fluids. Despite the initial euphoria, the revenues of the enormous investments in biomarker discovery are moderate, scientifically and commercially. In addition, biomarker discovery in veterinary science is hampered by lack of appropriate tissue banks with proper clinical data, the high costs for initial proteome analysis, and the high costs for the establishment and evaluation of subsequent diagnostic tests.

In terms of data analyses, supervised and unsupervised clustering analysis are the dominating approaches to identify disease-associated gene expression. Supervised clustering allows the identification of prognostic gene sets that may predict disease and treatment outcome and has already been successfully applied in veterinary science. It is based on the comparison of gene expression profiles of tissue samples with a known disease outcome. In contrast, unsupervised clustering is used to elucidate molecular mechanisms behind morphologically and clinically similar diseases. Application of this approach on veterinary diseases will certainly refine or even change our perception of many diseases. Hypothesis-driven gene expression profiling is a less frequently used but promising approach which experimentally derived expression profiles to identify molecular pathways with relevance in clinical tissue samples.

In summary, "-omics" technology has made it to a standard method in human and to a minor extend also in veterinary biomedical research. They are useful tools for the explorative studies and allow the analysis of complex gene expression patterns. Given that the costs for these methods will further drop, it can be expected that the results of numerous transcriptomics and proteomics studies will contribute to the understanding of several veterinary diseases in the near future.

Acknowledgments

The preparation of this paper has been supported be the German Research Council (DFG KL 2240/1). The authors thank Patricia Klose for providing the figure of the 2D-gel electrophoresis and Dido Lenze for preparation of the figure of the microarray cluster analysis.

References

[1] K. Kubo, S. Matsuyama, K. Katayama et al., "Frequent expression of the c-kit proto-oncogene in canine malignant mammary tumor," *Journal of Veterinary Medical Science*, vol. 60, no. 12, pp. 1335–1340, 1998.

[2] B. Vogelstein and K. W. Kinzler, "The multistep nature of cancer," *Trends in Genetics*, vol. 9, no. 4, pp. 138–141, 1993.

[3] V. E. Velculescu, L. Zhang, W. Zhou et al., "Characterization of the yeast transcriptome," *Cell*, vol. 88, no. 2, pp. 243–251, 1997.

[4] M. R. Wilkins, C. Pasquali, R. D. Appel et al., "From proteins to proteomes: large scale protein identification by two-dimensional electrophoresis and amino acid analysis," *Biotechnology*, vol. 14, no. 1, pp. 61–65, 1996.

[5] S. G. Oliver, M. K. Winson, D. B. Kell, and F. Baganz, "Systematic functional analysis of the yeast genome," *Trends in Biotechnology*, vol. 16, no. 9, pp. 373–378, 1998.

[6] T. Feizi, "Progress in deciphering the information content of the "glycome"—a crescendo in the closing years of the millennium," *Glycoconjugate Journal*, vol. 17, no. 7-9, pp. 553–565, 2000.

[7] R. C. Lee, R. L. Feinbaum, and V. Ambros, "The C. elegans heterochronic gene lin-4 encodes small RNAs with antisense complementarity to lin-14," *Cell*, vol. 75, no. 5, pp. 843–854, 1993.

[8] U. Maskos and E. M. Southern, "Oligonucleotide hybridisations on glass supports: a novel linker for oligonucleotide synthesis and hybridisation properties of oligonucleotides synthesised in situ," *Nucleic Acids Research*, vol. 20, no. 7, pp. 1679–1684, 1992.

[9] H. J. Lee, T. T. Goodrich, and R. M. Corn, "SPR imaging measurements of 1-D and 2-D DNA microarrays created from microfluidic channels on gold thin films," *Analytical Chemistry*, vol. 73, no. 22, pp. 5525–5531, 2001.

[10] J. G. Hacia, J. B. Fan, O. Ryder et al., "Determination of ancestral alleles for human single-nucleotide polymorphisms using high-density oligonucleotide arrays," *Nature Genetics*, vol. 22, no. 2, pp. 164–167, 1999.

[11] D. Shalon, S. J. Smith, and P. O. Brown, "A DNA microarray system for analyzing complex DNA samples using two-color fluorescent probe hybridization," *Genome Research*, vol. 6, no. 7, pp. 639–645, 1996.

[12] Y. Zhang, J. Szustakowski, and M. Schinke, "Bioinformatics analysis of microarray data," *Methods in Molecular Biology*, vol. 573, pp. 259–284, 2009.

[13] Y. F. Leung and D. Cavalieri, "Fundamentals of cDNA microarray data analysis," *Trends in Genetics*, vol. 19, no. 11, pp. 649–659, 2003.

[14] I. Priness, O. Maimon, and I. Ben-Gal, "Evaluation of gene-expression clustering via mutual information distance measure," *BMC Bioinformatics*, vol. 8, article 111, 2007.

[15] L. Li, "Dimension reduction for high-dimensional data," *Methods in Molecular Biology*, vol. 620, pp. 417–434, 2010.

[16] J. H. Do and D. K. Choi, "Clustering approaches to identifying gene expression patterns from DNA microarray data," *Molecules and Cells*, vol. 25, no. 2, pp. 279–288, 2008.

[17] A. Brazma, P. Hingamp, J. Quackenbush et al., "Minimum information about a microarray experiment (MIAME)-toward standards for microarray data," *Nature Genetics*, vol. 29, no. 4, pp. 365–371, 2001.

[18] L. Shi, L. H. Reid, W. D. Jones et al., "The MicroArray Quality Control (MAQC) project shows inter- and intraplatform reproducibility of gene expression measurements," *Nature Biotechnology*, vol. 24, no. 9, pp. 1151–1161, 2006.

[19] R. Kothapalli, S. J. Yoder, S. Mane, and T. P. Loughran, "Microarray result: how accurate are they?" *BMC Bioinformatics*, vol. 3, article 22, 2002.

[20] Z. Wang, M. Gerstein, and M. Snyder, "RNA-Seq: a revolutionary tool for transcriptomics," *Nature Reviews Genetics*, vol. 10, no. 1, pp. 57–63, 2009.

[21] M. Meyerson, S. Gabriel, and G. Getz, "Advances in understanding cancer genomes through second-generation sequencing," *Nature Reviews Genetics*, vol. 11, no. 10, pp. 685–696, 2010.

[22] D. A. Wheeler, M. Srinivasan, M. Egholm et al., "The complete genome of an individual by massively parallel DNA sequencing," *Nature*, vol. 452, no. 7189, pp. 872–876, 2008.

[23] T. J. Ley, E. R. Mardis, L. Ding et al., "DNA sequencing of a cytogenetically normal acute myeloid leukaemia genome," *Nature*, vol. 456, no. 7218, pp. 66–72, 2008.

[24] R. D. Morin, M. Bainbridge, A. Fejes et al., "Profiling the HeLa S3 transcriptome using randomly primed cDNA and massively parallel short-read sequencing," *BioTechniques*, vol. 45, no. 1, pp. 81–94, 2008.

[25] C. A. Maher, C. Kumar-Sinha, X. Cao et al., "Transcriptome sequencing to detect gene fusions in cancer," *Nature*, vol. 458, no. 7234, pp. 97–101, 2009.

[26] N. Cloonan, A. R. R. Forrest, G. Kolle et al., "Stem cell transcriptome profiling via massive-scale mRNA sequencing," *Nature Methods*, vol. 5, no. 7, pp. 613–619, 2008.

[27] S. J. Emrich, W. B. Barbazuk, L. Li, and P. S. Schnable, "Gene discovery and annotation using LCM-454 transcriptome sequencing," *Genome Research*, vol. 17, no. 1, pp. 69–73, 2007.

[28] P. Milos, "Helicos BioSciences," *Pharmacogenomics*, vol. 9, no. 4, pp. 477–480, 2008.

[29] M. Margulies, M. Egholm, W. E. Altman et al., "Genome sequencing in microfabricated high-density picolitre reactors," *Nature*, vol. 437, no. 7057, pp. 376–380, 2006.

[30] E. R. Mardis, "Next-generation DNA sequencing methods," *Annual Review of Genomics and Human Genetics*, vol. 9, pp. 387–402, 2008.
[31] S. C. Schuster, "Next-generation sequencing transforms today's biology," *Nature Methods*, vol. 5, no. 1, pp. 16–18, 2008.
[32] A. Valouev, J. Ichikawa, T. Tonthat et al., "A high-resolution, nucleosome position map of C. elegans reveals a lack of universal sequence-dictated positioning," *Genome Research*, vol. 18, no. 7, pp. 1051–1063, 2008.
[33] J. C. Vera, C. W. Wheat, H. W. Fescemyer et al., "Rapid transcriptome characterization for a nonmodel organism using 454 pyrosequencing," *Molecular Ecology*, vol. 17, no. 7, pp. 1636–1647, 2008.
[34] J. Shendure, "The beginning of the end for microarrays?" *Nature Methods*, vol. 5, no. 7, pp. 585–587, 2008.
[35] A. Mortazavi, B. A. Williams, K. McCue, L. Schaeffer, and B. Wold, "Mapping and quantifying mammalian transcriptomes by RNA-Seq," *Nature Methods*, vol. 5, no. 7, pp. 621–628, 2008.
[36] B. T. Wilhelm, S. Marguerat, S. Watt et al., "Dynamic repertoire of a eukaryotic transcriptome surveyed at single-nucleotide resolution," *Nature*, vol. 453, no. 7199, pp. 1239–1243, 2008.
[37] Y. Chen, J. A. L. Gelfond, L. M. McManus, and P. K. Shireman, "Reproducibility of quantitative RT-PCR array in miRNA expression profiling and comparison with microarray analysis," *BMC Genomics*, vol. 10, article 1471, p. 407, 2009.
[38] S. Griffiths-Jones, H. K. Saini, S. Van Dongen, and A. J. Enright, "miRBase: tools for microRNA genomics," *Nucleic Acids Research*, vol. 36, no. 1, pp. D154–D158, 2008.
[39] S. Griffiths-Jones, R. J. Grocock, S. van Dongen, A. Bateman, and A. J. Enright, "miRBase: microRNA sequences, targets and gene nomenclature," *Nucleic Acids Research*, vol. 34, pp. D140–D144, 2006.
[40] S. Griffiths-Jones, "The microRNA registry," *Nucleic Acids Research*, vol. 32, pp. D109–D111, 2004.
[41] M. Dufva, J. Petersen, and L. Poulsen, "Increasing the specificity and function of DNA microarrays by processing arrays at different stringencies," *Analytical and Bioanalytical Chemistry*, vol. 395, no. 3, pp. 669–677, 2009.
[42] S. Sharbati-Tehrani, B. Kutz-Lohroff, R. Bergbauer, J. Scholven, and R. Einspanier, "MiR-Q: a novel quantitative RT-PCR approach for the expression profiling of small RNA molecules such as miRNAs in a complex sample," *BMC Molecular Biology*, vol. 9, article 34, 2008.
[43] C. Chen, D. A. Ridzon, A. J. Broomer et al., "Real-time quantification of microRNAs by stem-loop RT-PCR," *Nucleic Acids Research*, vol. 33, no. 20, p. e179, 2005.
[44] R. Klopfleisch and A. D. Gruber, "Derlin-1 and Stanniocalcin-1 are Differentially Regulated in Metastasizing Canine Mammary Adenocarcinomas," *Journal of Comparative Pathology*, vol. 141, no. 2-3, pp. 113–120, 2009.
[45] R. Klopfleisch and A. D. Gruber, "Differential expression of cell cycle regulators p21, p27 and p53 in metastasizing canine mammary adenocarcinomas versus normal mammary glands," *Research in Veterinary Science*, vol. 87, no. 1, pp. 91–96, 2009.
[46] R. Klopfleisch and A. D. Gruber, "Increased expression of BRCA2 and RAD51 in lymph node metastases of canine mammary adenocarcinomas," *Veterinary Pathology*, vol. 46, no. 3, pp. 416–422, 2009.
[47] D. Greenbaum, C. Colangelo, K. Williams, and M. Gerstein, "Comparing protein abundance and mRNA expression levels on a genomic scale," *Genome Biology*, vol. 4, no. 9, article 117, 2003.
[48] J. M. Gilmore and M. P. Washburn, "Advances in shotgun proteomics and the analysis of membrane proteomes," *Journal of Proteomics*, vol. 73, no. 11, pp. 2078–2091, 2010.
[49] T. Kislinger and A. O. Gramolini, "Proteome analysis of mouse model systems: a tool to model human disease and for the investigation of tissue-specific biology," *Journal of Proteomics*, vol. 73, no. 11, pp. 2205–2218, 2010.
[50] P. H. O'Farrell, "High resolution two dimensional electrophoresis of proteins," *Journal of Biological Chemistry*, vol. 250, no. 10, pp. 4007–4021, 1975.
[51] J. Klose, "Protein mapping by combined isoelectric focusing and electrophoresis of mouse tissues. A novel approach to testing for induced point mutations in mammals," *HUMANGENETIK*, vol. 26, no. 3, pp. 231–243, 1975.
[52] B. Bjellqvist, K. Ek, P. Giorgio Righetti et al., "Isoelectric focusing in immobilized pH gradients: principle, methodology and some applications," *Journal of Biochemical and Biophysical Methods*, vol. 6, no. 4, pp. 317–339, 1982.
[53] U. K. Laemmli, "Cleavage of structural proteins during the assembly of the head of bacteriophage T4," *Nature*, vol. 227, no. 5259, pp. 680–685, 1970.
[54] T. S. Meyer and B. L. Lamberts, "Use of coomassie brilliant blue R250 for the electrophoresis of microgram quantities of parotid saliva proteins on acrylamide-gel strips," *Biochimica et Biophysica Acta*, vol. 107, no. 1, pp. 144–145, 1965.
[55] T. Rabilloud, G. Carpentier, and P. Tarroux, "Improvement and simplification of low-background silver staining of proteins by using sodium dithionite," *Electrophoresis*, vol. 9, no. 6, pp. 288–291, 1988.
[56] K. Berggren, T. H. Steinberg, W. M. Lauber et al., "A luminescent ruthenium complex for ultrasensitive detection of proteins immobilized on membrane supports," *Analytical Biochemistry*, vol. 276, no. 2, pp. 129–143, 1999.
[57] M. Berth, F. M. Moser, M. Kolbe, and J. Bernhardt, "The state of the art in the analysis of two-dimensional gel electrophoresis images," *Applied Microbiology and Biotechnology*, vol. 76, no. 6, pp. 1223–1243, 2007.
[58] M. Ünlü, M. E. Morgan, and J. S. Minden, "Difference gel electrophoresis: a single gel method for detecting changes in protein extracts," *Electrophoresis*, vol. 18, no. 11, pp. 2071–2077, 1997.
[59] M. Stessl, C. R. Noe, and B. Lachmann, "Influence of image-analysis software on quantitation of two-dimensional gel electrophoresis data," *Electrophoresis*, vol. 30, no. 2, pp. 325–328, 2009.
[60] D. B. Friedman, S. Hoving, and R. Westermeier, "Chapter 30 isoelectric focusing and two-dimensional gel electrophoresis," *Methods in Enzymology*, vol. 463, no. C, pp. 515–540, 2009.
[61] M. Mann, P. Hojrup, and P. Roepstorff, "Use of mass spectrometric molecular weight information to identify proteins in sequence databases," *Biological Mass Spectrometry*, vol. 22, no. 6, pp. 338–345, 1993.
[62] F. Hillenkamp, M. Karas, R. C. Beavis, and B. T. Chait, "Matrix-assisted laser desorption/ionization mass spectrometry of biopolymers," *Analytical Chemistry*, vol. 63, no. 24, pp. 1193A–1203A, 1991.
[63] W. J. Henzel, T. M. Billeci, J. T. Stults, S. C. Wong, C. Grimley, and C. Watanabe, "Identifying proteins from two-dimensional gels by molecular mass searching of peptide fragments in protein sequence databases," *Proceedings of the National*

Academy of Sciences of the United States of America, vol. 90, no. 11, pp. 5011–5015, 1993.

[64] R. Klopfleisch, P. Klose, C. Weise et al., "Proteome of metastatic canine mammary carcinomas: similarities to and differences from human breast cancer," *Journal of Proteome Research*, vol. 9, no. 12, pp. 6380–6391, 2010.

[65] S. P. Gygi, G. L. Corthals, Y. Zhang, Y. Rochon, and R. Aebersold, "Evaluation of two-dimensional gel electrophoresis-based proteome analysis technology," *Proceedings of the National Academy of Sciences of the United States of America*, vol. 97, no. 17, pp. 9390–9395, 2000.

[66] M. Fountoulakis, M. F. Takács, P. Berndt, H. Langen, and B. Takács, "Enrichment of low abundance proteins of Escherichia coli by hydroxyapatite chromatography," *Electrophoresis*, vol. 20, no. 11, pp. 2181–2195, 1999.

[67] C. L. Corthals, V. C. Wasinger, D. F. Hochstrasser, and J. C. Sanchez, "The dynamic range of protein expression: a challenge for proteomic research," *Electrophoresis*, vol. 21, no. 6, pp. 1104–1115, 2000.

[68] M. Oh-Ishi, M. Satoh, and T. Maeda, "Preparative two-dimensional gel electrophoresis with agarose gels in the first dimension for high molecular mass proteins," *Electrophoresis*, vol. 21, no. 9, pp. 1653–1669, 2000.

[69] V. Santoni, M. Molloy, and T. Rabilloud, "Membrane proteins and proteomics: un amour impossible?" *Electrophoresis*, vol. 21, no. 6, pp. 1054–1070, 2000.

[70] M. P. Washburn, D. Wolters, and J. R. Yates, "Large-scale analysis of the yeast proteome by multidimensional protein identification technology," *Nature Biotechnology*, vol. 19, no. 3, pp. 242–247, 2001.

[71] P. Mauri and M. Scigelova, "Multidimensional protein identification technology for clinical proteomic analysis," *Clinical Chemistry and Laboratory Medicine*, vol. 47, no. 6, pp. 636–645, 2009.

[72] M. L. Fournier, J. M. Gilmore, S. A. Martin-Brown, and M. P. Washburn, "Multidimensional separations-based shotgun proteomics," *Chemical Reviews*, vol. 107, no. 8, pp. 3654–3686, 2007.

[73] V. Sanz-Nebot, E. Balaguer, F. Benavente, C. Neusüß, and J. Barbosa, "Characterization of transferrin glycoforms in human serum by CE-UV and CE-ESI-MS," *Electrophoresis*, vol. 28, no. 12, pp. 1949–1957, 2007.

[74] K. G. Kline, G. L. Finney, and C. C. Wu, "Quantitative strategies to fuel the merger of discovery and hypothesis-driven shotgun proteomics," *Briefings in Functional Genomics and Proteomics*, vol. 8, no. 2, pp. 114–125, 2009.

[75] J. Z. Bereszczak and F. L. Brancia, "Offline and online liquid chromatography mass spectrometry in quantitative proteomics," *Combinatorial Chemistry and High Throughput Screening*, vol. 12, no. 2, pp. 185–193, 2009.

[76] B. Zybailov, M. K. Coleman, L. Florens, and M. P. Washburn, "Correlation of relative abundance ratios derived from peptide ion chromatograms and spectrum counting for quantitative proteomic analysis using stable isotope labeling," *Analytical Chemistry*, vol. 77, no. 19, pp. 6218–6224, 2005.

[77] H. Liu, R. G. Sadygov, and J. R. Yates, "A model for random sampling and estimation of relative protein abundance in shotgun proteomics," *Analytical Chemistry*, vol. 76, no. 14, pp. 4193–4201, 2004.

[78] K. G. Kline, B. Frewen, M. R. Bristow, M. J. MacCoss, and C. C. Wu, "High quality catalog of proteotypic peptides from human heart," *Journal of Proteome Research*, vol. 7, no. 11, pp. 5055–5061, 2008.

[79] Y. Oda, K. Huang, F. R. Cross, D. Cowburn, and B. T. Chait, "Accurate quantitation of protein expression and site-specific phosphorylation," *Proceedings of the National Academy of Sciences of the United States of America*, vol. 96, no. 12, pp. 6591–6596, 1999.

[80] C. C. Wu, M. J. MacCoss, K. E. Howell, D. E. Matthews, and J. R. Yates, "Metabolic labeling of mammalian organisms with stable isotopes for quantitative proteomic analysis," *Analytical Chemistry*, vol. 76, no. 17, pp. 4951–4959, 2004.

[81] K. Michael, B. G. Klupp, T. C. Mettenleiter, and A. Karger, "Composition of pseudorabies virus particles lacking tegument protein US3, UL47, or UL49 or envelope glycoprotein E," *Journal of Virology*, vol. 80, no. 3, pp. 1332–1339, 2006.

[82] S. P. Gygi, B. Rist, S. A. Gerber, F. Turecek, M. H. Gelb, and R. Aebersold, "Quantitative analysis of complex protein mixtures using isotope-coded affinity tags," *Nature Biotechnology*, vol. 17, no. 10, pp. 994–999, 1999.

[83] P. L. Ross, Y. N. Huang, J. N. Marchese et al., "Multiplexed protein quantitation in Saccharomyces cerevisiae using amine-reactive isobaric tagging reagents," *Molecular and Cellular Proteomics*, vol. 3, no. 12, pp. 1154–1169, 2004.

[84] V. Kulasingam and E. P. Diamandis, "Strategies for discovering novel cancer biomarkers through utilization of emerging technologies," *Nature Clinical Practice Oncology*, vol. 5, no. 10, pp. 588–599, 2008.

[85] G. I. Abelev, S. D. Perova, N. I. Khramkova, Z. A. Postnikova, and I. S. Irlin, "Embryonal serum alpha- globulin and its synthesis by transplantable mouse hepatomas," *Biokhimiia*, vol. 28, pp. 625–634, 1963.

[86] P. Gold and S. O. Freedman, "Demonstration of tumor-specific antigens in human colonic carcinomata by immunological tolerance and absorption techniques," *The Journal of Experimental Medicine*, vol. 121, pp. 439–462, 1965.

[87] C. J. Henry, "Biomarkers in veterinary cancer screening: applications, limitations and expectations," *Veterinary Journal*, vol. 185, no. 1, pp. 10–14, 2010.

[88] K. Lindblad-Toh, C. M. Wade, T. S. Mikkelsen et al., "Genome sequence, comparative analysis and haplotype structure of the domestic dog," *Nature*, vol. 438, no. 7069, pp. 803–819, 2005.

[89] D. W. Burt, "The chicken genome," *Genome Dynamics*, vol. 2, pp. 123–137, 2006.

[90] R. L. Tellam, D. G. Lemay, C. P. Van Tassell, H. A. Lewin, K. C. Worley, and C. G. Elsik, "Unlocking the bovine genome," *BMC Genomics*, vol. 10, p. 193, 2009.

[91] W. J. Murphy, "The feline genome," *Genome Dynamics*, vol. 2, pp. 60–68, 2006.

[92] B. P. Chowdhary and T. Raudsepp, "The horse genome," *Genome Dynamics*, vol. 2, pp. 97–110, 2006.

[93] B. Matharoo-Ball, A. K. Miles, C. S. Creaser, G. Ball, and R. Rees, "Serum biomarker profiling in cancer studies: a question of standardisation?" *Veterinary and Comparative Oncology*, vol. 6, no. 4, pp. 224–247, 2008.

[94] T. Reynolds, "Validating biomarkers: early detection research network launches first phase III study," *Journal of the National Cancer Institute*, vol. 95, no. 6, pp. 422–423, 2003.

[95] L. A. Liotta, M. Ferrari, and E. Petricoin, "Clinical proteomics: written in blood," *Nature*, vol. 425, no. 6961, p. 905, 2003.

[96] P. Wang, J. R. Whiteaker, and A. G. Paulovich, "The evolving role of mass spectrometry in cancer biomarker discovery," *Cancer Biology and Therapy*, vol. 8, no. 12, pp. 1083–1094, 2009.

[97] S. A. Carr and L. Anderson, "Protein quantitation through targeted mass spectrometry: the way out of biomarker purgatory?" *Clinical Chemistry*, vol. 54, no. 11, pp. 1749–1752, 2008.

[98] N. L. Anderson, N. G. Anderson, T. W. Pearson et al., "A human proteome detection and quantitation project," *Molecular and Cellular Proteomics*, vol. 8, no. 5, pp. 883–886, 2009.

[99] D. S. A. Nuyten and M. J. van de Vijver, "Using microarray analysis as a prognostic and predictive tool in Oncology: focus oVn breast cancer and normal tissue toxicity," *Seminars in Radiation Oncology*, vol. 18, no. 2, pp. 105–114, 2008.

[100] L. J. van't Veer, H. Dai, M. J. Van de Vijver et al., "Gene expression profiling predicts clinical outcome of breast cancer," *Nature*, vol. 415, no. 6871, pp. 530–536, 2002.

[101] R. Klopfleisch, P. Klose, and A. D. Gruber, "The combined expression pattern of BMP2, LTBP4, and DERL1 discriminates malignant from benign canine mammary tumors," *Veterinary Pathology*, vol. 47, no. 3, pp. 446–454, 2010.

[102] R. Klopfleisch, D. Lenze, M. Hummel, and A. D. Gruber, "Metastatic canine mammary carcinomas can be identified by a gene expression profile that partly overlaps with human breast cancer profiles," *BMC Cancer*, vol. 10, article 618, 2010.

[103] S. Michiels, S. Koscielny, and C. Hill, "Prediction of cancer outcome with microarrays: a multiple random validation strategy," *Lancet*, vol. 365, no. 9458, pp. 488–492, 2005.

[104] R. Klopfleisch, D. Lenze, M. Hummel, and A. D. Gruber, "The metastatic cascade isreflected in the transcriptome of metastatic canine mammary carcinomas," *Veterinary Journal*. In press.

[105] P. Uva, L. Aurisicchio, J. Watters et al., "Comparative expression pathway analysis of human and canine mammary tumors," *BMC Genomics*, vol. 10, article 135, 2009.

[106] M. Krol, K. M. Pawlowski, J. Skierski et al., "Transcriptomic profile of two canine mammary cancer cell lines with different proliferative and anti-apoptotic potential," *Journal of Physiology and Pharmacology*, vol. 60, supplement 1, pp. 95–106, 2009.

[107] N. A.S. Rao, M. E. Van Wolferen, A. Gracanin et al., "Gene expression profiles of progestin-induced canine mammary hyperplasia and spontaneous mammary tumors," *Journal of Physiology and Pharmacology*, vol. 60, supplement 1, pp. 73–84, 2009.

[108] N. A. S. Rao, M. E. Van Wolferen, R. Van Den Ham et al., "cDNA microarray profiles of canine mammary tumour cell lines reveal deregulated pathways pertaining to their phenotype," *Animal Genetics*, vol. 39, no. 4, pp. 333–345, 2008.

[109] D. L. McCaw, A. S. Chan, A. L. Stegner et al., "Proteomics of canine lymphoma identifies potential cancer-specific protein markers," *Clinical Cancer Research*, vol. 13, no. 8, pp. 2496–2503, 2007.

[110] P. Klose, C. Weise, A. Bondzio et al., "Is there a malignant progression associated with a linear change in protein expression levels from normal canine mammary gland to metastatic mammary tumors?" *Journal of Proteome Research*, vol. 10, no. 10, pp. 4405–4415, 2011.

[111] C. M. Perou, T. Sørile, M. B. Eisen et al., "Molecular portraits of human breast tumours," *Nature*, vol. 406, no. 6797, pp. 747–752, 2000.

[112] T. Sørlie, C. M. Perou, R. Tibshirani et al., "Gene expression patterns of breast carcinomas distinguish tumor subclasses with clinical implications," *Proceedings of the National Academy of Sciences of the United States of America*, vol. 98, no. 19, pp. 10869–10874, 2001.

[113] H. Y. Chang, J. B. Sneddon, A. A. Alizadeh et al., "Gene expression signature of fibroblast serum response predicts human cancer progression: similarities between tumors and wounds," *PLoS Biology*, vol. 2, no. 2, p. E7, 2004.

[114] H. F. Dvorak, "Tumors: wounds that do not heal: similarities between tumor stroma generation and wound healing," *New England Journal of Medicine*, vol. 315, no. 26, pp. 1650–1659, 1986.

[115] H. Y. Chang, D. S. A. Nuyten, J. B. Sneddon et al., "Robustness, scalability, and integration of a wound-response gene expression signature in predicting breast cancer survival," *Proceedings of the National Academy of Sciences of the United States of America*, vol. 102, no. 10, pp. 3738–3743, 2005.

Use of Spineless Cactus (*Opuntia ficus indica f. inermis*) for Dairy Goats and Growing Kids: Impacts on Milk Production, Kid's Growth, and Meat Quality

M. Mahouachi,[1] N. Atti,[2] and H. Hajji[2,3]

[1] *Ecole Supérieure d'Agriculture du Kef, Le Kef 7119, Tunisia*
[2] *INRA-Tunisie, Laboratoire des Productions Animales et Fourragères, Rue Hédi Karray, Ariana 2080, Tunisia*
[3] *Institut National Agronomique de Tunis, Tunis 2019, Tunisia*

Correspondence should be addressed to M. Mahouachi, mehouachi_mokhtar@hotmail.com

Academic Editor: Rouf M. Mian

The objective of this study was to determine the effect of spineless cactus incorporation in food of dairy goats and growing kids on milk production and composition and on kid's growth and meat characteristics. Two experiments were conducted on Tunisian local goats. In the first, 30 females were divided into two groups; goats of Control group were reared on grazing pasture receiving indoor 0.5 kg of hay and 0.4 kg of concentrate. Goats for the second group (Cac-FL) were kept in feedlot and fed cactus ad libitum more 0.5 kg of hay and 0.4 kg of concentrate. In the second experiment, 14 kids were divided into 2 groups receiving 600 g of hay. The Control group received ad libitum a concentrate containing 130 g crude protein (CP) per kg of dry matter. The second group received cactus ad-libitum plus the half concentrate quantity of control one with 260 g CP/kg DM (Cactus). The daily milk production averaged 485 ml for Control group and 407 ml for Cac-FL one. The milk fat content was significantly higher for Control than Cac-FL group. In the second experiment, animals in Control and Cactus groups had similar growth rate. Carcass fat was significantly lower in Cactus than in the Control group. Cactus in the diet was associated with more C18:2 and conjugated linoleic acid as well as a higher proportion of PUFA than Control ones.

1. Introduction

The arid and semiarid areas are characterized by limited food resources, and the production of green fodder is rare, particularly during the hot and dry season (summer) when the animals are strongly complemented by food concentrate [1]. To face these critical periods, the search for other natural resources is needed to better sustain the dairy production and the growth of the young animals and to preserve breeding continuity. In some arid regions, the spineless cactus or prickly peartree (*Opuntia ficus indica f. inermis*), which is useful for ground conservation and reduction of streaming, is widely cultivated and could be used as green fodder in all seasons. The digestibility of the ration and the growth of the lambs nourished with cactus were studied [2] whereas works on meat quality or dairy ewe and goat fed cactus are rare [3]. The objective of this work is to study the production and the composition of the nursing goat's milk eating cactus in comparison with the production on pasture of the natural range and its effects on kid's growth and meat characteristics.

2. Material and Methods

2.1. Animals and Feeding. Two experiments were conducted on Tunisian local goats (Maure breed). In the first experiment, 30 adult goats were divided into two groups according to the parity, the milk production with the first control, and the number of nursed kids. Goats for Control group were reared on grazing pasture during 6 hours per day and received indoor per head and day 0.5 kg of oat hay and 0.4 kg of concentrate (180 g crude protein (CP) per kg dry matter (DM)). Goats for the second group (Cac-FL) were kept in feedlot and fed spineless cactus ad libitum plus 0.5 kg of the same hay and 0.4 kg of the same concentrate. In the second experiment, 14 kids (17.4 kg live weight) and two kinds of concentrates were used. The concentrates C130 and C260 contained 130 and 260 g CP/kg DM, respectively. Animals were divided into 2 groups receiving 600 g of oat hay. The first group (Control) received 600 g of C130 concentrate, while the second group (Cactus) received cactus ad libitum plus 300 g of C260 concentrate. Animals were allowed 84 days in this trial and then were slaughtered.

2.2. Animal Performance Recording and Sampling. For the first experiment, the goats and kids were weighed weekly before eating. Dairy control was bi monthly. For this control and during the suckling phase, the kids were separated from their mothers during 8 hours; the goats were then milked and the quantity of milk obtained was multiplied by 3 to have the total daily milk production. For each control, an individual milk sample was reserved for the chemical analysis. For the second experiment, kids were weighed weekly before eating. After slaughter, carcasses were weighed then split into two halves. The left sides were separated into five joints, which were dissected into fat, muscles, and bones. Samples of the *longissimus dorsi* muscles were taken for chemical meat analysis.

2.3. Chemical Analysis. The individual milk samples were kept (4°C) and analyzed for milk fat (MF) and protein (MP) using a MilkoScan 4000 (FOSS ELECTRIC, Integrated Milk Testing). For chemical composition of the Muscle *longissimus dorsi*, DM was determined by lyophilisation, mineral content by ashing at 600°C for 8 h and Nitrogen by Kjeldahl method ($CP = N \times 6.25$). Meat lipids were calculated as DM minus the sum of protein and ash. The fatty acid composition of the intramuscular (i.m.) fat was analyzed after extraction and methylation with K-OH on chromatograph (HP-5890) equipped with a flame ionization detector and split (1 : 24) injector.

2.4. Statistical Analysis. Statistical analysis was performed by analysis of variance using the GLM procedure of SAS (1989). The effect of dietary treatment was analyzed on milk production and composition for the first experiment and on kid growth and carcass and meat quality for the second.

3. Results and Discussion

3.1. First Experiment

3.1.1. Milk Production. Daily milk production was not significantly affected by diet treatment (Table 1). The peak of lactation was observed towards the 4th week for Ca-FL group and the 6th week for the Control group. The increase in milk production was associated with a decrease in goats' weight underlining the mobilization of the body reserves. Then the production level dropped with a persistence coefficient of 0.85. The milk production level remained relatively low; the limited concentrate supply (maximum 400 g) with cactus or pasture in dry year may be the reason of this weak production, since the performances of the same herd are higher (600 to 800 ml/j) with other diets [1].

Table 1: Milk production and composition.

Parameter	Pasture	Cac-FL	stat
Daily milk production (mL)	485 ± 42	403 ± 43	ns
Fat content (%)	3.9 ± 0.17	3.7 ± 0.17	*
Protein content (%)	2.8 ± 0.09	2.8 ± 0.09	ns

* $P < 0.05$; ns: not significant ($P < 0.05$).

3.1.2. Chemical Milk Composition. The protein content had the same value during all the experimental period without significant difference between the experimental groups (Table 1). The evolution of the milk fat shows more fluctuations than that of protein. The milk fat rate was higher for pasture group than Cac-FL (Table 1), particularly at the end of the lactation. The variability of the grazed species would result in ingestion of plants rich in the most widespread fatty acids precursor in the goat's milk. The fat content increased considerably at the end of the lactation which corresponds to the period of milk production decrease confirming the negative correlation between the dairy production and the fat content rate [4, 5].

3.2. Second Experiment

3.2.1. Kid's Growth. The use of cactus, despite the reduction of concentrate, tends to improve the ADG from 35 g/day (Control) to 55 g/day (Cactus); this result is in relationship with the high energy and protein intake of groups fed cactus diets, which characterized by a high DM intake and digestibility. These results confirmed partially those of Negesse et al. [6] and Titi et al. [7] who observed a linear increase in weight gain for Saanen kids and Black goat kids, fed with higher levels of diet CP. These results showed clearly that cactus, largely used in arid and semiarid areas for rangeland rehabilitation, is also a potential cost-effective fodder for weaned kids in semiarid areas. However, the slight difference in growth rates among treatments would suggest that the nutritive value of diets was not the only limiting factor but reflects also the low potential growth rate of this local breed.

3.2.2. Carcass and Meat Composition. The results concerning slaughter BW, carcass weight, and importance of fat and muscle tissues were presented in Table 2. The muscle weight was similar for both groups. For this similar amount of muscle, the fat amount was 150% for Control group compared to Cactus one ($P < 0.001$). As proportions of carcass weight, there were significant effects ($P < 0.001$) of diet on muscle and fat values, carcasses of kids given cactus diet presented relatively less fat (105 g/kg) and more muscle (62 g/kg) than those fed control diet (135 g/kg fat and 58 g/kg muscle). It is necessary to point out that cactus supply decreased the fat tissue weight and proportion and increased muscle proportion in the carcass suggesting that carcasses of fed cactus goats were leaner than carcasses produced on grain diets, which confirmed other results [3]. Hence, cactus acts on carcass composition as a green forage confirming

Table 2: Slaughter BW, carcass weight, and importance of fat and muscle tissues for kids receiving cactus or conventional diets.

	Control	Cactus	stat
SBW, kg	21.2	21.4	ns
Cold carcass weight, kg	9.1	9.4	ns
Muscle, g	5109	5114	ns
Muscle, g/kg	570^a	622^b	***
Fat, g	1275^a	810^b	***
Fat, g/kg	142^a	101^b	***
Protein, g/kg DM	800	858	ns
Fat, g/kg DM	151	91	*

*** $P < 0.001$; * $P < 0.05$; ns: not significant ($P > 0.05$).

Table 3: Average fatty acid (FA) profile in meat fat of kids, g/kg.

Measurement	C130	C260-Cac	P
C16	188	196	ns
C16:1	27.0	23.5	ns
C18	140	175	ns
C18:1	547	504	ns
C18:2n-6	22.8	23.8	ns
C18:3n-3	1.5	1.8	ns
CLA (cis-9, trans-11)	1.5^A	2.2^A	***
C20:4	8.1	10.2	ns
EPA (C20:5n-3)	0.3	0.9	*
DPA (C22:5n-3)	0.17^A	1.7^B	***
SFA	366	400	ns
MUFA	588	539	ns
PUFA	37.2	44.4	ns

SFA: sum of saturated fatty acids: C14:0 + C15:0 + C16:0 + C17:0 + C18:0.
MUFA: sum of monounsaturated fatty acids: C14:1 + C16:1 + C17:1 + C18:1 + C20:1.
PUFA: sum of polyunsaturated fatty acids: C18:2 + C18:3 + CLA + C20:2 + C20:3 + C20:4 + EPA + DP.
*** $P < 0.001$; * $P < 0.05$; ns: not significant ($P > 0.05$).

other results where animals (steers, beef and lambs) raised on pasture displayed a greater proportion of muscle and a lower percentage of fat compared to concentrate fed animals [8–10].

Results of chemical characteristics determined on LD muscles were shown in Table 2. No significant differences were found for moisture, crude protein, and ash contents between treatment groups. The crude fat decreased from 151 to 91 g/kg DM for Control and Cactus groups, respectively. So, meat of kids fed on cactus was leaner than that of Control.

3.2.3. Fatty Acid Composition. Results obtained for proportions of i.m. fatty acid composition for both groups (Table 3) were in concordance with Banskalieva et al. [11] for other goat breeds, showing the prevalence of oleic (C18:1), palmitic (C16:0), stearic (C18:0), and linoleic (C18:2) FA, which accounted for about 910 g/kg of total fatty acids. However, CLA and DPA (C22:5n-3), healthy FA, were significantly higher ($P < 0.001$) in the Cactus group than Control one (Table 3). These results are in accordance with other reports, which compared fatty acid composition of grass-fed to concentrate-fed lambs [12], steers or cattle [10, 13], and goats [3]. There was no significant influence of feeding ($P > 0.05$) on the SFA, PUFA, and the PUFA/SFA ratio.

4. Conclusions

The cactus used as basic food, in addition to moderate quantity of concentrate, could generate a dairy production of the goats comparable or slightly lower than those of the animals led on rangeland in average years. Moreover, the surface reserved for the production of cactus represents only the tenth of that reserved for the pasture, which makes cactus a solution for the stockbreeders who do not have sufficient rangeland.

Kids reared by cactus feeding produce meat with enhanced nutritional quality for the consumer due to lower carcass adiposity, lower intramuscular fat content, and a higher accumulation of beneficial fatty acids, n-3 FA, and CLA.

Given the increasing cost of concentrates, raising kids under cactus regimen could be more economic than the conventional regimen.

References

[1] H. Rouissi, M. Mahouachi, and N. Atti, "Effet de la complémentation énergétique sur les performances de la chèvre locale au cours de la phase d'allaitement," *Annales de l'INRA*, vol. 75, pp. 223–239, 2002.

[2] A. Nefzaoui and H. Ben Salem, "Opuntia-A strategic fodder and efficient tool to combat desertification *In* the WANA region," in *Cactus (Opuntia ssp.) as Forage*, vol. 169, pp. 73–90, 2003.

[3] N. Atti, M. Mahouachi, and H. Rouissi, "The effect of spineless cactus (Opuntia ficus-indica f. inermis) supplementation on growth, carcass, meat quality and fatty acid composition of male goat kids," *Meat Science*, vol. 73, no. 2, pp. 229–235, 2006.

[4] T. T. El-Gallad, E. A. Gihad, S. M. Allam, and T. M. El-Bedawy, "Effect of energy intake and roughage ratio on the lactation of Egyptian Nubian (Zaraibi) goats," *Small Ruminant Research*, vol. 1, no. 4, pp. 327–341, 1988.

[5] C. D. Lu, M. J. Potchoiba, T. Sahlu, and J. M. Fernandez, "Performance of dairy goats fed isonitrogenous diets containing soybean meal or hydrolyzed feather meal during early lactation," *Small Ruminant Research*, vol. 3, no. 5, pp. 425–434, 1990.

[6] T. Negesse, M. Rodehutscord, and E. Pfeffer, "The effect of dietary crude protein level on intake, growth, protein retention and utilization of growing male Saanen kids," *Small Ruminant Research*, vol. 39, no. 3, pp. 243–251, 2001.

[7] H. H. Titi, M. J. Tabbaa, M. G. Amasheh, F. Barakeh, and B. Daqamseh, "Comparative performance of Awassi lambs and Black goat kids on different crude protein levels in Jordan," *Small Ruminant Research*, vol. 37, no. 1-2, pp. 131–135, 2000.

[8] I. B. Mandell, J. G. Buchanan-Smith, and C. P. Campbell, "Effects of forage vs grain feeding on carcass characteristics, fatty acid composition, and beef quality in limousin-cross steers when time on feed is controlled," *Journal of Animal Science*, vol. 76, no. 10, pp. 2619–2630, 1998.

[9] N. Atti and H. Abdouli, "Effets du niveau du concentré sur les performances bouchères des agneaux de race Barbarine conduits au pâturage ou en bergerie," *Annales INRAT*, vol. 73, pp. 151–163, 2001.

[10] K. Nuernberg, D. Dannenberger, G. Nuernberg et al., "Effect of a grass-based and a concentrate feeding system on meat quality characteristics and fatty acid composition of longissimus muscle in different cattle breeds," *Livestock Production Science*, vol. 94, no. 1-2, pp. 137–147, 2005.

[11] V. Banskalieva, T. Sahlu, and A. L. Goetsch, "Fatty acid composition of goat muscles and fat depots: a review," *Small Ruminant Research*, vol. 37, no. 3, pp. 255–268, 2000.

[12] G. Demirel, H. Ozpinar, B. Nazli, and O. Keser, "Fatty acids of lamb meat from two breeds fed different forage: concentrate ratio," *Meat Science*, vol. 72, no. 2, pp. 229–235, 2006.

[13] P. French, E. G. O'Riordan, F. J. Monahan et al., "Meat quality of steers finished on autumn grass, grass silage or concentrate-based diets," *Meat Science*, vol. 56, no. 2, pp. 173–180, 2000.

12

Effects of Aflatoxin on Some Haematological Parameters and Protective Effectiveness of Esterified Glucomannan in Merino Rams

Nurcan Dönmez,[1] H. H. Dönmez,[2] E. Keskin,[3] and İ. Kısadere[1]

[1] *Department of Physiology, Faculty of Veterinary Medicine, University of Kyrgyzstan-Turkey Manas, Bishkek 720044, Kyrgyzstan*
[2] *Department of Histology and Embryology, Faculty of Veterinary Medicine, University of Kyrgyzstan-Turkey Manas, Bishkek 720044, Kyrgyzstan*
[3] *Department of Physiology, Faculty of Veterinary Medicine, Selçuk University, 42075 Konya, Turkey*

Correspondence should be addressed to Nurcan Dönmez, nurcandonmez@selcuk.edu.tr

Academic Editor: Daiji Endoh

The objective of the present study was to evaluate the toxic effects of aflatoxin on some hematological parameters and to determine the preventive effectiveness of added glucomannan. In the study, 32 Merino rams were used, and the rams were separated equally to four groups as control (C), glucomannan (G), glucomannan + aflatoxin (AG), and aflatoxin (A). Erythrocyte, leukocyte count, hemoglobin, and hematocrit levels were decreased in A group compared with the other groups, and there was a reduction in similar parameters in AG group compared to control values. On the other hand, these parameters were tended to increase in AG group compared to A group values. Aflatoxicosis caused the lymphocytopenia and monocytopenia but increased percentage of neutrophil counts. In conclusion, the results determined in the study might be important to demonstrate the effects of aflatoxicosis and glucomannan on some haematological parameters before the clinical symptoms appear.

1. Introduction

One of the most important problems that occurs as a result of unconditioned storage of food and foodstuff is toxications caused by mycotoxins [1]. Mycotoxins are toxic metabolic by-products, which are produced by fungi. Naturally fungi on crops produce mycotoxins in the fields, during harvest and in storage. Contamination of food or feedstuffs and their consumption can result in mycotoxicosis. In these mycotoxins, aflatoxins are the mostly seen and aflatoxin B1 is the most harmful one [2, 3]. Synthesis of aflatoxins in feeds are increased at temperatures above 27°C (80 F), humidity levels greater than 62%, and moisture levels in the feed above 14% [4]. Consumption of aflatoxin-contaminated food by human and animals causes important health problems together with important economical losses. All animal species are susceptible to aflatoxicosis, but outbreaks occur mostly in pigs, sheep, and cattle. Beef and dairy cattle are more susceptible to aflatoxicosis than sheep or horses [5]. Aflatoxicosis causes several defects in organs and tissues, decrease in growth rate, increase in death rate, immunosuppression, anemia, and increase in coagulation time and deteriorates lipid, carbohydrate, and protein metabolism [1, 6].

As a result of toxic effect of aflatoxin, biochemical and hematological parameters have been reported to be changed importantly. In chronic and subclinical aflatoxicosis case, changes in biochemical and hematological parameters occur before clinical symptoms develop [7, 8]. Significant changes in serum biochemical and hematological parameters are seen in aflatoxicosis cases, and these can assist in the diagnosis of toxications [9, 10].

Removing AF from contaminated food and foodstuffs remains a major problem, and there is a great demand for effective decontamination technology. Decontamination procedures have focused on degrading, destroying, inactivating, or removing AF by physical, chemical, or biological

Table 1: Body weight of groups before and after experiment (n = 8).

Groups	Before experiment	After experiment
C	57.65 ± 0.94	80.93 ± 1.51
G	57.70 ± 1.18	81.96 ± 1.86
A	57.90 ± 0.87	75.69 ± 3.46
AG	57.85 ± 1.32	80.65 ± 1.17

methods [10, 11]. Use of adsorbents (silicates) or chemicals (ammonia, sodium bisulfate) or biological agents (Saccharomyces cerevisiae) in animal feeds has been shown to minimize the untoward effect of aflatoxin. Esterified glucomannan (EG) showed very high binding ability (80–97%) with AF [9, 12]. The studies performed with EG at different concentrations of AF showed that EG partially or completely reversed the effect of AF on performance, biochemistry, hematology, and immune response [6, 7, 13].

In the present study, the effects of aflatoxin on some hematological parameters were determined in ram fed feed containing aflatoxin. Furthermore, the effect of adding glucomannan, which is a known aflatoxin binder, on the negative effects of aflatoxin was studied, as well.

2. Materials and Methods

In the present study, 32 healthy Merino rams (3 years old) were used. The rams were divided into 4 equal groups. Body weight of groups were close to each other and given in Table 1 before and after experiment.

During the experiment (12 weeks), the rams received clean water continuously and were fed *ad libitum* as follows.

Group 1 (C): fed with the normal diet for rams.

Group 2 (A): fed with the food containing 250 μg/day aflatoxin.

Group 3 (G): fed with the food containing 2 g/day glucomannan.

Group 4 (AG): fed with the food containing 250 μg/day aflatoxin + 2 g/day glucomannan.

Aflatoxin and glucomannan were given to rams by mixing to 100 gr diet before morning feeding. When the rams finished the mixed diet, the rest feed was given.

At the end of the experiment, blood samples were collected into tubes with added anticoagulant. The red blood cell (RBC), white blood cell (WBC), hematocrit values, haemoglobin levels, and differential leukocyte counts were determined. The red blood cell (RBC) and white blood cell (WBC) were determined by haematocytometer; haemoglobin amounts were determined by commercial kit (Biosystem), and differential leukocyte counts were determined in blood smears [14].

Statistical differences among the groups were tested by analysis of variance (ANOVA) which is followed by Duncan's test using SPSS for windows version 16.0 [15]. Significants were considered as $P < 0.05$.

3. Results and Discussion

Results obtained from all groups were given in Tables 2 and 3.

Chronic aflatoxicosis may be diagnosed by determining serum biochemical and hematological alterations before clinical symptoms become apparent [11]. Even small amounts of AF are dangerous for animal health because of detrimental effect on some biochemical and hematological values [16].

In the present study, erythrocyte count, leukocyte count, hemoglobin, and hematocrit levels were decreased in A group compared with the other groups. But this reduction was significantly ($P < 0.05$) important in RBC, WBC, and hemoglobin in A group compared with control, and there was a reduction in similar parameters in AG group compared to control values. On the other hand, these parameters were tended to increase in AG group compared to A group values (Table 2).

Keçeci et al. [16] have reported that the hematocrit and hemoglobin levels, MCH, and thrombocyte counts were depressed and increased the sedimentation rate by AF in broilers, and Oğuz et al. [11] reported that decreased were hematocrit and hemoglobin levels, MCV, erythrocyte, thrombocyte, and lymphocyte counts. Furthermore, in another study, it has been reported that AF caused decrease in hematocrit and hemoglobin levels, MCV, erythrocyte, thrombocyte, and lymphocyte counts, and glucomannan (1 g/kg) depressed these negative effects of AF in broilers [9]. Our findings supported statement of above studies, and Yousef et al. [17] and Abdel-Wahhab et al. [2] have reported similar changes to our data.

Abdel-Wahhab et al. [2] have reported that decrease in hemoglobin concentration and total red blood cell counts resulting in normocytic normochromic anaemia in aflatoxin application alone. This decrease in the hematological parameters may be due to many factors such as inhibition of protein synthesis as evidenced by lower serum albumin [18], decrease of the total iron binding capacity [19], and the hemopoietic cellular defects of AF [2, 20].

Furthermore, broiler chicks given 2,5 mg AF/kg diet have shown not only decreased hemoglobin, and hematocrit values, thrombocyte counts, percentage of lymphocyte and basophil counts but also increased percentage of heterophils [21]. Again, the researchers reported that aflatoxicosis caused the lymphocytopenia and monocytopenia but increased the WBC and percentage of heterophil counts [2, 9, 11, 22]. This increase in WBC and percentage of heterophil counts suggest that the toxin elicited an inflammatory response. However, the decreases in the other percentage of leukocyte types may be related with relative reduction [1, 16]. There was significant increase ($P < 0.05$) in percentage of neutrophil and decrease in percentage of lymphocyte and monocyte counts in A group compared to control in this study (Table 3).

The using of agents that act as antidotes or antagonize the effects of toxic substances such as AF has therapeutic and economic importance. The major advantages of these absorbents include expense, safety, and easy administration

Table 2: Effects of AF and glucomannan on some haematological parameters ($n = 8$, X ± SX).

Parameters	C	G	A	AG
Erythrocyte ($\times 10^6/mm^3$)	11.32 ± 2.86^a	11.10 ± 3.15^a	9.42 ± 3.60^b	10.90 ± 2.87^a
Leukocyte ($\times 10^3/mm^3$)	10.87 ± 6.01^a	10.40 ± 6.42^a	8.01 ± 7.09^b	9.38 ± 4.91^{ab}
Haematocrit (%)	29.62 ± 1.33	29.50 ± 1.73	25.50 ± 0.86	28.25 ± 1.68
Haemoglobin (gr/dL)	11.87 ± 0.21^a	11.58 ± 0.54^{ab}	9.58 ± 0.40^c	10.62 ± 0.25^{bc}

$^{a,b,c}P < 0.05$.

Table 3: Effects of AF and glucomannan on differential leukocyte counts ($n = 8$, X ± SX).

	C	G	A	AG
Neutrophile	33.0 ± 1.47^b	31.63 ± 1.03^b	40.63 ± 2.21^a	34.75 ± 2.16^b
Lymphocyte	63.13 ± 1.20^a	64.25 ± 0.99^a	57.50 ± 2.18^b	62.12 ± 2.20^{ab}
Monocyte	2.12 ± 0.35^a	1.87 ± 0.58^a	0.63 ± 0.26^b	1.75 ± 0.36^{ab}
Eosinophil	1.25 ± 0.31	1.75 ± 0.36	0.87 ± 0.29	1.00 ± 0.26
Basophile	0.50 ± 0.18	0.50 ± 0.18	0.37 ± 0.18	0.38 ± 0.18

$^{a,b}P < 0.05$.

through addition to foods [11], and glucomannan was selected for use in the present study. We considered that toxin absorption from the gastrointestinal tract can be prevented by formation of complex with AF. In the study, there were no significant differences in hematological parameters compared to control group (Tables 2 and 3).

In conclusion, AG group's levels being between G and A groups have showed that glucomannan at this level has moderate counteracts to this aflatoxin dosage in respect of these parameters. Thus, it needs the other studies in different aflatoxin and glucomannan levels. As a result, findings presented in this study contribute to the overall literature, and also chronic intoxications can be diagnosed before clinical signs occurrence. The effectiveness of glucomannan at this dose is believed to be important.

Acknowledgment

This study was supported by TUBITAK (Project no. 107O866).

References

[1] I. Çelik, H. Oguz, Ö. Demet et al., "Embryotoxicity assay of aflatoxin produced by Aspergillus parasiticus NRRL 2999," *British Poultry Science*, vol. 41, no. 4, pp. 401–409, 2000.

[2] M. A. Abdel-Wahhab, S. A. Nada, and F. A. Khalil, "Physiological and toxicological responses in rats fed aflatoxin-contaminated diet with or without sorbent materials," *Animal Feed Science and Technology*, vol. 97, no. 3-4, pp. 209–219, 2002.

[3] G. Eraslan, B. C. Liman, B. K. Güçlü, A.N. Atasever Koç, and L. Beyaz, "Evaluation of aflatoxin toxicity in Japanes quails given various doses of hidrated sodium calcium aluminosilicate," *Bulletin of the Veterinary Institute in Pulawy*, vol. 48, pp. 511–517, 2004.

[4] J. B. Royes and R. P. Yanong, *Molds in Fish Feeds and Aflatoxicosis*, University of Florida, Institute of Agricultural Sciences (UF/ IFAS), 2002.

[5] O. M. Rasostits, C. C. Gay, D. C. Blood, and K. W. Hinchcliff, *Veterinary Medicine*, W. B. Saunders Co., London, UK, 2000.

[6] M. V. L. N. Raju and G. Devegowda, "Influence of esterified-glucomannan on performance and organ morphology, serum biochemistry and haematology in broilers exposed to individual and combined mycotoxicosis (aflatoxin, ochratoxin and T-2 toxin)," *British Poultry Science*, vol. 41, no. 5, pp. 640–650, 2000.

[7] K. L. Arawind, V. S. Patil, G. Devegowda, B. Umakantha, and S. P. Ganpule, "Efficiacy of esterified glucomannan to counteract mycotoxicosis in naturally contaminated feed on performance and serum biochemical, haematological parameters in broilers," *Poultry Science*, vol. 82, pp. 571–576, 2003.

[8] N. Dönmez and E. Keskin, "The effects of aflatoxin and glucomannan on some antioxidants and biochemical parameters in rabbits," *Acta Veterinaria*, vol. 58, no. 4, pp. 308–313, 2008.

[9] H. Basmacioglu, H. Oguz, M. Ergul, R. Çöl, and Y. O. Birdane, "Effect of dietary esterified glucomannan on performance, serum biochemistry and haematology in broilers exposed to aflatoxin," *Czech Journal of Animal Science*, vol. 50, no. 1, pp. 31–39, 2005.

[10] N. Dönmez and E. Keskin, "The effects of aflatoxin and glucomannan on coagulation parameters in rabbits," *Veterinarski Arhiv*, vol. 79, no. 6, pp. 555–560, 2009.

[11] H. Oğuz, T. Keçeci, Y. O. Birdane, F. Önder, and V. Kurtoğlu, "Effect of clinoptilolite on serum biochemical and haematological characters of broiler chickens during aflatoxicosis," *Research in Veterinary Science*, vol. 69, no. 1, pp. 89–93, 2000.

[12] D. E. Diaz, W. M. Hagler, B. A. Hopkins, and L. W. Whitlow, "Aflatoxin binders I: in vitro binding assay for aflatoxin B1 by several potential sequestering agents," *Mycopathologia*, vol. 156, no. 3, pp. 223–226, 2002.

[13] E. Santin, A. C. Paulillo, A. Maiorka et al., "Evaluation of the efficacy of saccharomyces cerevisiae cell wall to ameliorate the toxic effects of aflatoxin in broilers," *International Journal of Poultry Science*, vol. 2, pp. 341–344, 2003.

[14] B. Yilmaz, *Fizyoloji*, Feryal Matbaacılık, Ankara, Turkey, 2nd edition, 2000.

[15] SPSS 16.0., SPSS Inc., 2007.

[16] T. Keçeci, H. Oguz, V. Kurtoglu, and Ö. Demet, "Effects of polyvinylpolyprolidone, synthetic zeolite and bentonite on serum biochemical and haematological characters of broiler

chickens during aflatoxicosis," *British Poultry Science*, vol. 39, pp. 452–458, 1998.

[17] M. I. Yousef, M. H. Salem, K. I. Kamel, G. A. Hassan, and F. D. El-Nouty, "Influence of ascorbic acid supplementation on the haematological and clinical biochemistry parameters of male rabbits exposed to aflatoxin B1," *Journal of Environmental Science and Health B*, vol. 38, no. 2, pp. 193–209, 2003.

[18] J. J. Kaneko, *Clinical Chemistry of Domestic Animals*, Academic Press, San Diego, Calif, USA, 4th edition, 1989.

[19] R. B. Harvey, L. F. Kubera, T. D. Phillips, D. E. Cornier, M. H. Ellisade, and W. E. Huff, "Dimunition of aflatoxin toxicity to growing lambs by dietary supplementation with HSCAS," *American Journal of Veterinary Research*, vol. 52, pp. 152–156, 1991.

[20] J. F. van Vleet and V. J. Ferrans, "Etiologic factors and pathologic alterations in selenium-vitamin E deficiency and excess in animals and humans," *Biological Trace Element Research*, vol. 33, no. 1, pp. 1–21, 1992.

[21] T. Keçeci, Ö. Demet, and H. Oguz, "Single and combination effects of dietary aflatoxin and adsorbent (Mycofix Plus) on some hematological and serum biochemical parameters of broiler chickens," *Journal of Veterinary Science*, vol. 11, pp. 95–101, 1995.

[22] I. Çelik, H. Oguz, Ö. Demet, H. H. Dönmez, M. Boydak, and E. Sur, "Efficacy of polyvinylpolypyrrolidone in reducing the immunotoxicity of aflatoxin in growing broilers," *British Poultry Science*, vol. 41, no. 4, pp. 430–439, 2000.

13

Effects of Elevated Ambient Temperature on Reproductive Outcomes and Offspring Growth Depend on Exposure Time

Huda Yahia Hamid,[1,2] Md Zuki Abu Bakar Zakaria,[2] Goh Yong Meng,[2] Abd. Wahid Haron,[3] and Noordin Mohamed Mustapha[4]

[1] *Department of Anatomy, Faculty of Veterinary Medicine, University of Khartoum, Khartoum 13314, Sudan*
[2] *Department of Veterinary Preclinical Sciences, Faculty of Veterinary Medicine, Universiti Putra Malaysia, Selangor, 43400 Serdang, Malaysia*
[3] *Department of Veterinary Clinical Studies, Faculty of Veterinary Medicine, Universiti Putra Malaysia, Selangor, 43400 Serdang, Malaysia*
[4] *Department of Veterinary Pathology & Microbiology, Faculty of Veterinary Medicine, Universiti Putra Malaysia, Selangor, 43400 Serdang, Malaysia*

Correspondence should be addressed to Md Zuki Abu Bakar Zakaria, zuki@vet.upm.edu.my

Academic Editors: L. H. Baumgard, M. S. Cupp, and J. L. Dunn

Reproductive performance has been shown to be greatly affected by changes in environmental factors, such as temperature. However, it is also crucial to identify the particular stage of pregnancy that is most adversely affected by elevated ambient temperature. The aims of this study were to determine the effect on reproductive outcomes of exposure to elevated ambient temperature during different stages of pregnancy and to determine the effect of prenatal heat stress on offspring growth. Sixty pregnant rats were used in this study. The rats were divided equally into four groups as group 1 (control), group 2 (exposed to elevated temperature following implantation), group 3 (exposed to elevated temperature during pre- and periimplantation), and group 4 (exposed to elevated temperature during pre- and periimplantation and following implantation). Groups 3 and 4 had prolonged gestation periods, reduced litter sizes, and male-biased sex ratios. Moreover, the growth patterns of group 3 and 4 pups were adversely affected by prenatal exposure to elevated temperature. The differences between group 1 and group 3 and between group 1 and group 4 were highly significant. However, no significant differences were observed between groups 1 and 2 in the gestation length, sex ratios, and growth patterns. Thus, it can be concluded that exposure to elevated ambient temperature during pre- and periimplantation has stronger adverse effects on reproductive outcomes and offspring growth than postimplantation exposure.

1. Introduction

Reproductive performance has been shown to be greatly affected by changes in environmental factors, such as temperature. The most economically important reproductive performance traits of farm animals may be endangered by high environmental temperature [1]. In tropical countries and in summer of temperate countries, the reproductive performance of dairy cattle is low [2, 3]. Bloemhof et al. [1] observed that the pregnancy outcomes of sow decrease in the hot weather. Furthermore, the reproductive efficiency of Holstein cows is lower in autumn than in winter, suggesting a late effect of high temperature during the summer [4]. Both male and female reproductive processes are sensitive to high temperature. High environmental temperature has adverse effect on spermatogenesis and oocyte development and maturation [5, 6]. Fortunately, the reduced quality of the sperm and ova during the hot season has been overcome to some extent by artificial insemination (AI) and embryo transfer techniques [6]. However, overcoming the problems resulting from exposure to elevated ambient temperatures during pregnancy is more complicated. Ealy et al. [7] reported that exposure to elevated temperatures at day 1 of pregnancy in cow compromises early embryonic

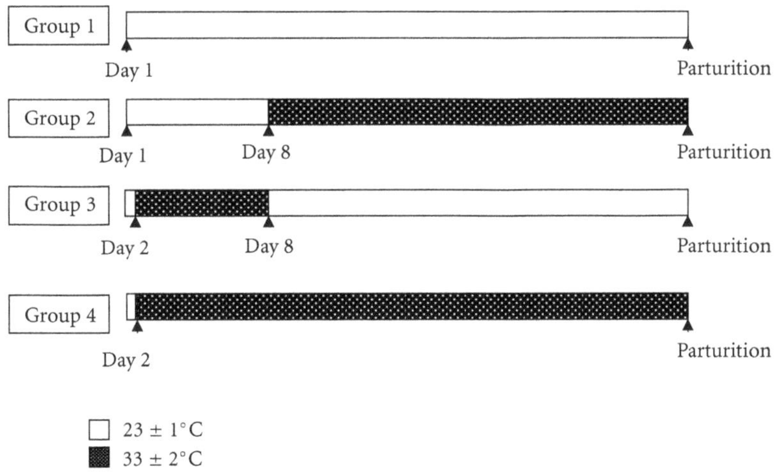

FIGURE 1: Schematic illustration of pregnancy period and time of exposure to elevated temperatures in the four groups.

development. In mice, several studies have shown that exposure to elevated temperatures for 12 h soon after mating disturbs normal embryonic development [8–11]. On the other hand, exposure of pregnant ewes to high temperatures during midgestation causes reduced foetal weights [12].

The recent climate changes and global warming have led to renewed interest in the study of the effects of exposure to elevated ambient temperatures on pregnancy outcomes and offspring growth with special attention to the time of exposure that leads to more deleterious effects on pregnancy outcomes. Determining the pregnancy stage that is most sensitive to heat exposure will assist in the design of environmental modification systems that provide an optimal temperature at critical period of pregnancy to improve the pregnancy rates and outcomes in hot climates. Therefore, the current study was intended to determine the effects of exposure to elevated ambient temperature during different pregnancy stages on reproductive outcomes and offspring growth and to determine the stage of pregnancy that is most sensitive to elevated temperature.

2. Materials and Methods

2.1. Animals. Sixty virgin female Sprague Dawley rats were used in this study. These in-house bred rats were 2-3 months old and weighed 200–220 g. The animals were maintained under a controlled lighting regime of 12 hours light and 12 hours dark; the lights were turned on at 0700 h and off at 1900 h. The rats were maintained under a temperature of 23 ± 1°C and relative humidity of 55–65%. The rats were allowed free access to chow and water. The animal care and handling throughout the study were approved by the Animal Care and Use Committee of the Faculty of Veterinary Medicine, Universiti Putra Malaysia, Malaysia.

Only females that showed at least two consecutive, regular four-day estrous cycles immediately before the study were used. Proestrus females were caged overnight with a male from the same strain with an age of 4-5 months, a weight of 400–500 g, and proven fertility. The presence of spermatozoa in a vaginal smear performed the next morning was used to detect successful copulation, and that day was designated as day 1 of the pregnancy.

2.2. Experimental Design. Parental influence was controlled by mating each male with four littermate females. On pregnancy day 1, each rat was randomly assigned to one of the following groups.

In group 1 (control, $n = 15$), the rats were maintained under optimal temperature (23 ± 1°C) from pregnancy day 1 until parturition.

In group 2 ($n = 15$), the rats were kept under optimal temperature (23 ± 1°C) during pre- and periimplantation, and, on day 8, they were transferred to a room without an air conditioner or fan and remained there until parturition. The temperature in the room was 33 ± 2°C, and the relative humidity was 80–86%.

In group 3 ($n = 15$), the rats were subjected to the elevated temperatures (33 ± 2°C) during pre- and periimplantation (from day 2 to day 7), and, on day 8, they were transferred to optimal conditions and remained there until parturition.

In group 4 ($n = 15$), the rats were maintained under elevated temperatures (33 ± 2°C) from day 2 of pregnancy until parturition.

After parturition, dams of groups 2 and 4 and their pups were returned to the room with optimal temperature (23 ± 1°C) and maintained there until the end of the study. The schematic illustration of experimental design is shown in Figure 1.

The length of gestation, litter sizes, neonatal deaths, sex ratios (male proportions), and body weights were recorded and compared among the four groups.

The body weight was measured immediately after birth and at one week, two weeks, and three weeks. Litters ($n = 6$) were culled to eight pups, with sex distribution kept as equal as possible in each litter. The mean weight of the male and female pups of each dam was recorded separately.

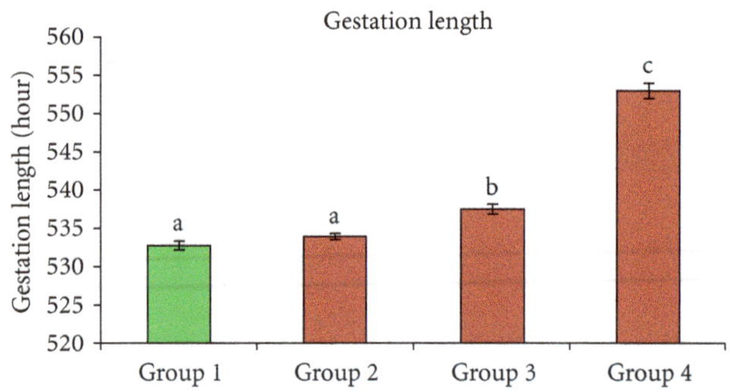

Figure 2: The gestation lengths of the control group (group 1) and groups exposed to elevated ambient temperature. The bars represent the mean ± SEM. Data labeled with different letters are significantly different at $P < 0.001$.

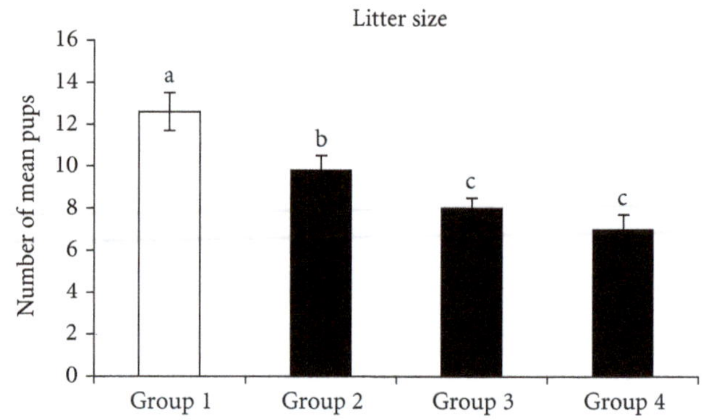

Figure 3: The litter sizes produced by the females of the control group (group 1) and groups exposed to elevated ambient temperature. The bars represent the mean ± SEM. Data labeled with different letters are significantly different at $P < 0.05$.

2.3. Statistical Analysis. The gestational length, litter size, and sex ratio in the different groups were compared using a one-way analysis of variance (ANOVA). The weights of the four groups' pups were compared using repeated measures ANOVA. Tukey's test was used for post hoc analyses. The statistical analysis was carried out using the PASW statistics 18 package (SPSS Inc., Chicago, IL, USA) with the significance level at $P < 0.05$. All the data are presented as the mean ± SEM.

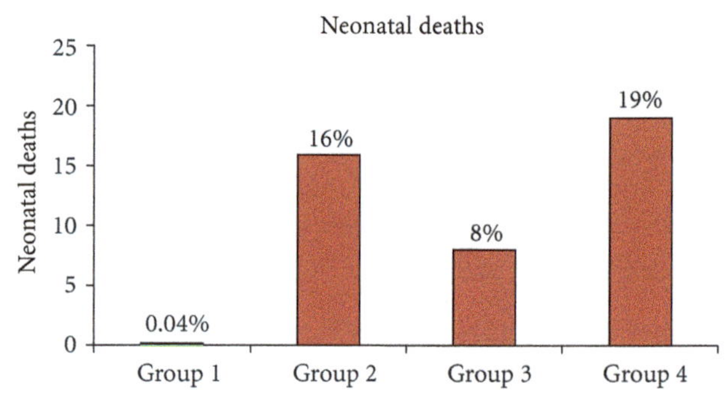

Figure 4: The percentages of neonatal deaths in the control group and in the three groups exposed to elevated temperature.

3. Results

3.1. Gestation Length and Time of Birth. Gestation length and time of birth were adversely affected by exposure to elevated temperatures. The longest gestation length was recorded in group 4. There was a significant increase ($P < 0.001$) in the gestation length of group 4 when compared with that of the control group (Figure 2). No significant difference was found between group 2 and the control group ($P > 0.05$), while group 3 had a significantly longer gestation length than the control group ($P = 0.001$) and group 2 ($P < 0.01$).

All of the females in the control group gave birth on day 23 of pregnancy before 11:00 h. In group 2, 87% of the females gave birth on day 23 before 11:00 h and the rest (13%) gave birth from 12:00 h to 13:30 h. The group 3 females gave birth later on day 23 of pregnancy, with 80% of the births occurring from 15:00 h to 18:00 h and 20% of births occurring from 12:00 h to 14:00 h. In group 4, the births occurred on day 24 of pregnancy, with 93% of the females giving birth in the early morning and 7% giving birth from 11:00 h to 12:00 h.

3.2. Litter Size. Results of litter sizes are shown in Figure 3. The largest litter size was recorded in the control group, while the smallest was found in group 4; the difference between the two was highly significant ($P < 0.001$). The litter size in group 2 was significantly smaller than that in the control group ($P < 0.05$), and group 3 showed a dramatic decrease in litter size compared with the control group ($P = 0.002$). However, no significant difference was observed between the litter sizes of group 3 and group 4 ($P > 0.05$) (Figure 3).

3.3. Neonatal Death. Neonatal deaths in all groups occurred within 24 h after parturition, mostly in the first 6 h. Neonatal death was increased in the groups exposed to elevated ambient temperatures (groups 2, 3, and 4) compared with the control group (Figure 4). The highest proportion of neonatal deaths was recorded in groups 2 and 4, while the lowest proportion was recorded in the control group.

3.4. Sex Ratio. More males were produced by the females of groups exposed to elevated ambient temperatures than those of the control group (Figure 5). Low and modest sex ratios were recorded in group 1 and group 2, respectively. The females in group 1 (control) produced offspring with 41% sex ratio, while the females in group 2 produced offspring with 49% sex ratio. By contrast, the sex ratios in group 3 and group 4 were biased toward males. The females in group 3 produced offspring with 57% sex ratio ($P < 0.001$), and the highest sex ratio was produced by the females in group 4, which delivered a significantly larger number of males (63%) than those of both group 1 ($P < 0.001$) and group 2 ($P < 0.01$). However, the sex ratios in groups 3 and 4 did not differ significantly ($P > 0.05$). Similarly, the sex ratios in group 1 (control) and group 2 were not significantly different ($P > 0.05$).

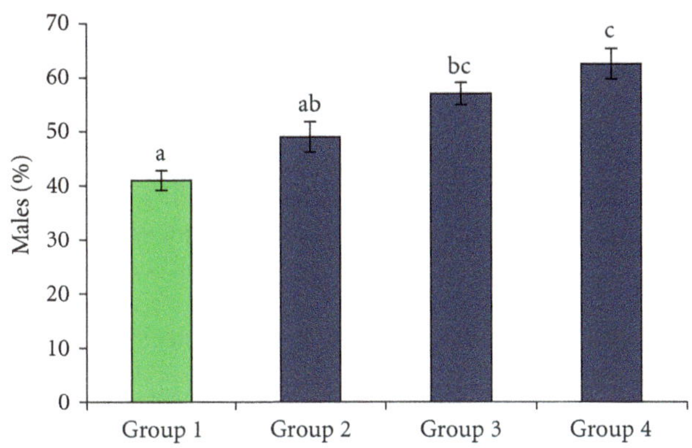

FIGURE 5: The percentages of males produced in the control group and in the three groups exposed to elevated temperature. Data represent the mean ± SEM. Data labeled with different letters are significantly different at $P < 0.01$.

3.5. Growth Patterns. The growth curves of the four groups are shown in Figure 6. No significant birth weight differences were observed between groups 1 and 3 and between groups 2 and 4 ($P > 0.05$). However, the group 2 pups showed significantly low birth weight compared with group 3 pups ($P < 0.001$).

The growth curves (Figures 6(a) and 6(b)) for both the male and female pups in group 1 (control) were significantly different from those of group 3 ($P < 0.01$) and group 4 ($P < 0.001$). No significant differences were observed between group 1 (control) and group 2 in the growth patterns of either the male or female pups ($P > 0.05$).

Surprisingly, the growth patterns of the group 3 and group 4 pups did not differ for either the males or females ($P > 0.05$). The growth pattern of the group 2 pups was significantly different from that of the group 3 pups ($P < 0.01$ for both males and females) and group 4 pups ($P < 0.001$ for both males and females).

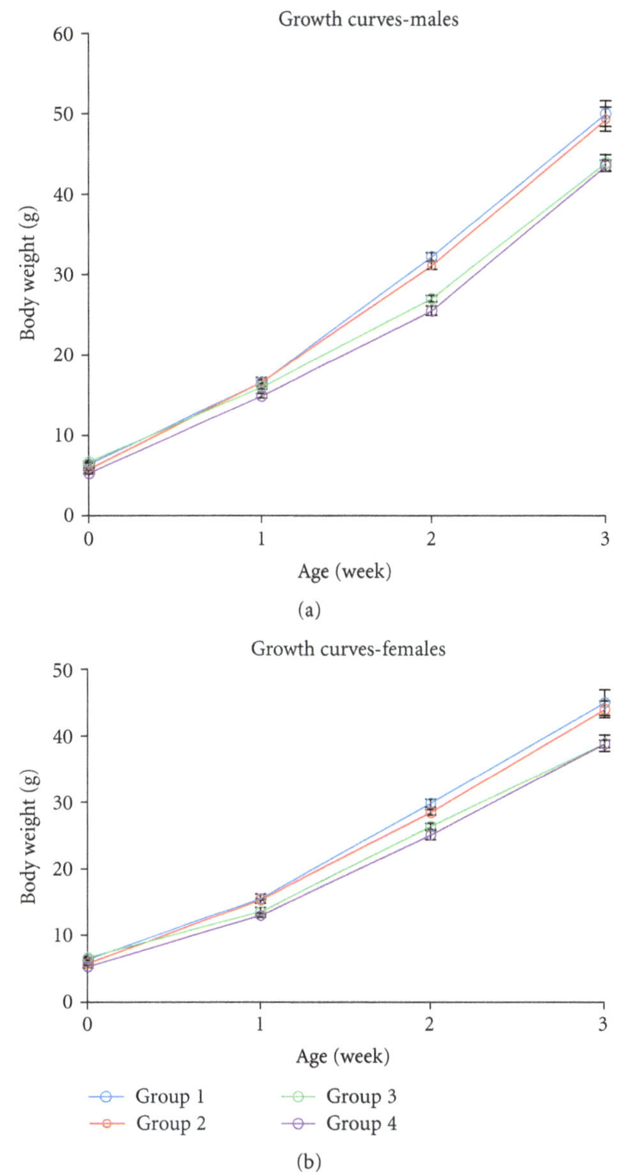

FIGURE 6: The growth curves for the male (a) and female (b) pups of the control group and the three groups exposed to elevated temperature from birth until weaning. Data represent the mean ± SEM.

4. Discussion

Maternal and paternal traits are strongly related to reproductive and productive efficiency. To control for parental factors, therefore, all of the rats used in this study were bred in our laboratory, and each of four littermate females were mated with the same male before being randomly assigned to one of the four groups.

In mammals, gestation can be lengthened by delayed fertilization (sperm storage), delayed implantation (embryonic diapause), or delayed development [13]. In this study, an increase in gestation length was observed in groups 3 and 4. In group 3, the prolonged gestation period may have been due to an implantation delay because our previous study has shown that exposure to elevated temperatures during pre- and periimplantation can delay the implantation in rats [14]. Furthermore, the increased gestation time in group 4 may have been due to both delayed implantation and delayed development. This possibility is supported by a previous finding [13] that the fetal development may become slower in response to environmental cues, such as temperature. However, the gestation length of the group 2 rats was not significantly affected by the exposure to elevated temperatures during the developmental stages. This result suggests that rat embryos that undergo a delay in implantation are more susceptible to developmental delays than are normally implanted embryos.

Elevated ambient temperature during pregnancy decreased the litter size in all of the groups, but it appears that the harmful effect strongly depended on in which stage of pregnancy the exposure occurred. Although the litter sizes of the three groups exposed to elevated temperature were reduced, the litter size of group 2 would still be considered large (mean = 9.8), suggesting that exposure to elevated temperature following implantation may not have a severe effect on litter size. By contrast, exposure to elevated temperature during pre- and periimplantation resulted in reduced litter size, as was noted in groups 3 and 4. Reduced litter size is likely a consequence of early embryonic loss because elevated temperature compromises embryonic survival during the developmental stages prior to the morula stage [15] and can severely decrease the implantation rates [14]. The lack of a significant difference between the litter sizes of groups 3 and 4 indicates that preimplantation exposure to elevated temperature may reduce litter size more strongly than postimplantation exposure. Nevertheless, fetal loss during the postimplantation period was demonstrated by the variation between the litter sizes of groups 1 and 2.

Because the risk of neonatal death increases exponentially as birth weight decreases [16], the mortality of the neonatal rats in the exposed groups may be related to their low birth weights, with the highest rates of mortality being found among the group 2 and 4 pups. The high neonatal death rates in groups 2 and 4 confirm that the most detrimental effect of elevated ambient temperature on pup survival occurred when the pregnant rats were exposed to elevated temperature during the period from implantation to birth. In group 3, neonatal mortality among normal birth weight pups may be related to prolonged gestation period [17]. Therefore, the highest mortality rate in group 4 may have been due to both low birth weights and prolonged gestation.

In this study, more males were produced by the three groups exposed to elevated ambient temperature. Skewed sex ratios have been a topic of great interest for more than a century. Many studies have been conducted to identify the causes associated with variations in sex ratios within and between populations. The causes of such changes are difficult to identify, although numerous demographic and environmental factors have been shown to be related to skewed sex ratios. These factors include maternal psychological stress, maternal diet, latitude, ambient temperature, and season [18–24]; however, the results concerning temperature are conflicting.

Our finding of a male-skewed sex ratio following exposure to elevated temperature supports previous reports suggesting that a warm climate may increase sex ratios [19–21]. However, Navara [22] has reported that in countries at tropical latitudes, which have the highest average ambient temperatures, the sex ratios are lower than in countries at temperate and subarctic latitudes.

Variations in the sex ratio at birth are assumed to result from sex-biased fetal mortality [25], and increased mortality of the female fetuses in utero appears to have been responsible for the sex ratio bias toward males in this study. Although group 2 had a somewhat lower sex ratio, the proportion of males produced was still higher than in the control group. At the same time, the group 3 and 4 sex ratios were markedly biased toward males. The decrease in the proportion of females and reduced litter size in group 2 relative to the control group indicates that female fetuses were lost in the period between implantation and parturition because of exposure to elevated temperature.

It is clear that elevated ambient temperature can effectively increase the proportion of males, particularly if the exposure occurs during early pregnancy. The sex ratios in groups 2 and 3 confirm the findings of Evdokimova et al. [26], who observed that embryos aborted during the early stages of development are biased toward females (31% males), in contrast to late abortions (77% males).

The pups from groups 2 and 4 exhibited low birth weights. Surprisingly, the birth weight of pups from group 3 was not affected by prenatal heat exposure. The reduced birth weights of the group 2 and 4 pups may have been due to exposure to elevated ambient temperature during the developmental stages, which may have impaired the fetal growth [27].

In this study, no growth differences were observed between the pups of control and those of group 2 or between the pups of group 3 and those of group 4. The similarity in the growth patterns of the group 1 (control) and group 2 pups, regardless of their weight at birth, indicates the great importance of environmental conditions during early pregnancy for postnatal growth, at least in rats. This finding is confirmed by the similarity of the growth curves for the group 3 and 4 pups.

No differences were observed between the male and female growth patterns in any of the groups; this result indicates that the implications of exposure to elevated ambient temperature have no relationship with the sex.

In conclusion, elevated environmental temperature adversely affects reproductive performance. Exposure to elevated ambient temperature can lead to prolonged gestation time. This finding should be considered when making inferences about pregnancy due dates in the tropics and other regions with hot weather. Additionally, ambient temperature affects litter size, sex ratio, and the body weight. Exposure to elevated temperature during the early stages of pregnancy (the pre- and periimplantation stages) has stronger adverse effects on pregnancy outcomes and offspring growth than does exposure during the mid and late stages of pregnancy.

Acknowledgment

This work was supported by the Fundamental Research Grant Scheme (FRGS; no.01-11-08652FR), Malaysia.

References

[1] S. Bloemhof, E. H. van der Waaij, J. W. M. Merks, and E. F. Knol, "Sow line differences in heat stress tolerance expressed in reproductive performance traits," *Journal of Animal Science*, vol. 86, no. 12, pp. 3330–3337, 2008.

[2] E. R. Jordan, "Effects of heat stress on reproduction," *Journal of Dairy Science*, vol. 86, supplement 1, pp. E104–E114, 2003.

[3] B. Kornmatitsuk, P. Chantaraprateep, S. Kornmatitsuk, and H. Kindahl, "Different types of postpartum luteal activity affected by the exposure of heat stress and subsequent reproductive performance in holstein lactating cows," *Reproduction in Domestic Animals*, vol. 43, no. 5, pp. 515–519, 2008.

[4] D. Wolfenson, Z. Roth, and R. Meidan, "Impaired reproduction in heat-stressed cattle: basic and applied aspects," *Animal Reproduction Science*, vol. 60-61, pp. 535–547, 2000.

[5] P. J. Hansen, "Effects of heat stress on mammalian reproduction," *Philosophical Transactions of the Royal Society B*, vol. 364, no. 1534, pp. 3341–3350, 2009.
[6] P. J. Hansen, M. Drost, R. M. Rivera et al., "Adverse impact of heat stress on embryo production: causes and strategies for mitigation," *Theriogenology*, vol. 55, no. 1, pp. 91–103, 2001.
[7] A. D. Ealy, M. Drost, and P. J. Hansen, "Developmental changes in embryonic resistance to adverse effects of maternal heat stress in cows," *Journal of Dairy Science*, vol. 76, no. 10, pp. 2899–2905, 1993.
[8] M. Ozawa, M. Hirabayashi, and Y. Kanai, "Developmental competence and oxidative state of mouse zygotes heat-stressed maternally or in vitro," *Reproduction*, vol. 124, no. 5, pp. 683–689, 2002.
[9] M. Ozawa, Y. Yamasaki, M. Hirabayashi, and Y. Kanai, "Viability of maternally heat-stressed mouse zygotes in vivo and in vitro," *Animal Science Journal*, vol. 74, no. 3, pp. 181–185, 2003.
[10] T. Matsuzuka, M. Ozawa, A. Nakamura, A. Ushitani, M. Hirabayashi, and Y. Kanai, "Effects of heat stress on the redox status in the oviduct and early embryonic development in mice," *Journal of Reproduction and Development*, vol. 51, no. 2, pp. 281–287, 2005.
[11] N. Sakamoto, M. Ozawa, K. Yokotani-Tomita et al., "DL-α-tocopherol acetate mitigates maternal hyperthermia-induced pre-implantation embryonic death accompanied by a reduction of physiological oxidative stress in mice," *Reproduction*, vol. 135, no. 4, pp. 489–496, 2008.
[12] J. M. Wallace, T. R. H. Regnault, S. W. Limesand, W. W. Hay Jr., and R. V. Anthony, "Investigating the causes of low birth weight in contrasting ovine paradigms," *Journal of Physiology*, vol. 565, no. 1, pp. 19–26, 2005.
[13] M. B. Renfree and G. Shaw, "Diapause," *Annual Review of Physiology*, vol. 62, pp. 353–375, 2000.
[14] H. Y. Hamid, A. B. Z. Zuki, N. Yimer, A. W. Haron, M. M. Noordin, and Y. M. Goh, "Effects of elevated ambient temperature on embryo implantation in rats," *African Journal of Biotechnology*, vol. 11, no. 24, pp. 6624–6632, 2012.
[15] L. Hui-Hui, T. Wen-Ru, Z. Zhi-Hong, Z. Qi-Yao, and G. Shan-Song, "Oxidative damage of heat-stressed mouse oocytes and preimplantation embryos and their environments," *Scientia Agricultura Sinica*, vol. 42, pp. 2244–2249, 2009.
[16] K. P. Stillerman, D. R. Mattison, L. C. Giudice, and T. J. Woodruff, "Environmental exposures and adverse pregnancy outcomes: a review of the science," *Reproductive Sciences*, vol. 15, no. 7, pp. 631–650, 2008.
[17] T. A. Bruckner, Y. W. Cheng, and A. B. Caughey, "Increased neonatal mortality among normal-weight births beyond 41 weeks of gestation in California," *American Journal of Obstetrics and Gynecology*, vol. 199, no. 4, pp. 421.e1–421.e7, 2008.
[18] A. Lerchl, "Seasonality of sex ratio in Germany," *Human Reproduction*, vol. 13, no. 5, pp. 1401–1402, 1998.
[19] A. Lerchl, "Sex ratios at birth and environmental temperatures," *Naturwissenschaften*, vol. 86, no. 7, pp. 340–342, 1999.
[20] R. Catalano, T. Bruckner, and K. R. Smith, "Ambient temperature predicts sex ratios and male longevity," *Proceedings of the National Academy of Sciences of the United States of America*, vol. 105, no. 6, pp. 2244–2247, 2008.
[21] S. Helle, S. Helama, and J. Jokela, "Temperature-related birth sex ratio bias in historical Sami: warm years bring more sons," *Biology Letters*, vol. 4, no. 1, pp. 60–62, 2008.
[22] K. J. Navara, "Humans at tropical latitudes produce more females," *Biology Letters*, vol. 5, no. 4, pp. 524–527, 2009.
[23] K. E. Ruckstuhl, G. P. Colijn, V. Amiot, and E. Vinish, "Mother's occupation and sex ratio at birth," *BMC Public Health*, vol. 10, article 269, 2010.
[24] C. S. Rosenfeld, "Periconceptional influences on offspring sex ratio and placental responses," *Reproduction, Fertility and Development*, vol. 24, no. 1, pp. 45–48, 2012.
[25] C. S. Rosenfeld and R. M. Roberts, "Maternal diet and other factors affecting offspring sex ratio: a review," *Biology of Reproduction*, vol. 71, no. 4, pp. 1063–1070, 2004.
[26] V. N. Evdokimova, T. V. Nikitina, I. N. Lebedev, N. N. Sukhanova, and S. A. Nazarenko, "About the sex ratio in connection with early embryonic mortality in man," *Ontogenez*, vol. 31, no. 4, pp. 251–257, 2000.
[27] D. T. Yates, *Measurement of Physiological Stress Response, Effects of Stress on Reproduction, and Management Practices for Avoiding Embryonic Wastage [M.S. thesis]*, New Mexico State University, Las Cruces, NM, USA, 2010.

14

Neuronal Ceroid Lipofuscinosis in Border Collie Dogs in Japan: Clinical and Molecular Epidemiological Study (2000–2011)

Keijiro Mizukami,[1] Takuji Kawamichi,[2] Hiroshi Koie,[3] Shinji Tamura,[4] Satoru Matsunaga,[5] Shigeki Imamoto,[6] Miyoko Saito,[7] Daisuke Hasegawa,[8] Naoaki Matsuki,[9] Satoshi Tamahara,[9] Shigenobu Sato,[10] Akira Yabuki,[1] Hye-Sook Chang,[1] and Osamu Yamato[1]

[1] *Laboratory of Clinical Pathology, Department of Veterinary Medicine, Kagoshima University, 1-21-24 Korimoto, Kagoshima, Kagoshima 890-0065, Japan*
[2] *Japan Border Collie Health Network, 1-14-8 Manabigaoka, Tarumi-ku, Hyogo, Kobe 655-0004, Japan*
[3] *Department of Veterinary Medicine, College of Bioresource Sciences, Nihon University, 1866 Kameino, Kanagawa, Fujisawa 252-0880, Japan*
[4] *Tamura Animal Clinic, 7-16 Yoshimien, Saeki-ku, Hiroshima, Hiroshima 731-5132, Japan*
[5] *Japan Animal Referral Medical Center, 2-5-8 Kuji, Takatsu-ku, Kanagawa, Kawasaki 213-0032, Japan*
[6] *Shinjo Animal Hospital, 104-1 Katsuragi, Nara, Katsuragi 639-2144, Japan*
[7] *Laboratory of Veterinary Surgery II, School of Veterinary Medicine, Azabu University, 1-17-71 Fuchinobe, Kanagawa, Sagamihara 229-8501, Japan*
[8] *Department of Veterinary Science, Nippon Veterinary and Life Science University, 1-7-1 Kyounan-chou, Tokyo, Musashino 180-8602, Japan*
[9] *Department of Veterinary Clinical Pathobiology, Graduate School of Agricultural and Life Sciences, The University of Tokyo, 1-1-1 Yayoi, Tokyo, Bunkyo-ku 113-8657, Japan*
[10] *Sato Animal Hospital, 6-38-20 Goinishi, Chiba, Ichihara 290-0038, Japan*

Correspondence should be addressed to Osamu Yamato, osam@vet.kagoshima-u.ac.jp

Academic Editors: M. F. Landoni and E. J. Thompson

Neuronal ceroid lipofuscinosis (NCL) is an inherited, neurodegenerative lysosomal disease that causes premature death. The present study describes the clinical and molecular epidemiologic findings of NCL in Border Collies in Japan for 12 years, between 2000 and 2011. The number of affected dogs was surveyed, and their clinical characteristics were analyzed. In 4 kennels with affected dogs, the dogs were genotyped. The genetic relationships of all affected dogs and carriers identified were analyzed. The survey revealed 27 affected dogs, but there was a decreasing trend at the end of the study period. The clinical characteristics of these affected dogs were updated in detail. The genotyping survey demonstrated a high mutant allele frequency in examined kennels (34.8%). The pedigree analysis demonstrated that all affected dogs and carriers in Japan are related to some presumptive carriers imported from Oceania and having a common ancestor. The current high prevalence in Japan might be due to an overuse of these carriers by breeders without any knowledge of the disease. For NCL control and prevention, it is necessary to examine all breeding dogs, especially in kennels with a high prevalence. Such endeavors will reduce NCL prevalence and may already be contributing to the recent decreasing trend in Japan.

1. Introduction

Neuronal ceroid lipofuscinosis (NCL) is a rare group of inherited, neurodegenerative lysosomal storage diseases characterized histopathologically by the abnormal accumulation of ceroid- or lipofuscin-like autofluorescent lipopigments in neurons, retinal cells, and other visceral cells throughout the body [1–4]. NCL shares certain clinical features in both human beings and animals, including behavioral abnormalities, such as personality changes and aggressiveness, mental retardation and/or dementia; motor disturbances, such as ataxia and incoordination; visual problems leading to central and/or retinal blindness; premature death, but these differ in degree based on the causative gene, of which there are currently at least 8, all recessively inherited [4]. NCL has been described in several domestic species and occurs most commonly in dogs [1, 2, 5].

NCL in Border Collies was first identified in Australia in the 1980s [6–8], and a sporadic case with the disease was also reported in the USA in the 1990s [9]. A diagnosis of the first case in Japan was made in a Border Collie that was born in 2000 [10]. The pathogenic mutation was reported in 2005 to be a nonsense mutation (c.619C>T) in exon 4 in the canine *CLN5* gene [11], which enabled a DNA-based genotyping of affected dogs and carriers. Recently, several types of rapid genotyping assays for this mutation were developed, and the carrier frequency (8.1%) in Japan was determined by a genotyping survey using these assays, suggesting the mutant allele frequency of NCL in Border Collies is high enough in Japan that measures to control and prevent the disease would be warranted [5].

The present study describes the clinical and molecular epidemiologic findings of NCL in Border Collies in Japan for 12 years, between 2000 and 2011. This study also discusses the control and prevention of the disease based on the results of these analyses.

2. Materials and Methods

2.1. Dogs Affected with NCL. The number of affected dogs was surveyed based on the records in our laboratory, which have been exclusively supporting the diagnosis of the disease in Japan. Among 27 affected dogs identified in the present study, NCL was diagnosed definitively in 25 dogs by a genetic test [5] using their specimens containing DNA, but in the remaining 2 dogs that died without any specimens before the genetic test got available, NCL was strongly suspected based on their typical clinical history and blood relationship with molecularly defined affected littermates and/or carrier parents. The clinical characteristics were analyzed and summarized using information about all of the affected dogs, which was gleaned from interviews and questionnaires of their owners and veterinarians. Some of the affected dogs were examined using the following prediagnostic tests: magnetic resonance image (MRI) scan in 7 dogs, including a previously reported dog [10]; computed tomography (CT) scan in 2 dogs; ophthalmologic examination in 3 dogs. The findings of these examinations were also analyzed and summarized.

2.2. Genotyping Survey. Border Collies belonging to 4 special kennels (A, B, C, and D), which generated one or more affected dogs, were surveyed between 2008 and 2010 using a genetic test with the breeders' cooperation. The number of dogs examined was 82, including 23, 20, 29, and 10 in kennels A, B, C, and D, respectively. Whole blood or saliva specimens were collected from these dogs using the Flinders Technology Associates filter paper (FTA card, Whatman International). Genotyping was performed as reported previously [5].

2.3. Pedigree Analysis. Pedigree analysis was performed to elucidate the genetic relationships of affected and carrier dogs identified in Japan and to deduce the pathway of transmission and distribution of the mutant allele. The genetic relationships among affected and carrier dogs found in the present study were analyzed using the pedigree papers issued by the Japan Kennel Club (http://www.jkc.or.jp/) and the Kennel Club of Japan (http://www.kcj.gr.jp/). The pedigree information of carrier dogs identified in the previous random survey in Japan [5] was analyzed and added to the results of the present study. The pedigree information of the dogs was used under the informed consent of their owners. The ancestry in Oceania was traced using pedigree information of carrier dogs provided by the New South Wales Border Collie Club (http://www.mybcsite.com/bccnswwebfiles/bccnswframe.htm), which was also disclosed via the website of the Japan Border Collie Health Network (http://www.jbchn.net/cl_carrier.htm), a volunteer breeders' association for the healthy breeding of Border Collies. Pedigree information published in the Border Collie Database (http://db.kennel.dk/) was used to supplement the information about the ancestor dogs in Oceania.

All animals were cared for and were used in the experiments in accordance with the guidelines for proper conduct of animal experiments issued by the Science Council of Japan (http://www.scj.go.jp/en/animal/index.html). All experimental procedures using animals and their specimens were performed in accordance with the guidelines regulating animal use at Kagoshima University.

3. Results

3.1. The Number and Clinical Characteristics of Border Collies with NCL. The survey revealed that there were 27 affected dogs (13 males and 14 females) in the 12 years from 2000 to 2011 in Japan (Table 1). The first case, born in 2000, was diagnosed with NCL histopathologically [10], which was confirmed molecularly using the stored liver specimen. Since this case, several affected dogs from a single or a few litters were diagnosed nearly every year up until recently in Japan. However, currently there seems to be a decreasing trend based on the observation that only 1 affected dog was identified since 2009.

The clinical features of the affected dogs are summarized and listed in Table 2. They were divided into 3 stages, that is, early (15–20 months of age), middle (19–23 months of age), and late-to-terminal stages (22–32 months of age). The overlaps in age between adjacent stages were due to individual variability in the onset and progression rate of the disease. The features at the early stage were mainly behavioral problems that most owners of the dogs did not regard as pathological changes. The features at the middle stage included serious behavioral abnormalities, visual impairments, and slight motor disorders, which prompted

Table 1: Number of Border Collies with neuronal ceroid lipofuscinosis and the number of litters that included affected dogs during the 12 years between 2000 and 2011 in Japan.

Year of birth	Number of affected dogs (male and female)	Number of litters
2000	2 (2, 0)	1
2001	6 (3, 3)	3
2002	0 (0, 0)	0
2003	4 (3, 1)	3
2004	4 (1, 3)	2
2005	2 (1, 1)	2
2006	1 (0, 1)	1
2007	2 (1, 1)	2
2008	5 (2, 3)	4
2009	1 (0, 1)	1
2010–present*	0 (0, 0)	0
Total	27 (13, 14)	19

*June 2012.

Table 2: Summary of clinical features in Border Collies with neuronal ceroid lipofuscinosis*.

Stage (months of age)	Clinical signs
Early (15–20)	Altered characteristics; disregard for owner's commands; loss of interest in play and other dogs; morbid fear of noise, humans, and unspecified things; hallucination; disorientation; biting; averse to going up and down stairs (especially down)
Middle (19–23)	Fly-biting behavior; continuous shaking of the head; sudden halts during walks; uncooperativeness with other dogs; head tilt; chomping without food; tooth grinding; leg jerking; visual impairments (fear of darkness, unawareness of things such as food, and frequently hitting obstacles); aggressiveness; excitation; staggering; falling; toileting accidents; myoclonus; myoclonic seizure
Late to terminal (22–32)	Wandering; hair-pulling disorder; circadian rhythm disorder; acoustic and cutaneous hyperesthesia; cognitive and emotional impairments; blindness; dysmetria; gait deficiency; convulsive seizure; face and mouth tic; chewing difficulty; lethargy; stupor; death (mean age 26.7 months, ranging from 23 to 32 months)†

*Data summarized from the information of 27 affected dogs.
†Data from 17 affected dogs that died naturally without euthanasia.

the owners to consult veterinarians. The features at the late-to-terminal stage included serious motor, visual, psychointellectual, and vital dysfunctions due to a wide spectrum of brain dysfunctions. The mean life span of the 23 affected dogs examined was 26.4 months of age. Of these, 17 died naturally at a mean age of 26.7 months, ranging from 23 to 32 months. The other 6 dogs were euthanized at the terminal stage an average of 25.6 months. Although there were few specific changes before 15 months of age, some of the owners had an impression that their dogs had unusual characteristics and behaviors and low learning ability in the puppy and juvenile years. There was no abnormal change on general clinicopathological examinations. No abnormal vacuoles in the cytoplasm of leukocytes were observed in blood smear examinations.

3.2. MRI, CT, and Ophthalmologic Examinations. MRI, CT, and ophthalmologic examinations were performed in affected dogs in the middle-to-late stage (at approximately 2 years of age). The common findings of MR and CT images were ventricular enlargement and well-demarcated cerebral sulci (Figure 1). Dilation of cerebellar fissures was also observed at a sagittal section of the MRI scan (Figure 1(c)). No other organic lesion was detected in MRI and CT scans. In the affected dogs examined ophthalmologically, slight narrowing of blood vessels in the retina was commonly observed in ophthalmoscopy (Figure 2(a)), but this ophthalmoscopic finding was evaluated within the normal range by veterinary ophthalmologists. An examination using a slit lamp detected no abnormal finding, such as clouding of the cornea and lens (Figure 2(b)).

3.3. Genotyping Survey. The results of the genotyping survey in the 4 specific kennels are shown in Table 3. The frequencies of carriers (32.9%), affected dogs (18.3%), and the mutant allele (34.8%) were markedly high in the 4 kennels.

3.4. Pedigree Analysis. The pedigree analysis was performed mainly using the pedigree information of the 27 affected dogs and 58 carriers identified so far in Japan (Figure 3). These dogs were related to at least 13 possible carriers imported from Oceania to Japan in the middle 1990s, which ultimately revealed an ancestry from a male dog born in 1944 in Australia through 9 carriers reported by the New South Wales Border Collie Club. As a result, this analysis revealed that all dogs carrying the mutant allele in Japan share a blood relationship and a single common ancestor in Australia.

The pedigree analysis also revealed that breeding was repeated using a small number of carriers and their offspring in the 4 kennels surveyed in the present study. The breeders of these kennels were not aware of NCL in Border Collies before the genotyping survey. As a result, these kennels had markedly high frequencies of the mutant allele.

4. Discussion

The present study revealed 27 Border Collies (13 males and 14 females) with NCL in Japan during 2000–2011 (Table 1), although there might have been additional affected dogs elsewhere that had no opportunity to be diagnosed. Since the first affected dog, born in 2000, was diagnosed in 2002 [10], several affected dogs from a single or a few litters have been diagnosed nearly every year up until recently, but currently there seems to be a decline in the frequency of NCL. The decreasing trend may be due to the publication of the pathogenic mutation in 2005 [11], the subsequent

TABLE 3: Results of the genotyping survey carried out in 4 kennels that generated affected dogs*.

Kennel	Number of			Frequency (%)		
	Dogs examined	Carriers	Affected dogs	Carriers	Affected dogs	Mutant allele
A	23	9	8	39.1	34.8	54.3
B	20	11	2	55.0	10.0	37.5
C	29	6	2	20.7	6.7	17.2
D	10	1	3	10.0	30.0	35.0
Total	82	27	15	32.9	18.3	34.8

*These genotyping surveys were carried out between 2008 and 2010.

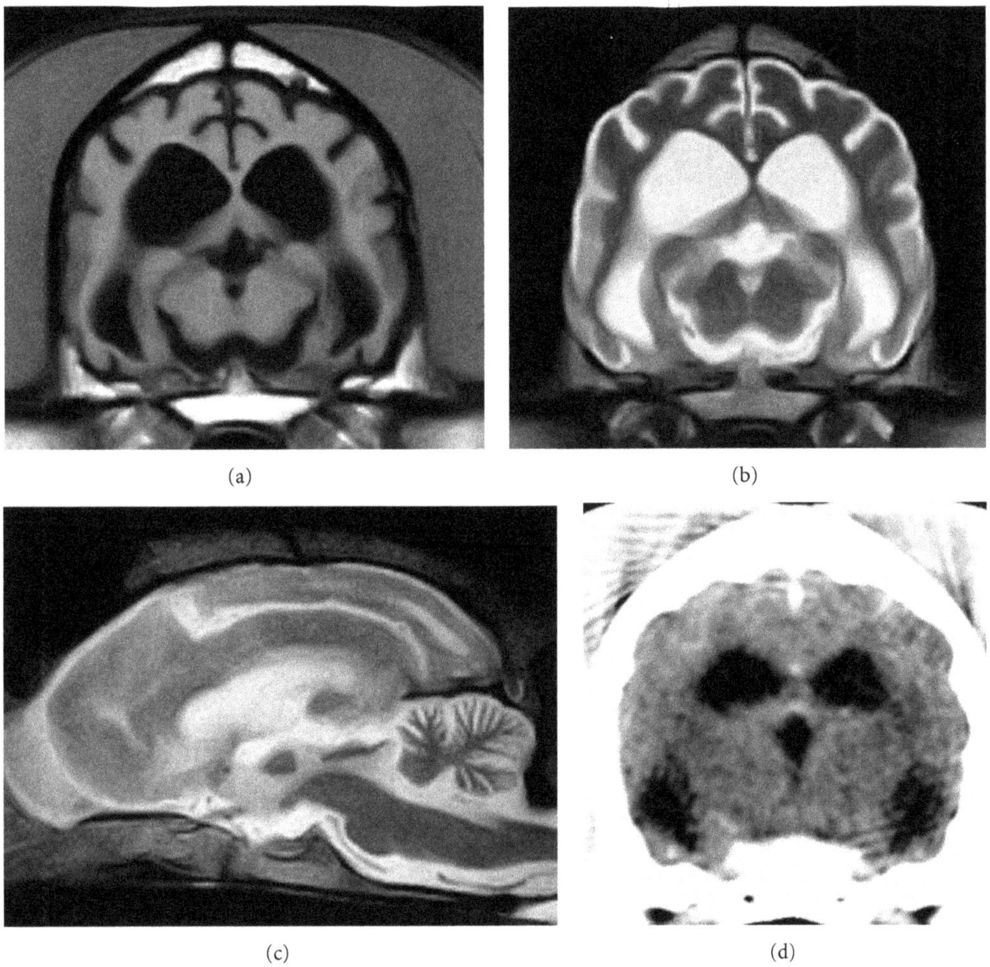

FIGURE 1: Representative magnetic resonance (MR) and computed tomography (CT) images of the brain of Border Collies with neuronal ceroid lipofuscinosis. MR images were obtained using a 0.3-tesla system (AIRIS2-comfort, Hitachi Medical Corporation) in a 24-month-old dog under general anesthesia. CT images were obtained using a multislice CT system (ECLOS, Hitachi Medical Corporation) in another 24-month-old dog under general anesthesia. (a) MR T1-weighted image (TR/TE = 500/20 ms) of a transverse section at the level of the thalamus, (b) MR T2-weighted image (TR/TE = 4,000/120 ms) of a transverse section at the level of the thalamus, (c) MR T2-weighted image of a sagittal section, and (d) CT image of a transverse section at the level of the thalamus. These images show enlarged ventricles and dilated cerebral and cerebellar sulci, suggesting forebrain atrophy.

development of a variety of genetic testing methods [5], and genotyping surveys in a random population of breeding Border Collies [5] and in a few specific kennels that generated affected dog(s) (present study). These events may have contributed to the prevention and control of the disease through the education of related breeders and fanciers of Border Collies.

Based on information from the owners and veterinarians of the affected dogs, their characteristic clinical features were determined (Table 2), although there were individual differences in the onset and progression rate of the disease and the symptoms, as reported previously [6]. Mild clinical signs, such as behavioral problems, begin at 15 months of age at the earliest, but the onset is usually a few months later

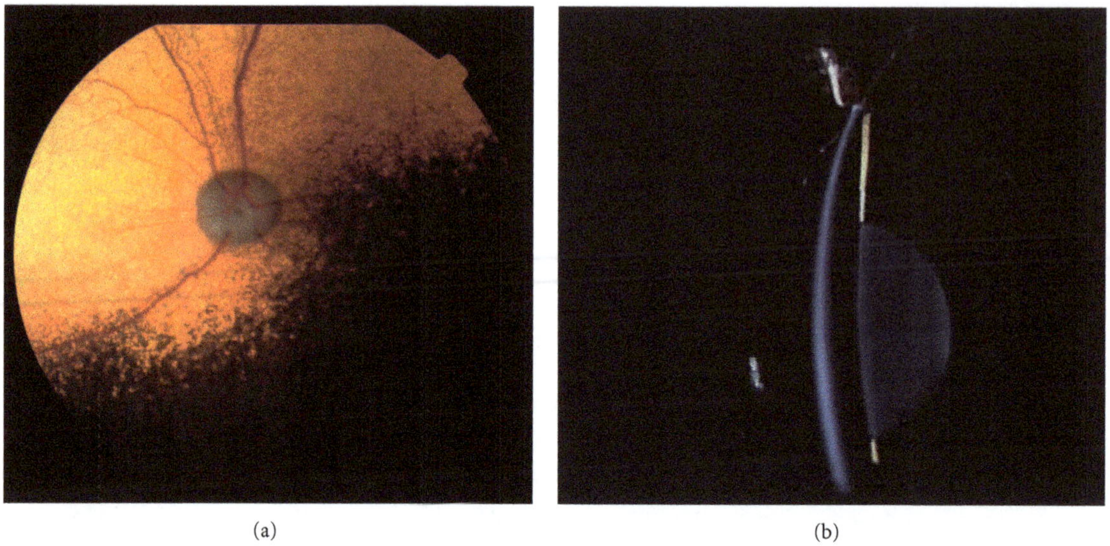

FIGURE 2: Photographs of ophthalmoscopic and slit-lamp examinations of the right eye in a 21-month-old Border Collie with neuronal ceroid lipofuscinosis. (a) Slight narrowing of blood vessels in the retina is observed, but (b) there is no abnormal finding in the slit-lamp examination.

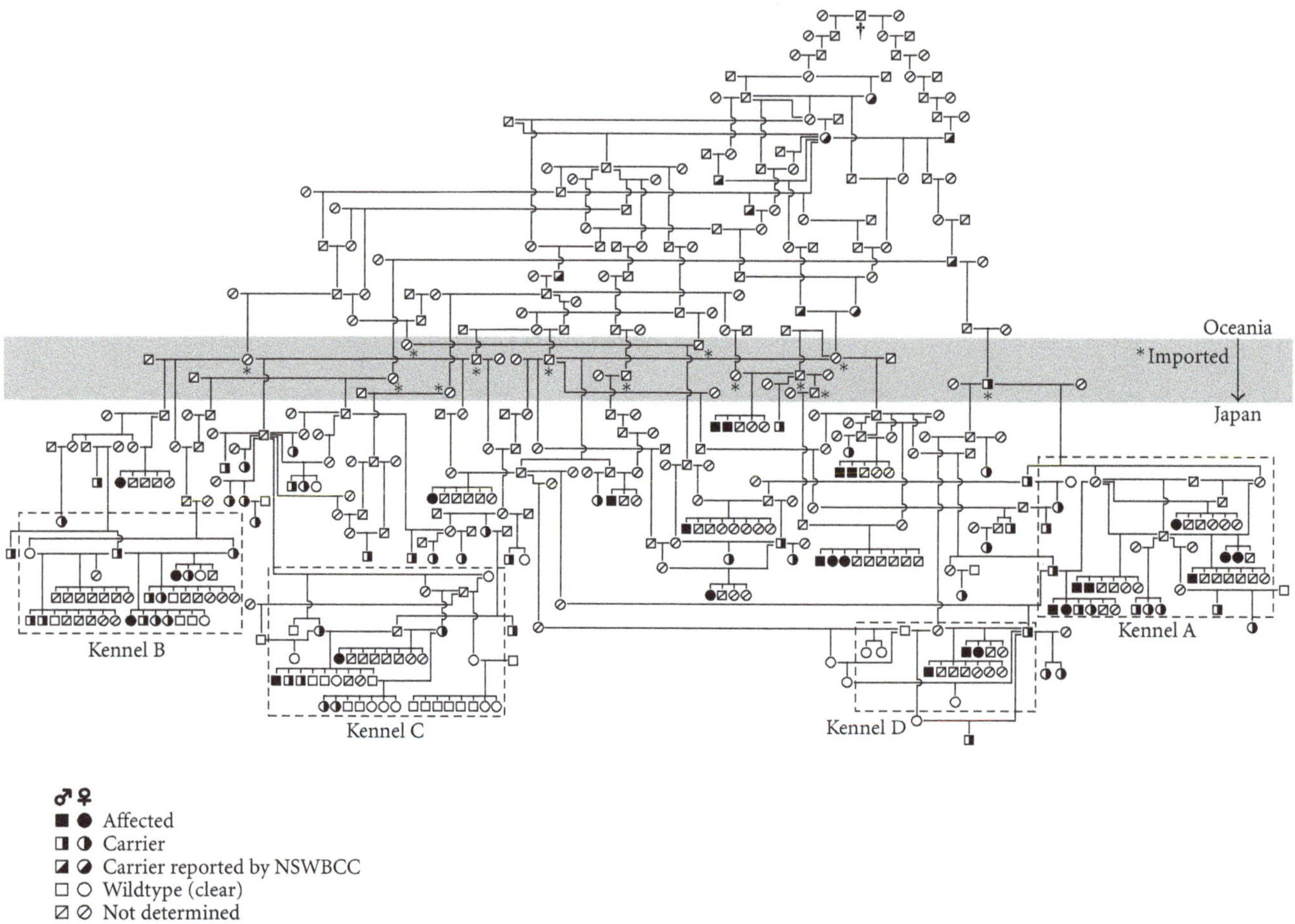

FIGURE 3: Genetic relationship of affected and carrier dogs identified in Japan between 2000 and 2011. The analysis was carried out using pedigree papers issued by the Japan Kennel Club and the Kennel Club of Japan and information reported by the New South Wales Border Collie Club (NSWBCC) and the Border Collie Database. The gray area indicates a border between Oceania and Japan. Dogs imported from Oceania to Japan were marked with an asterisk (*). All dogs carrying the mutant allele shared a common ancestor (†) born in 1944 in Australia. Areas surrounded by a dashed line indicate the 4 kennels surveyed using a genotyping test.

(approximately 18 months of age) at the early stage. The earliest age of onset in the present study is consistent with that in a previous report [8]. Clinical signs observed at the early stage (15–20 months of age) are mainly mild behavioral abnormalities that the owners, without any knowledge of NCL, hardly regard as pathological. Visual disorders become unambiguous and behavioral abnormalities increase in severity at the middle stage (19–23 months of age). Serious clinical signs, such as convulsive seizure and motor disorders, appear at the late-to-terminal stage (older than 22 months of age). The mean life span of affected dogs was 26.7 months of age in the present study. The life span was 26.4 months of age in the dogs that died naturally, ranging from 23 to 32 months of age. This is longer than the 23.1-month life span of affected Border Collies in a previous report in Australia [7]. The difference could be attributed to the fact that many Japanese pet owners feel that euthanasia is inhumane and do not want to kill animals before they die naturally.

The characteristic clinical features determined in the present study are similar to those in previous reports [6, 7]. However, a previously reported clinical sign, mania [7], was not observed in the present study. In addition, some affected dogs had unusual characteristics and behaviors and low learning ability in the puppy and juvenile years, which was not reported previously. These clinical characteristics, updated in detail, will be of further help for the diagnosis of NCL in Border Collies.

In the MRI examination, ventricular enlargement and dilated cerebral and cerebellar sulci were common findings in affected dogs (Figure 1). The CT examination also demonstrated ventricular enlargement. These characteristic findings suggest atrophy of the forebrain, which was similarly observed in previous MRI [10] and CT examinations [9]. The changes suggesting brain atrophy developed as early as the middle stage, when affected dogs were usually referred to animal hospitals. Similar changes have been observed in other types of NCL [12, 13] and other lysosomal storage diseases, such as GM1 gangliosidosis [14] and GM2 gangliosidosis [15–17] in dogs and cats. The brain atrophy usually develops as a specific and severe change even at the middle stage in NCL but as a secondary and mild change in the late-to-terminal stage in other lysosomal diseases. Therefore, the atrophic changes would be useful as an adjunct to the diagnosis of NCL. No other organic lesion was detected in MRI scans in Border Collies with NCL, although hyperintensity in T2-weighted images of the cerebral white matter is observed in GM1 and GM2 gangliosidoses in dogs and cats [14, 16–19]. Meningeal thickening, reported in Chihuahuas with NCL [13], was not observed in Border Collies with NCL.

Visual impairments appeared to various degrees in all affected dogs, especially at the middle stage (Table 2). Previous reports have not described any abnormal changes on ophthalmoscopic examination [7, 10]. In the present study, the affected dogs examined had slight narrowing of blood vessels in the retina (Figure 2(a)), but this ophthalmoscopic finding was considered within the normal range by veterinary ophthalmologists (Figure 2). In humans with NCL, there is a pronounced loss of photoreceptors in the end stage of the disease, but in NCL in English Setters only minimal structural damage is observed in the retina [20]. In Border Collies with NCL, inclusions with variable ultrastructure are common in all cells of the retina, but the pigment accumulation does not damage the retinal architecture [8]. The retinal lesions in the Border Collies are similar to those in the English Setters but are much less severe than in juvenile NCL in humans. The narrowing of retinal blood vessels observed in affected Border Collies may be an indication of mild retinal degeneration, but this feature cannot be used as a valuable diagnostic for NCL.

Based on data of the pedigree analysis, affected dogs and carriers identified in Japan share a blood relationship and a single common ancestor born in 1944 in Australia via some presumptive carriers in Oceania (Figure 3). Although it is impossible to demonstrate whether this ancestor was a founder of NCL in Border Collies, there is a possibility that the mutant allele was transmitted from Oceania to Japan in this way mainly in the middle of the 1990s, when the causative mutation had not been identified yet. The recent increase in prevalence of the disease in Japan is likely due to an overuse of imported carriers and their offspring as breeding dogs without any knowledge of the disease. Hereafter, dogs that will be bred should be genotyped beforehand.

The pedigree analysis also suggests that breeding has been repeated using a small number of carriers and their offspring in the 4 kennels that generated affected dogs (Figure 3). There was a trend toward inbreeding in these kennels. In addition, the breeders of the kennels were not aware of the disease until they were informed of the generation of affected dogs in their kennels. These issues may have caused the high frequencies of carriers (32.9%) and the mutant allele (34.8%) in the 4 kennels (Table 3), compared to the carrier (8.1%) and mutant allele frequencies (4.1%) in the random population of Border Collies [5]. Fifteen (55.6%) of the 27 affected dogs identified so far in Japan were generated in these 4 kennels. It is thought that affected dogs are generated in a small proportion of kennels, which have a high frequency of the mutant allele. Therefore, it is important for prevention of the disease to rapidly genotype all breeding dogs in kennels that have had an opportunity to generate affected dogs. This type of examination helps the kennels not only stop generating additional affected dogs but also stop spreading carriers to other kennels. In addition, a genotyping test using specimens from a random population of breeding Border Collies should be continued [5] to detect sporadic carriers and prevent them from being used as breeding dogs. These approaches would gradually decrease the number of dogs carrying the mutant allele. These active and continuous preventive measures may be necessary to eliminate NCL in Border Collies.

Acknowledgments

The authors are grateful to Ms. Kasukawa (the first affected dog's owner), all other affected dogs' owners, and all veterinarians associated with the dogs for providing their specimens and information about them. The authors are also grateful to all members of the Japan Border Collie Health Network for their help with the collection of information about affected and carrier Border Collies. This study was supported financially by grants (nos. 14560258, 1680210, 20380173, 20-08112, and 21658109, O. Yamato) from the Ministry of Education, Culture, Sports, Science and Technology of Japan.

References

[1] R. D. Jolly, D. N. Palmer, R. H. Studdert et al., "Canine ceroid-ipofuscinoses: a review and classification," *Journal of Small Animal Practice*, vol. 35, no. 6, pp. 299–306, 1994.

[2] R. D. Jolly and D. N. Palmer, "The neuronal ceroid-lipofuscinoses (Batten disease): comparative aspects," *Neuropathology and Applied Neurobiology*, vol. 21, no. 1, pp. 50–60, 1995.

[3] S. L. Hofmann and L. Petronen, "The neuronal ceroid lipofuscinoses," in *The Metabolic and Molecular Bases of Inherited Disease*, C. Scriver, A. Beaudet, W. Sly, and D. Valle, Eds., pp. 3877–3894, McGraw-Hill, New York, NY, USA, 8th edition, 2001.

[4] A. Jalanko and T. Braulke, "Neuronal ceroid lipofuscinoses," *Biochimica et Biophysica Acta*, vol. 1793, no. 4, pp. 697–709, 2009.

[5] K. Mizukami, H.-S. Chang, A. Yabuki et al., "Novel rapid genotyping assays for neuronal ceroid lipofuscinosis in Border Collie dogs and high frequency of the mutant allele in Japan," *Journal of Veterinary Diagnostic Investigation*, vol. 23, no. 6, pp. 1131–1139, 2011.

[6] R. M. Taylor and B. R. H. Farrow, "Ceroid-lipofuscinosis in Border Collie dogs," *Acta Neuropathologica*, vol. 75, no. 6, pp. 627–631, 1988.

[7] V. P. Studdert and R. W. Mitten, "Clinical features of ceroid lipofuscinosis in Border Collie dogs," *Australian Veterinary Journal*, vol. 68, no. 4, pp. 137–140, 1991.

[8] R. M. Taylor and B. R. H. Farrow, "Ceroid lipofuscinosis in the Border Collie dog: retinal lesions in an animal model of juvenile Batten disease," *American Journal of Medical Genetics*, vol. 42, no. 4, pp. 622–627, 1992.

[9] J. N. Franks, C. W. Dewey, M. A. Walker, and R. W. Storts, "Computed tomographic findings of ceroid lipofuscinosis in a dog," *Journal of the American Animal Hospital Association*, vol. 35, no. 5, pp. 430–435, 1999.

[10] H. Koie, H. Shibuya, T. Sato et al., "Magnetic resonance imaging of neuronal ceroid lipofuscinosis in a Border Collie," *Journal of Veterinary Medical Science*, vol. 66, no. 11, pp. 1453–1456, 2004.

[11] S. A. Melville, C. L. Wilson, C. S. Chiang, V. P. Studdert, F. Lingaas, and A. N. Wilton, "A mutation in canine CLN5 causes neuronal ceroid lipofuscinosis in Border Collie dogs," *Genomics*, vol. 86, no. 3, pp. 287–294, 2005.

[12] M. Kuwamura, R. Hattori, J. Yamate, T. Kotani, and K. Sasai, "Neuronal ceroid-lipofuscinosis and hydrocephalus in a chihuahua," *Journal of Small Animal Practice*, vol. 44, no. 5, pp. 227–230, 2003.

[13] Y. Nakamoto, O. Yamato, K. Uchida et al., "Neuronal ceroid-lipofuscinosis in longhaired chihuahuas: clinical, pathologic, and MRI findings," *Journal of the American Animal Hospital Association*, vol. 47, no. 4, pp. e64–e70, 2011.

[14] D. Hasegawa, O. Yamato, Y. Nakamoto et al., "Serial MRI features of canine GM1 gangliosidosis: a possible imaging biomarker for diagnosis and progression of the disease," *The Scientific World Journal*, vol. 2012, Article ID 250197, 2012.

[15] N. Matsuki, O. Yamato, M. Kusuda, Y. Maede, H. Tsujimoto, and K. Ono, "Magnetic resonance imaging of GM2-gangliosidosis in a golden retriever," *Canadian Veterinary Journal*, vol. 46, no. 3, pp. 275–278, 2005.

[16] D. Hasegawa, O. Yamato, M. Kobayashi et al., "Clinical and molecular analysis of GM2 gangliosidosis in two apparent littermate kittens of the Japanese domestic cat," *Journal of Feline Medicine and Surgery*, vol. 9, no. 3, pp. 232–237, 2007.

[17] S. Tamura, Y. Tamura, K. Uchida et al., "GM2 Gangliosidosis variant 0 (Sandhoff-like disease) in a family of toy poodles," *Journal of Veterinary Internal Medicine*, vol. 24, no. 5, pp. 1013–1019, 2010.

[18] E. M. Kaye, J. Alroy, S. S. Raghavan et al., "Dysmyelinogenesis in animal model of GM1 gangliosidosis," *Pediatric Neurology*, vol. 8, no. 4, pp. 255–261, 1992.

[19] R. A. Kroll, M. A. Pagel, S. Roman-Goldstein, A. J. Barkovich, A. N. D'Agostino, and E. A. Neuwelt, "White matter changes associated with feline G(M2) gangliosidosis (Sandhoff disease): correlation of MR findings with pathologic and ultrastructural abnormalities," *American Journal of Neuroradiology*, vol. 16, no. 6, pp. 1219–1226, 1995.

[20] N. Koppang, "The English setter with ceroid-lipofuscinosis: a suitable model for the juvenile type of ceroid-lipofuscinosis in humans," *American Journal of Medical Genetics*, vol. 5, pp. 117–125, 1988.

15

Altered Expression of Cellular Bcl-2 in the Progression of Hamster Cholangiocarcinogenesis

Byung-suk Jeon and Byung-IL Yoon

Laboratory of Histology and Molecular Pathogenesis, College of Veterinary Medicine and Institute of Veterinary Science, Kangwon National University, Chuncheon, 200-701, Republic of Korea

Correspondence should be addressed to Byung-IL Yoon, byoon@kangwon.ac.kr

Academic Editor: Roberto Agresti

Bcl-2 is an intracytoplasmic and membrane-associated apoptosis suppressor, and its overexpression is closely associated with survival of malignant tumors, in particular their aggressive behavior and poor prognosis. The role of Bcl-2 is, however, still controversial in cholangiocarcinogenesis because of the discrepancies in the expression of the protein. In the present study, alteration in the expression of Bcl-2 in cholangiocarcinogenesis was investigated by studying the immunoreactivities of this protein in normal, hyperplastic bile ducts with or without dysplastic changes, and neoplastic bile duct cells from a hamster cholangiocarcinoma (ChC) model. Cytoplasmic staining, which reflects high-Bcl-2 immunoreactivity, was negative to very weak in normal and hyperplastic bile ducts without dysplastic changes, while hyperplastic bile ducts with dysplasia indicated heterogeneously strong expression. On the other hand, most of the neoplastic cells of invasive cholangiocarcinomas were negative to weak as much as the level of normal bile ducts. The results suggest that the antiapoptotic factor Bcl-2 plays a limited role in the survival of highly proliferative, potentially dysplastic bile duct cells. However, the role of Bcl-2 in biliary cancer cells was not significant.

1. Introduction

Apoptosis, the so-called programmed cell death or cell suicide, is a key regulatory mechanism in the differentiation and maturation of an organism and during the development of cancer. Apoptosis is also essential for removing irreparable, damaged, and transformed cells in adults [1, 2]. Apoptosis is regulated by a variety of genes, including Bcl-2 and p53. p53 induces apoptosis to protect the body against cells that behave in a discoordinated fashion or have damaged DNA. The Bcl-2 oncogene inhibits apoptosis as a generalized cell death suppressor, thus allowing the accumulation and propagation of cells containing genetic alterations [3]. Altered expression of cell-survival genes such as Bcl-2 induces a malfunction in the apoptosis-regulating machinery and is therefore closely associated with carcinogenesis [4, 5]. Earlier studies reported aberrant Bcl-2 expression in a variety of tumors, such as adenocarcinoma of the prostate, bladder carcinoma, squamous cell carcinoma of the lung, nasopharyngeal carcinoma, and breast carcinoma [6–11].

Cholangiocarcinoma (ChC) is a highly malignant, generally fatal adenocarcinoma arising from bile-duct epithelial cells of the intrahepatic or extrahepatic biliary system. Although it is a relatively rare tumor, the incidence of ChC is increasing globally [12]. Despite advances in ChC diagnosis, surgery offers the only possibility of relatively long-term survival [13]. Nevertheless, the 5-year survival rate after curative resection is less than 30% [14]. The pathogenesis of biliary cancer remains unknown, but oxidative damage, oncogene activation, and impaired apoptosis may be involved [15]. In association with antiapoptosis, Bcl-2 overexpression has been implicated in carcinogenesis. However, data regarding Bcl-2 expression in human ChC are controversial, and the antiapoptotic mechanism in ChC cells remains unknown [8, 16–19]. Some studies have indicated that ChC expresses Bcl-2. Studies involving several hematological and solid

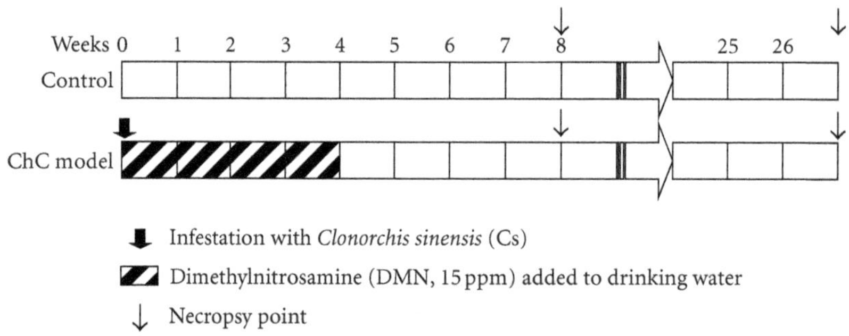

FIGURE 1: The time points of liver specimen collections in the hamster cholangiocarcinoma model. The liver specimens were respectively prepared at the precancerous phase (8 weeks after ChC model initiation) and the cancerous phase (27 weeks after the model initiation) as well as from the negative control hamsters. The hamster ChC model was composed of the initiation process by the treatment of dimethylnitrosamine (DMN) and infestation of 15 *Clonorchis sinensis* metacercariae as a strong promoter.

malignancies have identified a correlation between intense Bcl-2 or Bcl-X_L expression and poor patient response to cancer therapy and overall prognosis. A study by Charlotte et al. [8] reported that eight of 11 cases expressed Bcl-2 and suggested that the Bcl-2 protein could be a unique ChC marker. A study by Terada and Nakanuma [20] found Bcl-2 expression in one of 20 ChCs and suggested that a role of Bcl-2 is limited in ChC. These results correspond to the findings in experimental models.

We investigated altered Bcl-2 protein expression patterns during hamster cholangiocarcinogenesis to evaluate the role of Bcl-2 using immunohistochemical analyses.

2. Materials and Methods

2.1. Tissue Samples. Five paraffin-embedded tissue blocks of hamster livers with precancerous biliary lesions and ChC, as well as normal hamster livers, were prepared from hamster ChC models. The precancerous lesions were obtained from hamsters 8 weeks after inducing the hamster ChC model (interim phase of cholangiocarcinogenesis), and ChC tissues were obtained with tumor masses at 27 weeks (Figure 1). As described in a previous study, precancerous hamster livers were characterized by hyperplastic bile ducts with or without cellular dysplasia and intense surrounding inflammation; the ChCs were invasive tubular or tubulopapillary-type primary biliary cancers [21].

2.2. Bcl-2 Immunohistochemistry. The avidin-biotin complex method was used for Bcl-2 immunohistochemistry. After dewaxing with xylene and rehydration through a graded ethanol series, tissue sections were immersed in methanol (Daejung Chemicals and Metals, Siheung City, republic of Korea) containing 0.3% hydrogen peroxide (Showa Chemicals, Tokyo, Japan) for 30 min at room temperature to block endogenous peroxidase activity. Microwave antigen retrieval was performed using a preheated target-retrieval solution (0.01 M, pH 6.0; DakoCytomation, Carpinteria, CA, USA) followed by a 15 min incubation. This was followed by treatment with a detergent, which consisted of soaking the samples in phosphate-buffered saline (PBS) containing 0.05% Tween 20 (pH 7.2). After three 5 min washes in PBS, the tissue sections were incubated with normal blocking serum and prepared according to the manufacturer's instructions supplied in the Vectastain Elite ABC Kit (Vector Labs, Burlingame, CA, USA) for 1 h at room temperature. Avidin D and biotin blocking reagents (Vector Labs) were added to the sections according to the manufacturer's instructions to minimize background staining due to endogenous biotin or biotin-binding proteins, lectins, or nonspecific binding substances present within the tissue sections. The sections were then incubated with diluted primary antibody (rabbit polyclonal anti-human Bcl-2 IgG 1 : 50, Santa Cruz Biotechnology, Santa Cruz, CA, USA) overnight at 4°C. As a negative control, PBS was used instead of the primary antibody. Thereafter, the sections were washed with PBS and incubated with the appropriate biotinylated secondary antibody according to the Vectastain Elite ABC Kit for 40 min at room temperature, followed by a 30 min incubation with ABC reagent at room temperature. The sections were visualized with 3,3-diaminobenzidine tetrahydrochloride solution (DakoCytomation) containing 3% hydrogen peroxide and counterstained with Mayer's hematoxylin (Sigma-Aldrich, St. Louis, MO, USA). This was followed by routine dehydration in alcohol, clearing in xylene, and mounting.

2.3. Semiquantitative Evaluation of Bcl-2 Immunoreactivity. We counted the hyperplastic and dysplastic bile ducts in six hamster livers at 8 weeks and in 10 hamster livers at 27 weeks to semiquantitatively evaluate Bcl-2 immunoreactivity in the biliary cell populations during cholangiocarcinogenesis. Sections were evaluated at high-power magnification from a series of 10 randomly selected adjacent fields under a light microscope fitted with an ocular grid. In total, 100, 811, and 4890 biliary epithelial cells were counted in the hamster livers at normal, precancerous, and carcinogenic phases, respectively. Bcl-2 immunoreactivity in the biliary cell populations, including biliary cancer cells, was represented as the percentage of negative, weak (1+), moderate (2+), or strongly (3+) positive bile ducts or neoplastic cells for Bcl-2 to the total number of bile ducts or neoplastic cell numbers. Based on the criteria, a light microscopic examination of Bcl-2 immunoreactivity was performed blindly by two veterinary pathologists. Statistically significant differences between the biliary cell populations were detected using Student's t-test. Statistical significance was determined at $P < 0.05$.

2.4. Western Blot Assay. As the Bcl-2 antibody used for immunohistochemistry originated from human Bcl-2, the reactivity and specificity of the primary antibody against hamster Bcl-2 were tested by western blot assay. Additionally, Bcl-2 protein levels were respectively evaluated in precancerous hamster livers, the biliary tumor mass, and in normal livers.

Protein was extracted from the all liver tissues according to a previous study [21]. Briefly, the frozen hamster liver tissues were finely ground and dissolved by repeatedly passing them through a 26-gauge needle attached to a syringe containing protein extraction buffer (Intron, Chinju, Republic of Korea). After a 15 min incubation at 20°C, the suspension was centrifuged at 13,000 rpm for 5 min at 4°C. The protein extracts (20 μg) were subjected to 12% (w/v) SDS-polyacrylamide gel electrophoresis and transferred to PVDF membranes (Bio-Rad Lab., Hercules, CA, USA). After blocking the nonspecific binding sites by incubating the membranes with 5% nonfat dried milk and 0.1% Tween 20 in Tris-buffered saline (pH 7.4) for 1 h at room temperature, the membranes were incubated overnight at 4°C with diluted primary antihuman Bcl-2 antibody at a 1 : 200 dilution, followed by an incubation with secondary antibody for 50 min at room temperature. To visualize the bands, the membranes were treated with a detection reagent for 1 min, exposed to film, and then developed using a SEER medical film processor (SEER Technologies Inc., Seoul, Republic of Korea).

3. Results

High Bcl-2 expression was limited in some hyperplastic bile ducts with dysplastic changes during hamster cholangiocarcinogenesis. Most of the hyperplastic bile ducts were almost negative to weakly positive (Figure 2), and only 2.7% of the counted hyperplastic bile ducts showed high expression graded as >2+ (Figure 3). The hyperplastic bile ducts strongly expressing Bcl-2 were those with dysplastic changes, whereas the hyperplastic bile ducts without morphological transformation were all negative or very weakly positive (Figure 2). Hepatocytes in the precancerous hamster livers were generally negative. Sinusoidal, lymphocytes, eosinophils, macrophages, and plasma cells often showed strong Bcl-2 immunoreactivity.

The percentage of biliary cancer cells showing high Bcl-2 expression (above grade 2+) was much lower; it was less than 1% of the counted cancer cells in all of the ChCs examined (Figure 3). Hepatocytes in the cancerous phase did not express Bcl-2. In the normal hamster liver, all liver parenchymal cells including biliary epithelial cells and hepatocytes were negative for Bcl-2 (Figure 2).

We validated the specificity of the Bcl-2 antibody used for immunohistochemistry using a western blot assay because the antibody originated from human Bcl-2. As shown in Figure 4, clear bands were noted at 21 kD, corresponding to that of the Bcl-2 protein. The protein was prepared from the whole liver tissue which includes not only bile duct cells but also hepatocytes and other liver cell components. Thus, the results of western blotting could not absolutely reflect the expression of Bcl-2 in bile duct cells, but no notable changes in expression were found in precancerous liver tissues or in the ChC samples. Rather the expression of Bcl-2 was likely reduced in the ChC tissues, compared to normal tissues, which was a similar expression pattern to that of immunohistochemistry.

4. Discussion

Bcl-2 is a well-known general apoptosis suppressor that induces the formation and development of carcinomas and suppresses apoptosis. Bcl-2 is a critical factor in carcinogenesis [1], and Bcl-2 overexpression has been implicated in various tumors [6, 7, 9, 10, 19, 22]. However, Bcl-2 expression is controversial in normal liver cell components as well as in biliary cancers [8, 19]. A study by Charlotte et al. [8] reported the expression of the protein in epithelial cells of the intrahepatic small ducts, but not in hepatocytes or large bile duct cells, whereas a study by Okaro et al. [19] found no positive immunoreactivity in any of the biliary cell populations. Similarly, conflicting results have also been reported for Bcl-2 expression in association with ChC. Bcl-2 immunoreactivity occurred in more than 80% of the human ChC cases examined by Charlotte et al. [8], whereas no positive signal was found by Okaro et al. [19].

In the present study, the immunohistochemical Bcl-2 expression patterns were compared in samples obtained from hamster livers at serial cellular stages of cholangiocarcinogenesis as well as from normal livers. The results indicated heterogeneously strong expression of Bcl-2 in dysplastic bile ducts but negative to weak immunoreactivity in normal and hyperplastic small bile ducts. Despite such heterogeneous Bcl-2 expression in the biliary cell populations, overexpression of the protein in a limited number of dysplastic bile ducts suggests that it plays a role in ChC through survival of the transformed bile duct cells, which are presumably candidates for developing ChC. A high concentration of the antiapoptotic protein Bcl-2 within the biliary tree might allow cells that harbor growth promoting mutations, such as K-ras, c-erb-B-2, or c-myc mutations, to survive by evading apoptosis [15]. Furthermore, these expression patterns may explain the controversial Bcl-2 data generated by previous studies. Most studies investigating Bcl-2 expression in ChCs have reported varying degrees of Bcl-2 protein expression [8, 16, 18, 23, 24]. A study by Charlotte et al. [8] showed that the Bcl-2 protein is expressed by small bile duct epithelia in normal livers but not by hepatocytes or cells of the large duct. These authors suggested that the Bcl-2 protein is a diagnostic marker to distinguish ChC from hepatocellular carcinoma. A study by Skopelitou et al. [16] found Bcl-2 expression in normal small bile duct epithelia and in all cases of ChC, whereas it was not detected in neoplastic and dysplastic bile ducts, or normal hepatocytes. A study by Skopelitou et al. [16] also suggested that Bcl-2 appears to be a marker that distinguishes hepatocellular carcinoma from ChC. However, Bcl-2 expression in ChCs is also very controversial. A study

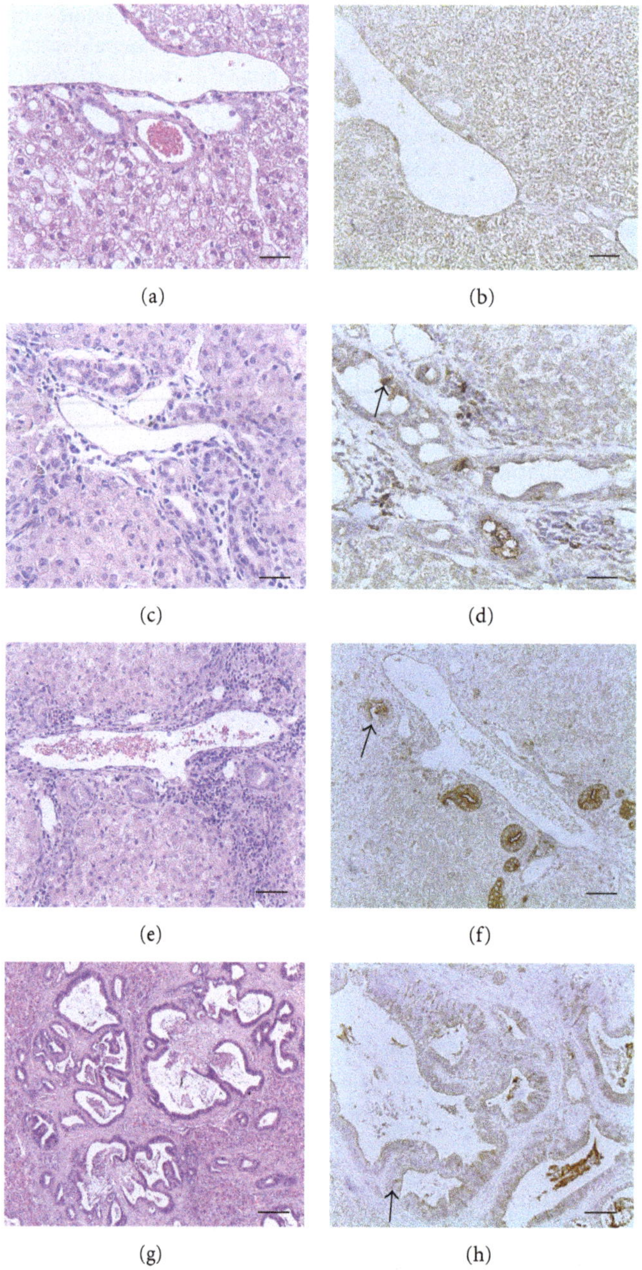

FIGURE 2: Immunohistochemistry for Bcl-2 in the liver tissue sections taken from cholangiocarcinoma (ChC) model and control group animals. (a) and (b) Normal bile ducts; (c) and (d) hyperplastic bile ducts; (e) and (f) dysplastic bile ducts; (g) and (h) cholangiocarcinoma. Bcl-2 staining was negative or weakly positive in normal and hyperplastic bile duct cells. Characteristically, Bcl-2 was heterogeneously expressed in the tissues (arrow in (d)). The Bcl-2 protein was strongly expressed in the cytoplasm of dysplastic biliary cells, although Bcl-2 expression was heterogeneous (arrow in (f)). Bcl-2 expression was negative or very weak in ChCs, similar to control levels (arrow in (h)). (a), (c), (e), and (g) hematoxylin and eosin stain; (b), (d), (f), and (h) Bcl-2 immunohistochemistry; (a)–(d) bars = 22.5 μm; (e)–(h) bars = 45 μm.

by Guo et al. [23] reported that 21 of 29 ChCs express the Bcl-2 protein (72.4%). In contrast, a study by Ito et al. [18] reported that only 31.7% (13/41) of ChCs are positive for Bcl-2 and that Bcl-2 expression was found in only 23.6% of ChCs and exhibited a strong association with tumor localization. Furthermore, some studies have reported that none of the ChC samples express Bcl-2 protein [17, 19, 20]. A study by Arora et al. [17] reported that most ChC cases did not express immunohistochemically detectable amounts of Bcl-2 protein and that its function could be performed by other proteins such as Bcl-X_L. A study by Terada and Nakanuma [20] also showed low or negative expression of Bcl-2 in bile duct epithelia and ChCs. In our paper, only 14.1% (690/4875) of small bile duct epithelia at the

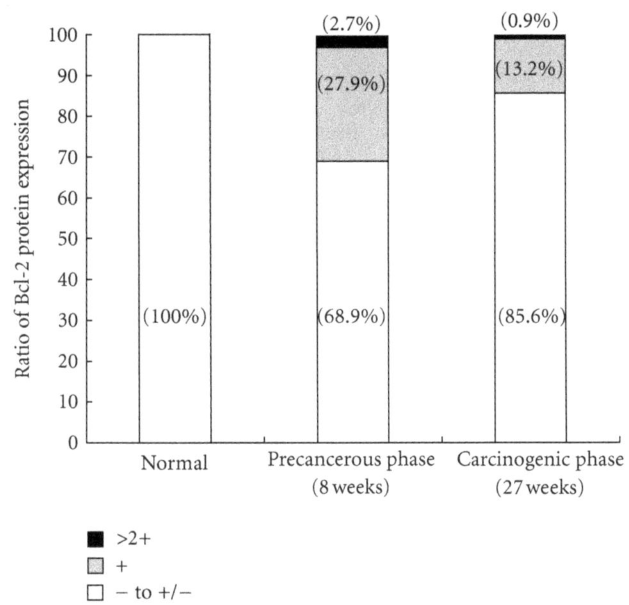

FIGURE 3: Semiquantitative analysis of Bcl-2 immunoreactivity in biliary cell populations at the precancerous and carcinogenic phases of cholangiocarcinogenesis in hamsters. The percentage of normal biliary cell populations with different grades of Bcl-2 immunoreactivity during cholangiocarcinogenesis in hamsters. The numbers on the columns represent the percentages of Bcl-2-positive cells. In total, 100, 811, and 4890 bile ducts were counted in the hamster livers at the normal, precancerous, and carcinogenic phases, respectively. Strong Bcl-2 immunoreactivity was found in some hyperplastic bile ducts with dysplastic changes at the precancerous phase. However, only <1.0% of neoplastic cells of cholangiocarcinomas indicated notable expression of Bcl-2. Normal and hyperplastic bile ducts without dysplastic changes were negative to very weak positive for Bcl-2.

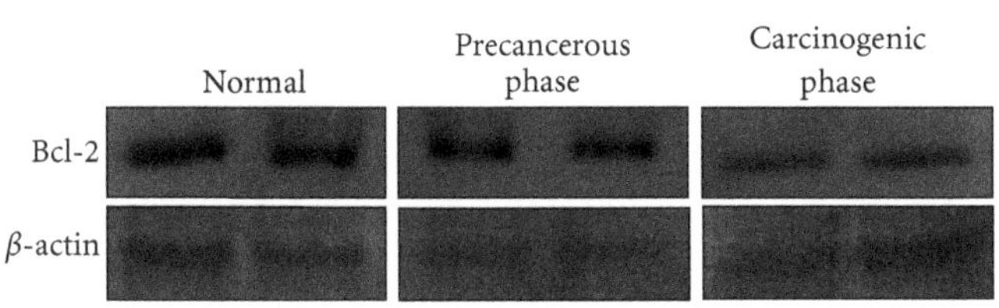

FIGURE 4: Western blot analysis for Bcl-2 in normal, precancerous, and neoplastic liver tissues in a hamster cholangiocarcinoma model. Note the specific bands made by the same antibody used for immunohistochemistry. No notable changes in the expression of Bcl-2 protein were found in the precancerous and cancerous liver tissues. The Bcl-2 expression was, compared to that of normal liver, more likely reduced in ChC tissues, which was in accordance with the results of immunohistochemistry.

carcinogenic phase were positive for Bcl-2, indicating that the role of Bcl-2 in ChCs is not very significant.

We were interested in determining what other molecules could play an important role in cancer cell survival and that are essential for tumor growth. Thus, we focused on the expression pattern of thioredoxin (Trx), a redox component and another apoptosis-inhibiting factor, during various stages of hamster and human cholangiocarcinogenesis [21]. Trx was heterogeneously expressed in hyperplastic bile ducts with morphological alterations, which was similar to the Bcl-2 expression pattern. However, unlike Bcl-2, high Trx expression continued consistently into the carcinogenic phase; Trx was overexpressed in hamster and human ChCs. We were unable to determine if an interacting relationship occurred between Bcl-2 and Trx during cholangiocarcinogenesis, but compensatory relationships between these two proteins were recently reported by Li et al. [25]. According to that study, Trx is correspondingly upregulated with Bcl-2 downregulation, following transfection of neuroblastoma cells with antisense Bcl-2. Further studies are needed to verify whether a similar relationship between Trx and Bcl-2 is involved in cholangiocarcinogenesis.

Why such a discrepancy in Bcl-2 expression is present in human ChCs as well as normal bile ducts in previous studies is still unclear but may have arisen because of the different methods used or differences in the ChC specimens. In our study, the same procedures were applied to all specimens, including fixation, tissue processing, and immunohistochemistry. The specificity of the Bcl-2 antibody used in the hamster livers was also validated by western blotting.

In summary, Bcl-2 was heterogeneously overexpressed in a limited number of dysplastic bile duct epithelial cells in a hamster ChC model, suggesting that the protein plays some role in cell survival of transformed bile duct cells. However, its role in the carcinogenic phase of ChCs was not significant in the present hamster ChC model.

Acknowledgment

This study was supported by the National Research Foundation of Korea (NRF) grant funded by the Korea government (MEST) (no. 2010-0009980) and partially by Institute of Veterinary Science of Kangwon National University.

References

[1] D. Heiser, V. Labi, M. Erlacher, and A. Villunger, "The Bcl-2 protein family and its role in the development of neoplastic disease," *Experimental Gerontology*, vol. 39, no. 8, pp. 1125–1135, 2004.

[2] N. C. Jhala, S. M. Vickers, P. Argani, and J. M. McDonald, "Regulators of apoptosis in cholangiocarcinoma," *Archives of Pathology and Laboratory Medicine*, vol. 129, no. 4, pp. 481–486, 2005.

[3] Y. Zhao, N. Zhang, and Q. Kong, "Does the cell-brain theory work in explaining carcinogenesis?" *Medical Hypotheses*, vol. 65, no. 4, pp. 708–715, 2005.

[4] A. Strasser, A. W. Harris, M. L. Bath, and S. Cory, "Novel primitive lymphoid tumours induced in transgenic mice by cooperation between myc and bcl-2," *Nature*, vol. 348, no. 6299, pp. 331–333, 1990.

[5] A. Strasser, A. W. Harris, and S. Cory, "E mu-bcl-2 transgene facilitates spontaneous transformation of early pre-B and immunoglobulin-secreting cells but not T cells," *Oncogene*, vol. 8, no. 1, pp. 1–9, 1993.

[6] T. J. McDonnell, P. Troncoso, S. M. Brisbay et al., "Expression of the protooncogene bcl-2 in the prostate and its association

with emergence of androgen-independent prostate cancer," *Cancer Research*, vol. 52, no. 24, pp. 6940–6944, 1992.

[7] Q. L. Lu, G. Elia, S. Lucas, and J. A. Thomas, "Bcl-2 proto-oncogene expression in Epstein-Barr-virus-associated nasopharyngeal carcinoma," *International Journal of Cancer*, vol. 53, no. 1, pp. 29–35, 1993.

[8] F. Charlotte, A. L'Hermine, N. Martin et al., "Immunohistochemical detection of bcl-2 protein in normal and pathological human liver," *The American Journal of Pathology*, vol. 144, no. 3, pp. 460–465, 1994.

[9] C. S. Papadimitriou, J. S. Costopoulos, B. P. Christoforidou et al., "Expression of Bcl-2 protein in human primary breast carcinomas and its correlation with multifocality, histopathological types and prognosis," *European Journal of Cancer, A*, vol. 33, no. 8, pp. 1275–1280, 1997.

[10] L. Nakopoulou, C. Vourlakou, A. Zervas, A. Tzonou, H. Gakiopoulou, and M. A. Dimopoulos, "The prevalence of bcl-2, p53, and Ki-67 immunoreactivity in transitional cell bladder carcinomas and their clinicopathologic correlates," *Human Pathology*, vol. 29, no. 2, pp. 146–154, 1998.

[11] G. Powis and W. R. Montfort, "Properties and biological activities of thioredoxins," *Annual Review of Biophysics and Biomolecular Structure*, vol. 30, pp. 421–455, 2001.

[12] T. Patel, "Cholangiocarcinoma," *Nature Clinical Practice. Gastroenterology & Hepatology*, vol. 3, no. 1, pp. 33–42, 2006.

[13] S. Isaji, Y. Kawarada, H. Taoka, M. Tabata, H. Suzuki, and H. Yokoi, "Clinicopathological features and outcome of hepatic resection for intrahepatic cholangiocarcinoma in Japan," *Journal of Hepato-Biliary-Pancreatic Surgery*, vol. 6, no. 2, pp. 108–116, 1999.

[14] A. Valverde, N. Bonhomme, O. Farges, A. Sauvanet, J. F. Flejou, and J. Belghiti, "Resection of intrahepatic cholangiocarcinoma: a western experience," *Journal of Hepato-Biliary-Pancreatic Surgery*, vol. 6, no. 2, pp. 122–127, 1999.

[15] F. Holzinger, K. Z'graggen, and M. W. Büchler, "Mechanisms of biliary carcinogenesis: a pathogenetic multi-stage cascade towards cholangiocarcinoma," *Annals of Oncology*, vol. 10, supplement 4, pp. S122–S126, 1999.

[16] A. Skopelitou, M. Hadjiyannakis, V. Alexopoulou, O. Krikoni, S. Kamina, and N. Agnantis, "Topographical immunohistochemical expression of bcl-2 protein in human liver lesions," *Anticancer Research*, vol. 16, no. 2, pp. 975–978, 1996.

[17] D. S. Arora, J. Ramsdale, J. P. A. Lodge, and J. I. Wyatt, "P53 but not bcl-2 is expressed by most cholangiocarcinomas: a study of 28 cases," *Histopathology*, vol. 34, no. 6, pp. 497–501, 1999.

[18] Y. Ito, T. Takeda, Y. Sasaki et al., "Bcl-2 expression in cholangiocellular carcinoma is inversely correlated with biologically aggressive phenotypes," *Oncology*, vol. 59, no. 1, pp. 63–67, 2000.

[19] A. C. Okaro, A. R. Deery, R. R. Hutchins, and B. R. Davidson, "The expression of antiapoptotic proteins Bcl-2, Bcl-X_L, and Mcl-1 in benign, dysplastic, and malignant biliary epithelium," *Journal of Clinical Pathology*, vol. 54, no. 12, pp. 927–932, 2001.

[20] T. Terada and Y. Nakanuma, "Utility of pancreatic digestive enzyme immunohistochemistry in the differential diagnosis of hepatocellular carcinoma, cholangiocarcinoma and metastatic adenocarcinoma of the liver," *Pathology International*, vol. 46, no. 3, pp. 183–188, 1996.

[21] B. I. Yoon, Y. H. Kim, J. Y. Yi et al., "Expression of thioredoxin during progression of hamster and human cholangiocarcinoma," *Cancer Science*, vol. 101, no. 1, pp. 281–288, 2010.

[22] F. Pezzella, H. Turley, I. Kuzu et al., "Bcl-2 protein in non-small-cell lung carcinoma," *The New England Journal of Medicine*, vol. 329, no. 10, pp. 690–694, 1993.

[23] L. L. Guo, S. Xiao, and Y. Guo, "Detection of bcl-2 and bax expression and bcl-2/JH fusion gene in intrahepatic cholangiocarcinoma," *World Journal of Gastroenterology*, vol. 10, no. 22, pp. 3251–3254, 2004.

[24] E. Karamitopoulou, L. Tornillo, I. Zlobec et al., "Clinical significance of cell cycle—and apoptosis-related markers in biliary tract cancer: a tissue microarray-based approach revealing a distinctive immunophenotype for intrahepatic and extrahepatic cholangiocarcinomas," *American Journal of Clinical Pathology*, vol. 130, no. 5, pp. 780–786, 2008.

[25] Y. Li, Z. Lu, F. Chen et al., "Antisense bcl-2 transfection upregulates anti-apoptotic and anti-oxidant thioredoxin in neuroblastoma cells," *Journal of Neuro-Oncology*, vol. 72, no. 1, pp. 17–23, 2005.

Pathogenesis and Tissue Distribution of Avian Infectious Bronchitis Virus Isolate IRFIBV32 (793/B Serotype) in Experimentally Infected Broiler Chickens

Zahra Boroomand,[1] Keramat Asasi,[1] and Ali Mohammadi[2]

[1] *Poultry Research Center, School of Veterinary Medicine, Shiraz University, Shiraz, Iran*
[2] *Department of Pathobiology, School of Veterinary Medicine, Shiraz University, Shiraz, Iran*

Correspondence should be addressed to Ali Mohammadi, mohammad@shirazu.ac.ir

Academic Editor: Marc E. Callebaut

Infectious bronchitis (IB) is one of the most important viral diseases of poultry. The aim of this study was to investigate the distribution of avian infectious bronchitis virus isolate IRFIBV32 (793/B serotype) in experimentally infected chicken. Ninety-one-day-old commercial broilers were divided randomly into two groups (seventy in the experimental and twenty in the control group). Chicks in the experimental group were inoculated intranasally with 10^5 ELD50/0.1 mL of the virus at three weeks of age. The samples from various tissues were collected at1, 2, 3, 5, 7, 11, 13, 15, and 20 days postinoculation. Chickens exhibited mild respiratory signs and depression. Viral RNA was detected in the kidney, lung and tracheas on days 1 to 13 PI, in the oviduct between, days 3 and 13, in testes between days 1 and 11 PI, and in the caecal tonsil consistently up to day 20 PI. The most remarkable clinical signs and virus detection appeared on day 1 PI. Data indicated that the number of infected chickens and viral RNA detection from tissues was reduced with increasing antibody titer on day 20 PI. The results demonstrated that the IRFIBV32 virus has wide tissue distribution for respiratory, urogenital, and digestive systems.

1. Introduction

Infectious bronchitis virus (IBV) is, by definition, the coronavirus of the domestic fowl. Although it does indeed cause respiratory disease, it also replicates at many nonrespiratory epithelial surfaces, where it may cause pathology, for example, kidney and gonads [1, 2]. Strains of the virus vary in the extent to which they cause pathology in nonrespiratory organs. Replication at enteric surfaces is considered to not normally result in clinical disease, although it does result in faecal excretion of the virus [3]. Infectious bronchitis (IB) is one of the most important diseases of chickens and continues to cause substantial economic losses to the industry. Infectious bronchitis is caused by IB virus (IBV), which is one of the primary agents of respiratory disease in chickens worldwide. All chickens are susceptible to IBV infection, and the respiratory signs include gasping, coughing, rales, and nasal discharge. Sick chicks usually huddle together and appear depressed. The severity of the symptoms in chickens is related to their age and immune status. Other signs of IB, such as wet droppings, are due to increased water consumption. The type of virus strain infecting a flock determines the pathogenesis of the disease, in other words, the degree and duration of lesions in different organs. The upper respiratory tract is the primary site of infection, but the virus can also replicate in the reproductive, renal, and digestive systems [4]. The conventional diagnosis of the IBV is based on virus isolation in embryonated eggs, followed by immunological identification of isolates. Since two or three blind passages are often required for successful primary isolation of IBV, this procedure could be tedious and time consuming [5]. Alternatively, IBV may be isolated by inoculation in chicken tracheal organ cultures. Furthermore, IBV may be detected directly in tissues of infected birds by means of immunohistochemistry [6, 7] or in situ hybridization [8]. The reverse transcription-polymerase chain reaction (RT-PCR) has proved useful in the detection of several RNA viruses [9, 10]. Outbreaks of the disease can

Table 1: RT-PCR primer sequences.

Target gene	Sequence	Size of amplicon (bp)
3′ UTR	UTR 1−: GCTCTAACTCTATACTAGCCTAT UTR 2+: AAGGAAGATAGGCATGTAGCTT	276

occur even in vaccinated flocks because there is little or no cross-protection between serotypes [2, 11]. The necessity of IB prevention in chicken regarding the nature of the virus with a high mutation rate in the S1 gene dictates the necessity to develop effective vaccines. The first step is to study the virus strains distributed in the geographical region and determine their antigenicity and pathogenicity in order to choose a suitable virus strain for vaccination. This virus was isolated from a flock suspected of IB suffering from severe respiratory distress and experiencing high mortality [12]. The objective of the present study was to clarify some aspects of pathogenesis of the disease caused by IRFIBV32 (793/B serotype) in experimentally infected broilers. RT-PCR test was performed to detect the presence of the virus in body tissues and samples. The clinical signs, gross lesions, and antibody response of the affected chicks were also monitored.

2. Materials and Methods

2.1. Virus. The virus isolate used in this study was IRFIBV32 (GenBank: HQ123359.1) [12]. It was obtained from Shiraz Veterinary University and was propagated two times in 9- to 11-day-old embryonated chicken eggs. The embryo lethal dose (ELD50) was calculated according to the Reed and Muench [13] formula.

2.2. Experimental Design. Ninety-one-day-old commercial broiler chicks were divided randomly into two groups (seventy chicks in the experimental and twenty chicks in the control group). They were reared separately in the Animal Research Unit of the Veterinary School of Shiraz University and received feed and water ad libitum during the experiment. All experiments were conducted after institutional approval of the animal use committee of Shiraz University. Prior to challenge, all birds were serologically tested using enzyme-linked immunosorbent assay (ELISA) and they were negative for antibodies to infectious bronchitis virus antigens. Furthermore, five birds from the experimental group were killed and their organs were investigated for virus detection. At the age of 20 days, all birds in the experimental group were challenged intranasally and with allantoic fluid containing 10^5 ELD50/0.1 mL of the virus. The remaining 20 birds were left as unchallenged control. All the chickens were monitored daily for 20 days for clinical signs, antibody responses to IBV, and mortality. On days 1, 2, 3, 5, 7, 11, 13, 15, and 20 postinoculation (PI), four chickens from the experimental group and two chickens from the control group were randomly selected and used for sample collection. All were bled before humanly euthanasia. Gross lesions were recorded, and their trachea, lungs, kidneys, caecal tonsil, testes, and oviduct were aseptically collected for virus detection using RT-PCR assay (Table 1). Sera of the birds were collected on 0, 5, 11, 15, and 20 days PI for ELISA test.

2.3. Extraction of Viral RNA. All tissue samples were immediately stored at −70°C until used. RNA of the samples was extracted using the Accuzol Userś Manual (BioNeer Corporation, Republic of Korea) according to the manufacturer's protocol. Briefly, appropriate tissue (50–100 mg of tissue) was homogenized with 1 mL of Accuzol, and then 200 μL chloroform was added into the mixture and the mixture was centrifuged at 12000 rpm at 4°C for 15 min. The upper phase was added to an equal volume of isopropyl alcohol and stored at −20°C for 10 min then centrifuged at 12000 rpm at 4°C for 10 min. After the washing step, by using 80% ethanol and centrifuging at 12000 rpm at 4°C for 5 min, the pellet was dissolved in a final volume of 50 μL distilled water (DW) and stored at −70°C until used.

2.4. RT-PCR. The cDNA was synthesized using AccuPowder RT PreMix kit (BioNeer Corporation, Republic of Korea) according to the manufacturer's instruction. The primers were specific for 3′ UTR gene [14]. Five μL of total RNA and one μL of each 10 pmol primer were used for cDNA preparation. PCR was performed to amplify a 276-bp fragment of the 3′ UTR gene of avian infectious bronchitis virus. The same primers were used in the PCR master mix containing: 2.5 μL PCR buffer 10X, 0.75 μL $MgCl_2$ (50 mM), 0.5 μL dNTPs (10 mM), 1 μL of each 10 pmol primer (UTR1 and UTR2), 3 μL cDNA, 15.75 μL water, and, at the end, 0.5 μL Taq DNA polymerase (5 IU/μL) was added. The program in Ependorf thermal cycler was 95°C for 3 min and 35 cycles including 95°C for 45 sec., 55.6°C for 45 sec, 72°C for 50 sec, and a postpolymerization step at 72°C for 7 min. The products were analyzed in 1% agarose gel containing ethidium bromide, using an ultraviolet transilluminator.

2.5. Serological Assay. The enzyme-linked immunosorbent assay (ELISA) technique was used to measure antibody levels to avian infectious bronchitis virus (IBV). Ten chickens in the inoculated and control groups were bled at days 0, 5, 11, 15, and 20 PI. Serum samples were collected and tested by Biochek Poultry Immunoassays Infectious Bronchitis Virus Antibody test kit (catalogue code CK119). Microtitre plates had been precoated with inactivated IBV antigen. Chicken serum samples were diluted and added to the microtitre wells where any anti-IBV antibodies and other serum proteins were then washed away. Anti-chicken IgG labeled with the enzyme alkaline phosphatase was then added to wells and bound to any chicken anti-IBV antibodies that had bound to the antigen. After another wash to remove unreacted conjugate, substrate was added in the form of

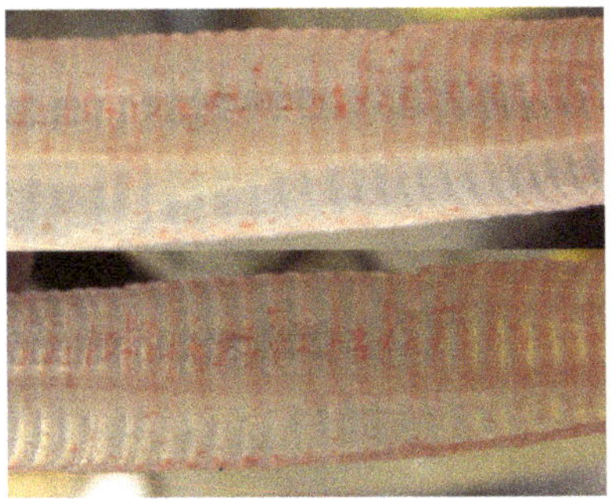

FIGURE 1: The tracheal mucosa shows slightly hyperemia and petechial hemorrhages on 1 day PI of the virus.

pNPP chromogen. A yellow color was developed if anti-IBV antibody was present, and the intensity was directly related to the amount of anti-IBV antibody present in the sample. The absorbance at 405 nm measured after 1 h in a ultra-microplate reader (Biotek, EL80).

2.6. Data Analysis. Descriptive statistics was used to summarize the data generated from the study. Data were presented as mean ± SE to compare antibody titers between the infected and the control group on different days following inoculation.

3. Results

3.1. Clinical Signs, Gross Lesions, and Mortality. Some chickens in the inoculated group showed mild tracheal rales, coughing, and gasping at 24 hours PI. The signs were less severe after 4 days PI. In addition, the birds appeared lethargic, reluctant to move from the 1st to the 4th day PI. No mortality was observed in any of the groups during the experiment. These symptoms disappeared at 4 days PI. On days 1, 2, 3, 5, 7, and 10 PI, two chickens from control group and four from test group were randomly selected; necropsied and gross lesions were recorded. Slight hyperaemia and oedema in tracheal mucosa were observed in the euthanased birds from 1 to 3 days PI (Figure 1). Pale and swollen kidneys were observed from 5 to 10 days PI. No gross lesions were observed in brain, gizzard, proventriculus, intestine, and heart muscle as well as liver and spleen. No clinical signs and gross lesions were observed in the uninfected control chickens.

3.2. Virus Distribution in Tissues following Virus Inoculation. The presence of the virus was checked in all samples obtained from the inoculated and control groups at different DPI. The RT-PCR test was performed for virus detection (Figure 2). No virus was detected from the birds killed before infection. Table 2 shows the virus distribution in tissues following virus inoculation. The virus was found in the trachea, lung, kidney, caecal tonsil consistently for 13 days PI, and also in the kidney, caecal tonsil at day 15, as well as being detected in the caecal tonsil at day 20 when the virus was not detected in any other tissue. The virus was also detected in the testes consistently for 11 days. The virus was detected on days between 3 and 13 PI from the ovary and oviduct. Virus was not found in any tissues of the control.

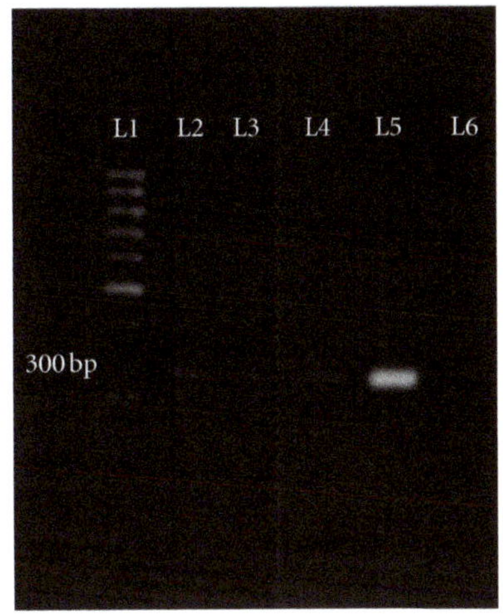

FIGURE 2: Results of the PCR assay. Amplifying 276-bp segment of 3′ UTR gene of IBV. Lane L1: DNA marker (50-bp), L5: positive control (RNA of the challenged IB virus), L6: negative control (RNA of negative chicken), L2, L3, L4, and L5: positive samples.

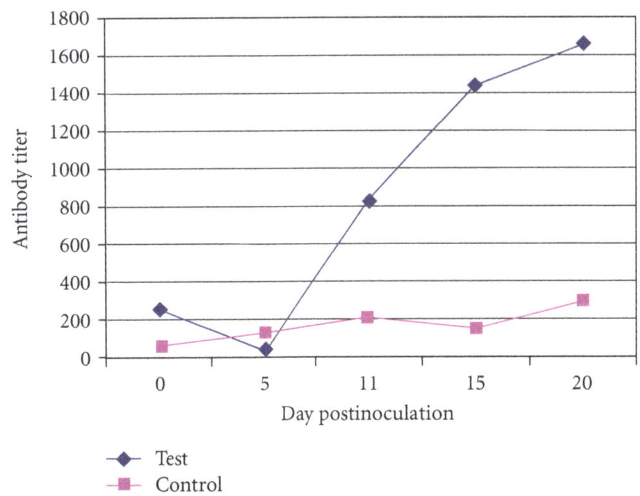

FIGURE 3: Representative graph of ELISA antibody titer against IBV of test and control group.

3.3. Serological Result. The sera from chickens of different groups were screened for antibodies levels against IBV using ELISA. For the result to be valid, the mean negative control absorbance should be read below 0.3 and the difference between the mean negative control and the mean positive control should be greater than 0.15 (titre range: 833 or less, negative antibody status, and 834 or greater, positive antibody status). Table 3 and Figure 3 show the mean antibody (Ab) titer in the challenged and control group. Increase of Ab titers occurred 11 days following inoculation. In the challenged group, sera were negative at 0, 5, and 11 days PI but they were positive (≥834) at 15 and 20 days. The Ab titer was 827.66 at 11 days, but it developed to 1657.87 at 20 days. Sera of the control was negative (≤833) on all of the days PI.

Table 2: Virus detection from various organs of chickens postinoculated (PI) of infectious bronchitis virus isolate IRFIBV32.

Time postinoculation (day)	Trachea	Lung	Kidney	Oviduct and ovary	Testis	Caecal tonsil
1	3/4*	1/4	1/4	0/2	1/2	4/4
2	4/4	3/4	2/4	0/2	2/2	4/4
3	4/4	4/4	4/4	1/2	2/2	4/4
5	4/4	4/4	4/4	2/2	1/2	4/4
7	4/4	3/4	4/4	2/2	1/2	4/4
11	4/4	3/4	4/4	1/2	2/2	4/4
13	4/4	3/4	2/4	1/2	0/2	4/4
15	0/4	0/4	2/4	0/2	0/2	3/4
20	0/4	0/4	0/4	0/2	0/2	2/4

*Number of positive/total samples.

Table 3: Comparisons of infectious bronchitis antibodies titers (ELISA) in infected and control group (mean ± SE).

Groups	DPI				
	0	5	11	15	20
Inoculated birds	245.51 ± 67.19	41.92 ± 15.62	827.66 ± 207.02	1440.14 ± 853.15	1657.87 ± 391.64
Control birds	63.30 ± 10.82	124.56 ± 41.39	205.71 ± 39.75	154.07 ± 127.67	294.67 ± 112.01

4. Discussion

In this study, the pathogenesis of the infectious bronchitis virus isolate IRFIBV32 which was recently isolated in Iran [12], tissue tropism, and dissemination of the virus throughout the body were evaluated following intranasal (IN) inoculation of commercial broiler chickens by RT-PCR.

After 24 hours postinoculation, the challenge infected chickens exhibited mild tracheal rales, coughing, and gasping. These signs were not visible from day 4 PI. In the present study, clinical signs and gross lesions were in agreement with the findings that have been described previously [15]. Twenty four hours after exposure, Purcell and McFerran [16] noted cloudy and edematous abdominal and posterior thoracic air sacs, which 3 days later thickened and filled with clear bubbly exudates. We did not observe any gross changes in the air sacs, which were thin, clear, and transparent. The lungs also appeared normal in all birds, similar to the observations of Grgić et al. [17]. In this study, IRFIBV32 induced mild lesions in trachea and kidneys. These findings are in accordance with some reported observations [17–19].

Terrigino et al. [20] reported that inoculated birds showed severe conjunctivitis, associated with abundant lacrimation, oedema, and cellulitis of the periorbital tissues at 48 hours following challenge with IBV. We observed predominant lesion in the trachea and kidneys. These results were similar to the findings that have been described previously [15, 20–22]. Diagnostic laboratories usually first isolate the virus in embryonated eggs and use the allantoic fluid to detect IBV specific RNA by RT-PCR. To reduce the time and labor needed for diagnosis, we first assessed the feasibility of the N-gene specific RT-PCR to detect the virus directly in tissues without virus isolation.

Stachowiak et al. [4] assessed the feasibility of the N-gene specific RT-PCR to detect the virus directly in tissues without virus isolation. Trachea, lung, kidney, and cecal tonsils from birds were analyzed. Representative RT-PCR results are shown, and, as expected, IB virus was detected more frequently in the tracheal tissues than in the lungs, kidney, or cecal tonsils. In the current experiment, the virus was detected from all organs of the infected birds except the oviduct at 24 hours PI. The virus was detected consistently in the trachea, lung, kidney, and caecal tonsil consistently for 13 days and persisted longer in the kidney and caecal tonsil than in the respiratory tissues. The virus disappeared from the kidney after 15 days, although it was found in the caecal tonsil and intestine consistently for 20 days PI. The virus was also detected in the testes consistently for 11 days. Previous studies confirmed IBV can also replicate in the testes [23]. The virus disappeared from the ovary and oviduct after 13 days, from testes after 11 days. These findings indicate IRFIBV32 isolate has a broad tissue distribution that includes respiratory, digestive, congenital, and urinary tract tissues; predominantly in urinary and digestive tracts. This result is in agreement with the previous studies about IBV distribution [6, 22, 24, 25]. Chen and Itakura [24] reported that the tracheal lesions recovered faster in IBV inoculated groups. The nephropathogenic property of their IBV was longer lasting than the respiratory involvement. In our investigation, virus was detected from kidneys more often than the tracheas.

Terrigino et al. [20] isolated virus from kidney, trachea, ovary, and oviduct following inoculation of the QX strain of infectious bronchitis virus. Mahdavi et al. [22] demonstrated the viral RNA antigen and tissue tropism of serotype 793/B (4/91) isolated in Iran, using the immunohistochemistry method. They reported that the 793/B serotype of IBV has a greater affinity and pathogenicity for the kidney than to other tissues, but, in our study, the distribution of viral RNA in caecal tonsils and guts was more than the other tissues. Virus detection in the caecal tonsil and intestine could indicate this isolate of IBV tropism for the digestive tract. However, in our experiment, no relevant gross lesions were detected in the digestive tract following IBV challenge. Cavanagh [3] also reported that infection of enteric tissues usually does not manifest itself clinically. Lucio and Fabricant [26] showed M41 strain can infect a variety of tissues and some isolates may be recovered frequently from the digestive tract. In another study, IBV was not detected from intestine and cecal tonsils using immunofluorescence technique [27]. Abdel-Moneim et al. [9] detected IBV antigen in the proventriculus, skin, sclera of the eye, spinal cord, and the central nervous system in infected embryos by immunohistochemistry. Lee et al. [28] investigated the tissue distribution of avian infectious bronchitis virus following in ovo inoculation of chicken embryos examined by in situ hybridization. Viral RNA was detected at 2 days after infection in epithelial cells of the trachea, lung, intestine, and bursa. In chickens, the virus has been routinely isolated from the trachea, lung, and caecal tonsils but the persistence of the virus in the bursa was of interest. Their results clearly confirm the strict epitheliotropic nature of IBV.

In this research, ELISA technique was used to measure antibody titer to IBV. ELISA detected moderate levels of the antibody to IBV on 11 days PI and high levels of antibody against IBV on day 20 PI. Sera were positive for IBV at 15 days PI. Ghadakchi et al. [29] showed that ELISA could be reliable, repeatable, and sensitive for monitoring vaccination schedules and the rapid detection of the early rise of antibodies against IB. Emikpe et al. [30] evaluated prevalence of antibodies to infectious bronchitis virus in southwestern Nigeria using ELISA. Their finding indicated that antibody titer to IBV increased following IBV infection.

Chen and Itakura [24] reported that the clinical signs and gross and histological lesions in the trachea and kidneys due to IBV infection were more severe and of longer duration in dually infected chicks (with infectious bursal disease virus and IBV) than in ones inoculated with IBV. Our field observation indicates that flocks that are infected by IBV have shown an increase in mortality in recent years that could be due to increased pathogenicity of the virus or due to other undetected field infections. This study demonstrated that IBV alone cannot cause severe and devastating disease, but IBV-infected birds can be susceptible to superinfectant bacteria and coinfection with endemic nonhighly H9N2 avian influenza virus. Future work should aim to determine if the available and used IB vaccines provide sufficient protection against this IBV isolate.

Acknowledgment

This research was funded by the Research Committee, School of Veterinary Medicine of Shiraz University, Shiraz, Iran.

References

[1] D. A. Boltz, M. Nakai, and J. M. Bahr, "Avian infectious bronchitis virus: a possible cause of reduced fertility in the rooster," *Avian Diseases*, vol. 48, no. 4, pp. 909–915, 2004.

[2] D. Cavanagh, "Severe acute respiratory syndrome vaccine development: experiences of vaccination against avian infectious bronchitis coronavirus," *Avian Pathology*, vol. 32, no. 6, pp. 567–582, 2003.

[3] D. Cavanagh, "Coronavirus avian infectious bronchitis virus," *Veterinary Research*, vol. 38, no. 2, pp. 281–297, 2007.

[4] B. Stachowiak, D. W. Key, P. Hunton, S. Gillingham, and É. Nagy, "Infectious bronchitis virus surveillance in Ontario commercial layer flocks," *Journal of Applied Poultry Research*, vol. 14, no. 1, pp. 141–146, 2005.

[5] J. K. H. Cook, J. H. Darbyshire, and R. W. Peters, "The use of chicken tracheal organ cultures for the isolation and assay of avian infectious bronchitis virus," *Archives of Virology*, vol. 50, no. 1-2, pp. 109–118, 1976.

[6] B. Y. Chen, S. Hosi, T. Nunoya, and C. Itakura, "Histopathology and immunohistochemistry of renal lesions due to infectious bronchitis virus in chicks," *Avian Pathology*, vol. 25, no. 2, pp. 269–283, 1996.

[7] K. Nakamura, J. K. A. Cook, K. Otsuki, M. B. Huggins, and J. A. Frazier, "Comparative study of respiratory lesions in two chicken lines of different susceptibility infected with infectious bronchitis virus: histology, ultrastructure and immunohistochemistry," *Avian Pathology*, vol. 20, pp. 241–257, 1991.

[8] E. W. Collisson, J. Li, L. W. Sneed, M. L. Peters, and L. Wang, "Detection of avian infectious bronchitis viral infection using in situ hybridization and recombinant DNA," *Veterinary Microbiology*, vol. 24, no. 3-4, pp. 261–271, 1990.

[9] A. S. Abdel-Moneim, P. Zlotowski, J. Veits, G. M. Keil, and J. P. Teifke, "Immunohistochemistry for detection of avian infectious bronchitis virus strain M41 in the proventriculus and nervous system of experimentally infected chicken embryos," *Virology Journal*, vol. 6, article 15, pp. 1–7, 2009.

[10] K. K. Chousalkar, B. F. Cheetham, and J. R. Roberts, "LNA probe-based real-time RT-PCR for the detection of infectious bronchitis virus from the oviduct of unvaccinated and vaccinated laying hens," *Journal of Virological Methods*, vol. 155, no. 1, pp. 67–71, 2009.

[11] D. Cavanagh, K. Mawditt, P. Britton, and C. J. Naylor, "Longitudinal field studies of infectious bronchitis virus and avian pneumovirus in broilers using type-specific polymerase chain reactions," *Avian Pathology*, vol. 28, no. 6, pp. 593–605, 1999.

[12] Z. Boroomand, I. Razeghian, K. Asasi, A. Mohammadi, and A. Hosseini, "Isolation and identification of a new isolate of avian infectious bronchitis virus IRFIBV32 and study of its pathogenicity," *Online Journal of Veterinary Research*, vol. 15, pp. 366–380, 2011.

[13] L. J. Reed and H. Muench, "A simple method of estimating fifty per cent endpoints," *American Journal of Epidemiology*, vol. 27, no. 3, pp. 493–497, 1938.

[14] A. Adzhar, K. Shaw, P. Britton, and D. Cavanagh, "Universal oligonucleotides for the detection of infectious bronchitis virus by the polymerase chain reaction," *Avian Pathology*, vol. 25, no. 4, pp. 817–836, 1996.

[15] S. Seifi, K. Asasi, A. Mohammadi, M. R. Shirzad, and M. Pourfallah, "Serological and gross findings in broilers with AIV and IBV," *Online Journal of Veterinary Research*, vol. 14, pp. 87–94, 2010.

[16] D. A. Purcell and J. B. McFerran, "The histopathology of infectious bronchitis in the domestic fowl," *Research in Veterinary Science*, vol. 13, no. 2, pp. 116–122, 1972.

[17] H. Grgić, D. B. Hunter, P. Hunton, and É. Nagy, "Pathogenicity of infectious bronchitis virus isolates from Ontario chickens," *Canadian Journal of Veterinary Research*, vol. 72, no. 5, pp. 403–410, 2008.

[18] M. A. Albassam, R. W. Winterfield, and H. L. Thacker, "Comparison of the nephropathogenicity of four strains of infectious bronchitis virus," *Avian Diseases*, vol. 30, no. 3, pp. 468–476, 1986.
[19] J. Ignjatovic, D. F. Ashton, R. Reece, P. Scott, and P. Hooper, "Pathogenicity of Australian strains of avian infectious bronchitis virus," *Journal of Comparative Pathology*, vol. 126, no. 2-3, pp. 115–123, 2002.
[20] C. Terregino, A. Toffan, M. Serena Beato et al., "Pathogenicity of a QX strain of infectious bronchitis virus in specific pathogen free and commercial broiler chickens, and evaluation of protection induced by a vaccination programme based on the Ma5 and 4/91 serotypes," *Avian Pathology*, vol. 37, no. 5, pp. 487–493, 2008.
[21] A. Gaba, H. Dave, J. K. Pal, and K. S. Prajapati, "Isolation, identification and molecular characterization of IBV variant from out break of visceral gout in commercial broilers," *Veterinary World*, vol. 3, pp. 375–377, 2010.
[22] S. Mahdavi, A. Tavasoly, S. A. Pourbakhsh, and R. Momayez, "Experimental histopathologic study of the lesions induced by serotype 793/B (4/91) infectious bronchitis virus," *Archives of Razi Institute*, vol. 62, pp. 15–22, 2007.
[23] F. Amjad, N. Hassan, and H. Arsalan, "Detection the 4/91 strain of infectious bronchitis virus in testicular tissue from experimentally infected rooster by reverse transcription-polymerase chain reaction," *African Journal of Agricultural Research*, vol. 4, no. 10, pp. 1093–1096, 2009.
[24] B. Y. Chen and C. Itakura, "Histopathology and immunohistochemistry of renal lesions due to avian infectious bronchitis virus in chicks uninoculated and previously inoculated with highly virulent infectious bursal disease virus," *Avian Pathology*, vol. 26, no. 3, pp. 607–624, 1997.
[25] D. A. Purcell, V. L. Tham, and P. G. Surman, "The histopathology of infectious bronchitis in fowls infected with a nephrotropic "T" strain of virus," *Australian veterinary journal*, vol. 52, no. 2, pp. 85–91, 1976.
[26] B. Lucio and J. Fabricant, "Tissue tropism of three cloacal isolates and Massachusetts strain of infectious bronchitis virus," *Avian Diseases*, vol. 34, no. 4, pp. 865–870, 1990.
[27] K. T. Chong and K. Apostolov, "The pathogenesis of nephritis in chickens induced by infectious bronchitis virus," *Journal of Comparative Pathology*, vol. 92, no. 2, pp. 199–211, 1982.
[28] C. W. Lee, C. Brown, and M. W. Jackwood, "Tissue distribution of avian infectious bronchitis virus following in ovo inoculation of chicken embryos examined by in situ hybridization with antisense digoxigenin-labeled universal riboprobe," *Journal of Veterinary Diagnostic Investigation*, vol. 14, no. 5, pp. 377–381, 2002.
[29] H. Ghadakchi, H. Dadras, S. A. Pourbakhsh, and S. M. H. Hosseini, "Standardization of an Enzyme-Linked Immunosorbent Assay for Detection of Infectious Bronchitis Virus Antibody," *Archives of Razi Institute*, vol. 59, pp. 75–83, 2005.
[30] B. O. Emikpe, O. G. Ohore, M. Olujonwo, and S. O. Akpavie, "Prevalence of antibodies to infectious bronchitis virus (IBV) in chickens in southwestern Nigeria," *African Journal of Microbiology Research*, vol. 4, no. 2, pp. 092–095, 2010.

17

Effects of Aflatoxin on Liver and Protective Effectiveness of Esterified Glucomannan in Merino Rams

Fatma Colakoglu and Hasan Hüseyin Donmez

Department of Histology and Embryology, Faculty of Veterinary Medicine, Selçuk University, 42075 Konya, Turkey

Correspondence should be addressed to Hasan Hüseyin Donmez, donmez68@hotmail.com

Academic Editors: J. F. Mee and W. Min

The effects of total aflatoxin (AF) given orally on liver in Merino rams were studied. In addition, this study was conducted in order to evaluate the efficacy of an esterified glucomannan (EG) for protection against aflatoxicosis. One-year-old 32 Merino rams were divided into four equal groups. The control group (C) was fed with the commercial feed. The AF group was fed with commercial feed plus 250 μg/day of total AF. The EG group was fed with commercial feed plus 2 g/day of EG. The AF + EG group was fed with commercial feed plus 250 μg/day of total AF and 2 g/day of EG. After feeding period, tissue samples were taken from the liver in order to perform histological analyses. Vacuolar degeneration with small and large droplets and hydropic degeneration in hepatocytes were observed in the AF group. The ceroid pigmentation was observed in macrophages in groups or one by one. It was observed that the fat rate in hepatocytes was 2.6% in the C group, 35.5% in the AF group, 2.9% in the EG group, and 9.6% in the AF + EG group. In conclusion, the adverse effects caused by aflatoxicosis on the liver could be ameliorated by adding EG to the ration.

1. Introduction

Mycotoxins are secondary metabolites of microscopic filamentous molds that have adverse effects on humans, animals, and crops that result in illnesses and economic losses [1]. Aflatoxins (AFs) are groups of structurally related mycotoxins produced as food-borne metabolites by toxigenic strains of *Aspergillus flavus* and *A. parasiticus* [2]. They are produced on cereal grains during growth, harvest, storage, or transportation [3]. It is well known that AFs are hepatotoxic, hepatocarcinogenic, teratogenic, mutagenic and immunosuppressive [4]. The AFs do not equally affect all animals. The environmental stress, sex, age, and breed differences play a significant role in toxicities. Some are more resistant, such as sheep and cattle, compared with swine, chickens, turkeys, and ducklings which are more susceptible [5]. The liver is the target organ following the ingestion of the toxin. High doses of AFs cause severe hepatocellular necrosis. On the other hand, prolonged low dosage leads to liver enlargements [6].

Prevention of feed and feedstuffs from possible mould growth and AF contamination is very important [7]. Practcial and cost-effective methods for detoxification of AF containing feed and feedstuff are in great demand [8]. Since the early 1990s, the adsorbent-based several studies have been performed to detoxify AF in contaminated food and foodstuffs and to minimize the deleterious effects of AF [4]. An approach to the problem has been the usage of nonnutritive and inert adsorbents in the diet to bind AF and reduce the absorption of AF from the gastrointestinal tract [9]. The nonnutritive clays such as aluminosilicates, zeolites, bentonites, and clinoptilolite were preferred by the researchers [4]. In the recent years, researchers suggested that the best approach for decontamination would be biological degradation [10]. Live yeast (*Saccharomyces cerevisiae*), initially used as a performance promoter in the early 1990s, was found to have beneficial effects on aflatoxicosis [11]. Esterified glucomannan (EG) showed considerably high binding ability (80–97%) with AF [8], and it has been preferred for detoxification of AF in poultry animals.

The aim of this study, the effects of total AF given orally on liver in Merino rams, was studied. In addition, this study was conducted in order to evaluate the efficacy of an EG for protection against aflatoxicosis.

2. Materials and Methods

2.1. Animals and Diet. Approval for the present study was obtained from the Animal Ethics Committee of the Faculty of Veterinary Medicine of the Selçuk University (2008/061). The study was created from the TUBITAK-TOVAG project entitled "Effects of Aflatoxin on Semen Quality, Testicular Histology, and Hyaluronidase Enzyme Activity, and Protective Effectiveness of Esterified Glucomannan in Ram."

Thirty-two Merino rams were approximately purchased 1-year old (12–14 months old). Animals were examined for general health. Antiparasitic ivermectin injection (Avromec-F, 1 mL/50 kg) and oxfendazole (Okzan-F, 1 tablet/50 kg) were performed. In addition, enterotoxemia (Pluritoxiven-8, 1 mL) and smallpox vaccines were performed. For adaptation to the environment and the new feeding implementation, it was applied the training program 15-days before starting the study. Individually weighted rams were divided into four equal groups. Experimental feeding was continued throughout the ninety-two days. The duration of treatment (92 days) was based on a possible cumulative toxicity and the duration of spermatogenesis and spermiogenesis in rams. The rams were fed a commercial food (Table 1). Water and alfalfa were given *ad libitum*. AF and EG that were mixed with 250 g commercial feed were given to animals before morning feeding and then morning feeding was continued.

2.2. Experimental Design. The experimental design consisted of four dietary treatments. The control group (C) was fed with the commercial feed. The AF group was fed with commercial feed plus 250 μg/day of total AF. The EG group was fed with commercial feed P 2 g/day of EG. The AF + EG groupwas fed with commercial feed plus 250 μg/day of total AF and 2 g/day of EG. The AF and EG doses which were given to animals throughout the study were calculated by pharmacologists.

2.3. Aflatoxin. The AF was produced (in the Department of Pharmacology and Toxicology, Faculty of Veterinary Medicine, Selçuk University, Konya, Turkey) from *Aspergillus parasiticus* NRLL 2999 culture (USDA, Agricultural Research Service, Peoria, IL, USA) via fermentation of rice by the method of Shotwell et al. [12] with minor modifications by Demet et al. [13]. Fermented rice was sterilized in autoclave, dried at 70°C, and ground to a fine powder. According to the method reported by Vicam [14], extraction and cleaning of AF in fermented rice was used in immunoaffinity column (Down Test; Vicam). The amount of AF measured by high performance liquid chromatography (HPLC) according to the method reported by Stroka et al. [15]. The amount of total AF in the fermented rice was found 73.96 ppm. The AF within the rice consisted of 84.15% AFB_1, 6.29% AFB_2, 9.13% AFG_1, and 4.25% AFG_2 (rate of return method 97.4%; sensitivity 0.4 ppb).

Table 1: Composition of the commercial feed.

Dry matter	88%
Crude protein	12%
Crude cellulous	12%
Crude ash	9%
Insoluble ash in HCL	1.0%
Ca	0.6–1.6%
P	0.4%
Na	0.1–0.4%
NaCl	1.0%
Metabolic energy	2750 kcal/kg
Vit A	7000 IU-kg
Vit D3	700 IU-kg
Vit E	25 mg/kg

2.4. Collection and Processing of Tissue Samples. At the end of the 92th day, liver tissue samples were taken from rams after scarification and were fixed in 10% neutralized buffered formaldehyde, embedded in paraffin wax, and then stained with Crosman's modification of trichrome stain in order to determine the histological structure [16]. In addition, in order to determine fat rate in hepatocytes, liver samples were determined along 16 hours in formol-calcium solution, at +4°C, and dark. Sections (12 μm) were taken from cryostat, and these were stained with Sudan Black B stain [17]. Fat rate in hepatocytes was determined with the method reported by Gaal et al. [18].

2.5. Statistical Analysis. The obtained results (ratio of fatty liver) were statistically analyzed using Duncan's multiple range test in SPSS software (version 17; SPSS Inc., Chicago, IL, USA). The level of significance was $P < 0.05$.

3. Results

Histopathologically, no specific lesion was observed in liver tissues from the C (Figure 1) and EG groups. In the AF group specific lesions were seen in liver. Vacuolar degeneration with small and large droplets (Figure 2) and hydropic degeneration (Figure 2) in hepatocytes, local hyperemia, marked sinusoidal contraction, and a few hepatocytes with pyknotic nuclei in lobules were noticed. Furthermore, the ceroid pigmentation (Figure 2) was observed in macrophages and local hemorrhage areas around central vein. In the AF+EG group was seen a mononuclear cell infiltration in portal areas (Figure 3). Specific lesions like ceroid pigmentation and vacuolar degeneration in this group were not seen. It was found that fat rate in hepatocytes (Table 2) was 2.6% in the C group, 35.5% in the AF group, 9.6% in the AF + EG group and 2.9% in the EG group.

TABLE 2: Fat rate in hepatocytes (%).

Groups ($n = 8$)	C	AF	EG	AF+EG
Fat rate (%)	2.63 ± 0.21^c	35.50 ± 0.65^a	2.94 ± 0.25^c	9.63 ± 0.98^b

C: control, AF: aflatoxin, EG: glucomannan, AF + EG: aflatoxin + glucomannan.
^{a,b,c}are significantly different ($P < 0.05$).

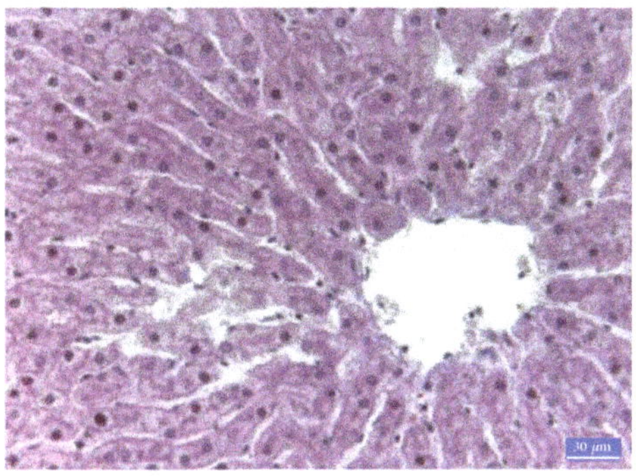

FIGURE 1: Normal histological appearance of the liver in the control group, 3rd region, trichrome staining.

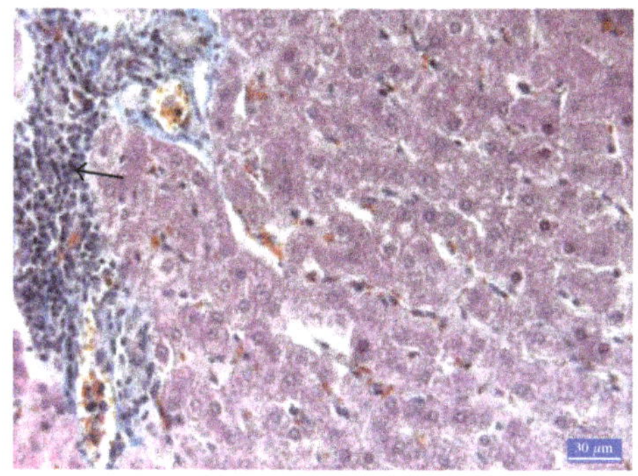

FIGURE 3: Mononuclear cell infiltration in portal areas in the AF + EG group (arrows), trichrome staining.

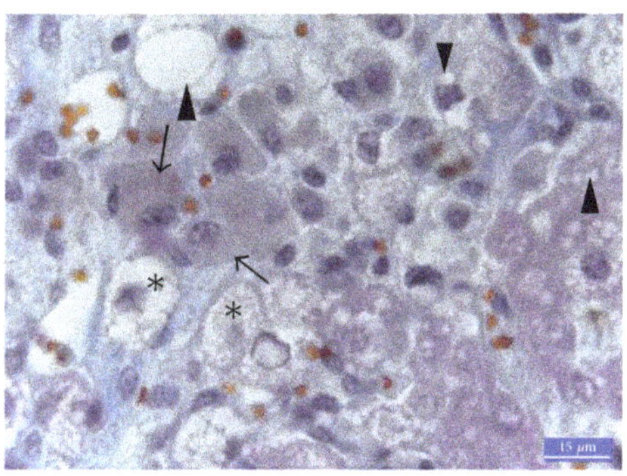

FIGURE 2: Liver histology from an animal contaminated with AF (250 μg/day of total AF, AF group). Macrophages containing ceroid pigment (arrows), severe vacuolar degeneration in hepatocytes (arrowheads), and hydropic degeneration (stars) in the AF group, 3rd region, trichrome staining.

4. Discussion

The liver is considered the main target organ for aflatoxicosis [10]. Lakkawar et al. [6] reported that liver was the most affected organ in rabbits fed an AFB_1 contaminated diet. The effects of AFs on histopathological changes are directly correlated with the concentration of AF and the duration of the exposure [19]. The vacuolar hepatocellular change in animals that were fed 1.6 ppm AFB_1 diet continuously throughout 40 weeks was more than animals that were fed diets that contained 0, 0.01, 0.04, 0.4, or 1.6 ppm AFB_1, using an intermittent dosing regimen, 4 weeks on and 4 weeks off AFB_1 [20]. In this study, it was observed that 250 μg/day AF caused significant histopathological changes in liver in 92 days.

Histopathological findings that were caused by AFs in liver were reported as enlarged nuclei, nuclear inclusions, and swollen hepatocytes [19]. Enlarged hepatocytes can arise from stored metabolism products as a result of shown activities when these cells perform metabolic activities [21], and the AF metabolites arising from the effects of some of the enzymes which react with hepatocyte DNA are thought to be caused by mutations in the nucleus [22]. Yıldırım et al. [10] saw that some hepatocytes nuclei were pyknotic and there was nucleus loss in some hepatocytes in the AF group. In this study, we also found a similar finding. A study of Ozen et al. [7] found apparently a dose-dependent mild to severe vacuolar degeneration with irregularly shaped vacuoles in hepatocytes; most of the hepatocytes also contained sharply edged vacuoles that were a sign of fatty accumulation. Kıran et al. [23] reported that hepatic lesions in broilers of the AF-treated group were characterized as diffuse and severe hydropic degeneration and periportal fibrosis. In this study, we also observed vacuolar and hydropic degeneration similar to previous studies [7, 23]. It was reported that vacuolar degeneration could be due to impaired lipid transport rather than increased lipid biosynthesis [24].

By histological examination of livers in the AF group, Lakkawar et al. [6] observed vascular congestion (up to 30 days), areas of coagulative necrosis around the central veins, and engorged portal areas (from the 40th day onwards) in rabbits. Abdel-Wahhab et al. [25] reported vascular dilation, congestion, and moderate hemorrhages in rats. Hemorrhages in animals of the AF group have also been reported in other studies [26, 27]. Although Salim et al. [28] reported dilated sinusoids depending on the hepatocytes necrosis as a result of aflatoxicosis, we observed sinusoidal contraction depending on the enlargement and swelling of hepatocytes. This finding was in agreement with that reported by Uopasai et al. [29]. Hyperemia was noted where there can be seen sinusoids. Dilation of arterioles causes hyperemia due to increased blood to the tissue depending on inflammation [30].

Some researchers have reported cellular disorganization characterized by the accumulation of pigments [19]. In cat's liver which has primary hepatic lipidosis, Gul et al. [31] have seen ceroid pigmentation which is Periodic Acid Schiff (PAS) positive, freely or shaped yellow large droplets in cytoplasm of hepatocyte/Kupffer cells, and more intense in the periportal areas of the liver. In the AF group, we also found hepatocytes and Kupffer's cells which were more intense around the central vein showing ceroid pigmentation. This station is a result of impaired lipid metabolism and severity steatosis [32].

AFs affect primarily the cellular immunity process in most animal species [4]. In the AF-exposed chickens, Yıldırım et al. [10] have declared mild mononuclear cell infiltration in the liver's portal areas. In this study, we also observed a similar finding in the AF + EG group. Small inflammatory cell infiltrates composed of lymphocytes, plasma cells, mononuclear cells, and few segmented neutrophils occur to respond to degenerate vacuolated hepatocytes [20].

In this study, histopathological findings obtained from the AF+EG group are close to the C group. This result has shown that EG is an important adsorbent in decreasing the detrimental effects of AFs. This finding was in agreement with the previous reports [8, 10, 19].

AF causes impaired lipid transport [24]. The data obtained from this study have also shown that AFs cause fatty liver in rams as in other animals [33]. Furthermore, it has been shown EG decreased significantly that fat rate in hepatocytes and the detrimental effects of AF.

5. Conclusion

In conclusion, the adverse effects AF impaired on histological structure of the liver that caus fatty liver could be ameliorated by adding EG to the ration. We conclude EG is an agent which can be used successfully to prevent aflatoxicosis.

Acknowledgments

The study was supported by TÜBİTAK-TOVAG (Project no. 107 O 866) and the Coordinatorship of Scientific Research Projects of Selcuk University (SU BAP Project no. 09202023).

References

[1] H. S. Hussein and J. M. Brasel, "Toxicity, metabolism, and impact of mycotoxins on humans and animals," *Toxicology*, vol. 167, no. 2, pp. 101–134, 2001.

[2] R. J. Verma, "Aflatoxin cause DNA damage," *International Journal of Human Genetics*, vol. 4, no. 4, pp. 231–236, 2004.

[3] M. H. Salem, K. I. Kamel, M. I. Yousef, G. A. Hassan, and F. D. El-Nouty, "Protective role of ascorbic acid to enhance semen quality of rabbits treated with sublethal doses of aflatoxin B1," *Toxicology*, vol. 162, no. 3, pp. 209–218, 2001.

[4] H. Oguz, H. H. Hadimli, V. Kurtoglu, and O. Erganis, "Evaluation of humoral immunity of broilers during chronic aflatoxin (50 and 100 ppb) and clinoptilolite exposure," *Revue de Medecine Veterinaire*, vol. 154, no. 7, pp. 483–486, 2003.

[5] J. L. Richard, "Discovery of aflatoxins and significant historical features," *Toxin Reviews*, vol. 27, pp. 171–201, 2008.

[6] A. W. Lakkawar, S. K. Chattopadhyay, and T. S. Johri, "Experimental aflatoxin B1 toxicosis in young rabbits-a clinical and patho-anatomical study," *Slovenian Veterinary Research*, vol. 41, no. 2, pp. 73–81, 2004.

[7] H. Ozen, M. Karaman, Y. Cigremis et al., "Effectiveness of melatonin on aflatoxicosis in chicks," *Research in Veterinary Sciences*, vol. 86, pp. 485–489, 2009.

[8] H. Basmacioglu, H. Oguz, M. Ergul, R. Col, and Y. O. Birdane, "Effect of dietary esterified glucomannan on performance, serum biochemistry and haematology in broilers exposed to aflatoxin," *Czech Journal of Animal Science*, vol. 50, no. 1, pp. 31–39, 2005.

[9] H. Oguz, "A review from experimental trials on detoxification of aflatoxin in poultry feed," *Eurasian Journal of Veterinary Sciences*, vol. 27, no. 1, pp. 1–12, 2011.

[10] E. Yıldırım, I. Yalcınkaya, M. Kanbur et al., "Effects of yeast glucomannan on performance, some biochemical parameters anf pathological changes in experimental aflatoxicosis in broilers chickens," *Revue de Medecine Veterinaire*, vol. 162, no. 8-9, pp. 413–420, 2011.

[11] V. G. Stanley, R. Ojo, S. Woldesenbet, D. H. Hutchinson, and L. F. Kubena, "The use of Saccharomyces cerevisiae to suppress the effects of aflatoxicosis in broiler chicks," *Poultry Science*, vol. 72, no. 10, pp. 1867–1872, 1993.

[12] O. L. Shotwell, C. W. Hasseltine, R. D. Stubblefield et al., "Production of aflatoxin on rice," *Applied Microbiology*, vol. 5, pp. 425–429, 1966.

[13] O. Demet, H. Oguz, I. Celik et al., "Pirincte aflatoksin uretilmesi," *Veteriner Bilimler Dergisi*, vol. 11, no. 1, pp. 19–23, 1995.

[14] L. P. Vicam, "Fluorometer USDA-FGIS prodecure for corn, corn meal, corn/soy blend, milled rice, popcorn, sorghum and soybeans," *Aflatest Instruction Manuel*, pp. 36–38, 1999.

[15] J. Stroka, R. V. Otterdijk, and E. Anklam, "Immunoaffinity column clean-up prior to thin-layer chromatography for the determination of aflatoxins in various food matrices," *Journal of Chromatography A*, vol. 904, no. 2, pp. 251–256, 2000.

[16] I. Ustunel and R. Demir, *Histolojik Boyama Teknikleri*, Palme Yayıncılık, Ankara, Turkey, 2001.

[17] K. L. Burdon, "Fatty material in bacteria and fungi revealed by staining dried, fixed slide preparations," *Journal of Bacteriology*, vol. 52, pp. 665–678, 1946.

[18] T. Gaal, I. M. Reid, and R. A. Collins, "Comparison of biochemical and histological methods of estimating fat content of liver of dairy cows," *Research in Veterinary Science*, vol. 34, no. 2, pp. 245–248, 1983.

[19] A. S. Baptista, A. L. Abdalla, C. L. Aguiar et al., "Utilization of diets amended with yeast and amino acids for the control of aflatoxicosis," *World Journal of Microbiology and Biotechnology*, vol. 24, no. 11, pp. 2547–2554, 2008.

[20] D. M. Hinton, M. J. Myers, R. A. Raybourne et al., "Immunotoxicity of aflatoxin B1 in rats: effects on lymphocytes and the inflammatory response in a chronic intermittent dosing study," *Toxicological Sciences*, vol. 73, no. 2, pp. 362–377, 2003.

[21] O. Nunez, J. D. Hendricks, and G. S. Bailey, "Enhancement of aflatoxin B1 and N-methyl-N'-nitro-N-nitrosoguanidine hepatocarcinogenesis in rainbow trout Salmo gairdneri by 17-β-estradiol and other organic chemicals," *Diseases of Aquatic Organisms*, vol. 5, pp. 185–196, 1988.

[22] H. M. Shen, C. N. Ong, and C. Y. Shi, "Involvement of reactive oxygen species in aflatoxin B1-induced cell injury in cultured rat hepatocytes," *Toxicology*, vol. 99, no. 1-2, pp. 115–123, 1995.

[23] M. M. Kıran, O. Demet, M. Ortatatlı et al., "The preventive effect of polyvinypolypyrrolidone on aflatoxicosis in broilers," *Avian Pathology*, vol. 27, no. 3, pp. 250–255, 1998.
[24] M. McLean and M. F. Dutton, "Cellular interactions and metabolism of aflatoxin: an update," *Pharmacology and Therapeutics*, vol. 65, no. 2, pp. 163–192, 1995.
[25] M. A. Abdel-Wahhab, S. A. Nada, and F. A. Khalil, "Physiological and toxicological responses in rats fed aflatoxin-contaminated diet with or without sorbent materials," *Animal Feed Science and Technology*, vol. 97, no. 3-4, pp. 209–219, 2002.
[26] D. C. Baker and R. A. Green, "Coagulation defects of aflatoxins in toxicated rabbits," *Veterinary Pathology*, vol. 24, pp. 62–70, 1987.
[27] R. Dafalla, A. Yagi, and S. Adam, "Experimental aflatoxicosis in hybro-type chicks: sequential changes in growth and serum constituents and histopathological changes," *Veterinary and Human Toxicology*, vol. 29, pp. 222–225, 1987.
[28] A. B. Salim, A. Zohair, A. E. S. Hegazy et al., "Effect of some strains of probiotic bacteria against toxicity induced by aflatoxins in vivo," *The Journal of American Science*, vol. 7, no. 1, pp. 1–12, 2011.
[29] S. Uopasai, K. Pimpukdee, B. Tengjaroenkul et al., "Effect of natural charcoal powder added in swine feeds as aflatoxin adsorbents on improving performance of swine production and histopathological changes of swine livers," *KKU Veterinary Journal*, vol. 18, no. 2, pp. 109–119, 2008.
[30] T. Unal, *Hemodinamik Bozukluklar*, Ege Üniversitesi Diş Hekimliği Fakültesi, 2012.
[31] Y. Gul, O. Kızıl, and A. O. Ceribası, "Bir kedide primer hepatik lipidozis olgusu," *Fırat Üniversitesi Sağlık Bilimleri Veteriner Dergisi*, vol. 20, no. 5, pp. 375–378, 2006.
[32] U. H. Milli and R. Hazıroglu, *Veteriner Patoloji*, Medisan, Ankara, Turkey, 2000.
[33] Z. Yener, I. Celik, F. Ilhan, and R. Bal, "Effects of Urtica dioica L. seed on lipid peroxidation, antioxidants and liver pathology in aflatoxin-induced tissue injury in rats," *Food and Chemical Toxicology*, vol. 47, no. 2, pp. 418–424, 2009.

18

Ultrasonograph and Clinical Quantitative Characterization of Tendinopathy by Modified Splitting in a Goat Model

A. Kavaguchi De Grandis, C. Boulocher, E. Viguier, T. Roger, and S. Sawaya

Université de Lyon et VetAgro Sup, Campus Vétérinaire de Lyon, UPSP ICE, 69280 Marcy l'Etoile, France

Correspondence should be addressed to A. Kavaguchi De Grandis, kavaguchi@gmail.com and C. Boulocher, caroline.boulocher@vetagro-sup.fr

Academic Editors: F. Frauscher, D. S. Gardner, H. Omoe, and V. Vindigni

A tendinopathy is a clinical condition characterized by activity-related pain, focal tendons tenderness, and intratendinous imaging changes. This study characterizes a surgically induced tendinopathy in a goat model with a noninvasive *in vivo* longitudinal followup based on physical examination and US. Cross-sectional area (CSA) is the most objective feature for the evaluation of tendinopathy in correlation with clinical findings. The deep digital flexor tendon (DDFT) of the left hind limb of six goats was isolated and scarified by a modified splitting. Pain and lameness at walk and trot were evaluated. External width and thickness of tendon region were measured by calipers. CSA and the ratio lesion/tendon CSA were obtained at days 0, 7, 21, 42, and 84 by US. The highest value of global functional score was obtained at day 7, then decreased until day 40 and was not significantly different from day 0 at the end of the study. The external width recovered a normal value at the end of the study, but the external thickness was still significantly increased ($P < 0.05$). Peritendinous oedema was observed at day 7, but intratendinous lesions were visible only at day 21 as a focal hypo to anechoic area. At day 84, two tendons still presented visible lesions. US examination was reproducible, specific, and provided complementary information to the global functional score. A standardized focal tendinopathy was induced in goats. This experimental model of focal tendinopathy could be used to study the effect of different treatments.

1. Background

A tendinopathy is a clinical condition characterised by activity-related pain, focal tendons tenderness, and intratendinous imaging changes requiring a recovery time of at least three to six months with first-line conservative management [1, 2].

In human and veterinary medicine, the musculoskeletal system is of special interest, as its damages are often fatal for adequate sportive performance. The incidence of tendinitis in sport horses has been reported to be between 11% and 46%, and recurrent injuries were found in 43 to 90% of the cases [3–5].

Injuries to the distal aspect of the limbs are common in horses and frequently involve injury of the flexor and/or extensor tendons [4, 6].

There is no consensus on a "gold standard" among the experimental models of tendinopathy: model requirements change as knowledge of the disease increases. Nonhuman primates, horses, goats, dogs, rabbits, rats, and mice have previously been used [1, 7]. Large animal models present the advantage to having naturally occurring tendonitis [1]. In addition, clinical examination and lameness assessment are easier to perform on large rather than on small animals.

Tendinopathies can be induced chemically by intratendinous injection of collagenase, PGE1, PGE2, corticosteroid, or cytokines [1, 7–9]. Recently new models have been developed *ex vivo*: cyclical loading, creep loading, and stress deprivation, and *in vivo*: electrical muscle stimulation, downhill and uphill treadmill running, fatigue loading, and disuse [7]. A surgical model (tenectomy) has been described in goats to study acute tendon rupture and healing [10].

In human and veterinary medicine, the usefulness of ultrasonography (US) in the diagnosis and in the characterisation of soft tissues injuries of the locomotor system has been widely demonstrated [11–15]. It is considered as an

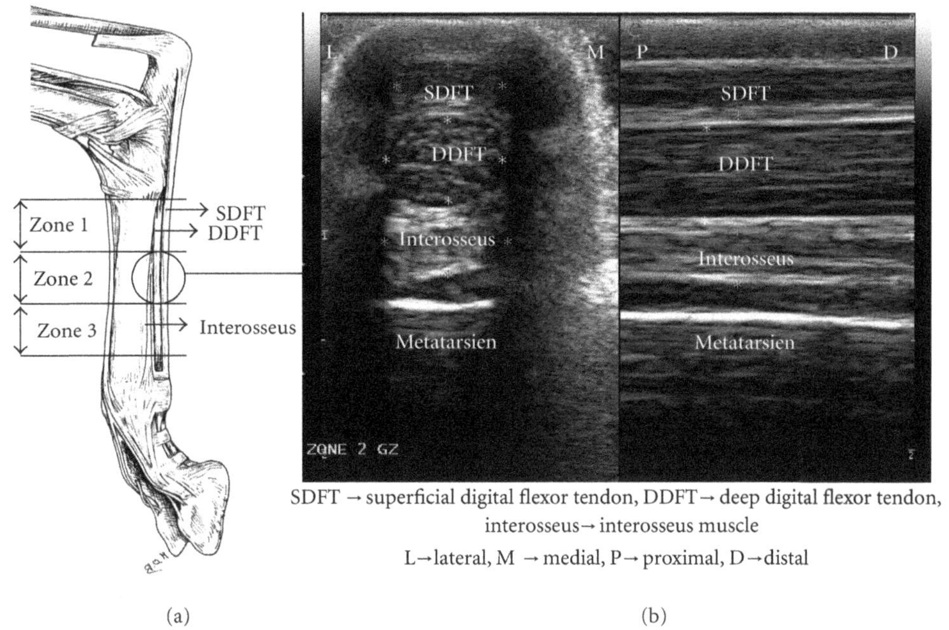

FIGURE 1: (a), anatomy of the goat's hind limb. (b), transversal and longitudinal US images of zone 2.

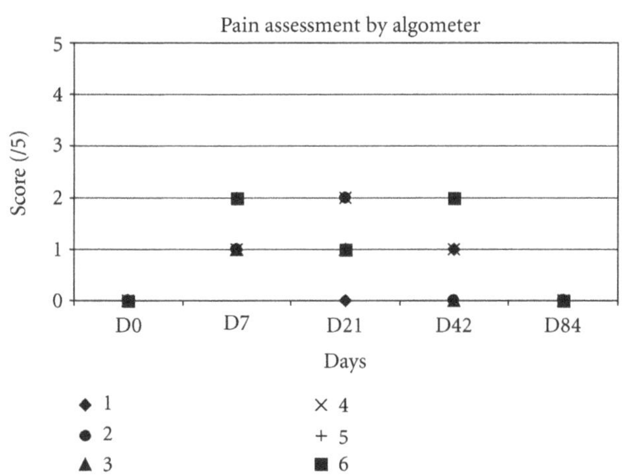

FIGURE 2: Pain assessment by algometer.

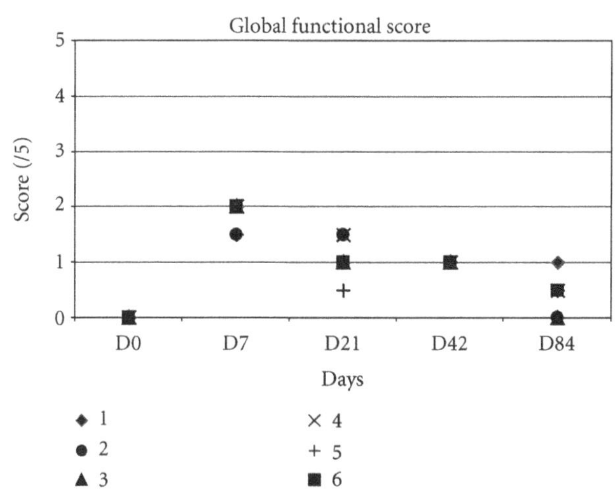

FIGURE 3: Global functional score of lameness.

essential imaging modality to evaluate the healing process of tendon lesions [15–17], and its real-time dynamic capability offers a major advantage compared with other imaging techniques [11]. US allows early detection of tendons lesions and the evaluation of their surrounding, in particular, synovial sheath lesions [18]. Analyses of US images use both quantitative and qualitative measurements to assess injuries, including echogenicity, fibre alignment, size, shape, margination, and tendon position. Cross-sectional area (CSA) is the most objective feature for the evaluation tendon pathology and can be assessed accurately with US [19–21].

US is also used to adjust exercises programmes during rehabilitation, with adaptation of the treatment for specific injuries [14] and to determine the readiness return to exercise and competition [12]. According to Reef 1998 [22], a CSA increase of more than 10% is suggestive of reinjury during the rehabilitation period. Nevertheless, the diagnostic values of imaging findings have to be correlated with the clinical findings [23].

The present study is part of a larger investigation on an experimental tendinopathy in a goat model. The objectives were to use US to establish the normal CSA of the metatarsal region of the goat model and to perform a noninvasive longitudinal followup of the tendon injury and healing (physical examination and US).

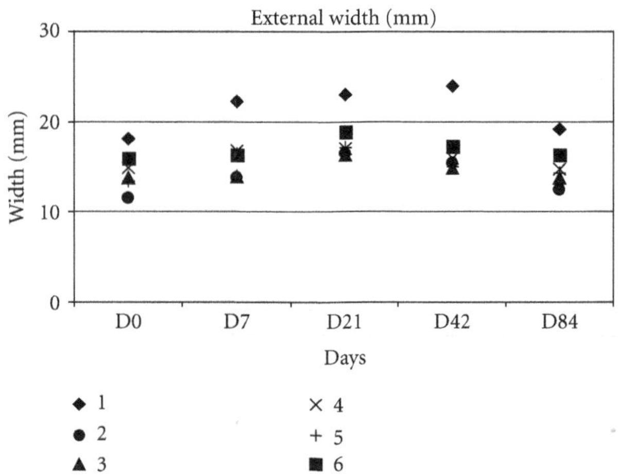

FIGURE 4: Change in external width.

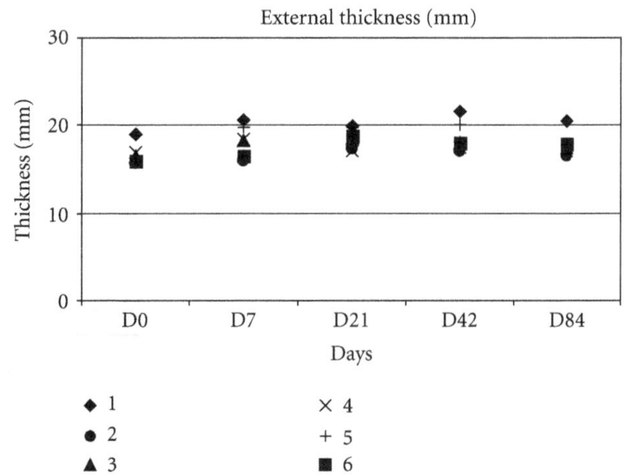

FIGURE 5: Change in external thickness.

2. Methods

The study was approved by the Ethical Committee on Animal Experiments of VetAgro Sup, Lyon, France (No. 1020/2010).

2.1. Animal Experimental Model. Six female adult goats weighing around 55 Kg and aged between 2 and 6 years old were used in the study. The goats were group-housed in a paddock at the Institut Claude-Bourgelat, Marcy l'Etoile, France, with hay and water ad libitum. Preentrance sanitary exams were performed to make certain goats not affected by any pathology which could interfere with the study. The acclimation period was of 21 days. Then, to induce a surgical focal tendinopathy, a modified splitting was performed on the left hindlimb deep digital flexor tendon (DDFT) in the metatarsal region.

2.2. Surgical Procedure. Goats were premedicated by subcutaneous injection of buprenorphine (0.02 mg/Kg). Anaesthesia was induced by intramuscular injection of a combination of xylazine (Rompun 2%, Bayer, 0.05 mg/kg) and ketamine (Imalgene 1000, Merial, 2.5 mg/kg) and maintained with isoflurane 2% in oxygen after intubation. Goats were given prophylactic antibiotic therapy prior to surgery by intramuscular injection of amoxicillin (15 mg/kg).

The left hind limb was operated on under sterile conditions. A three centimetre incision was made on the skin at the middle of the metatarsal region on the plantaro-lateral aspect. Then the DDFT was isolated and scarified as follows: 1/longitudinal splitting (1 cm) of the tendon and of the tendon sheath, 2/360 degrees rotation of the scalpel which created a "window" within the tendon fibres. All animals were operated on by the same person, using exactly the same technique.

The surgical wound was closed by separated points with Ethylon 2-0 and cleaned with vetedine solution (vetoquinol). The operated limb was then immobilized with a thick, well-packed compression bandage (Robert Jones type) for four days. The nonoperated limb was not immobilized. Goats were allowed free activity in their paddock and veterinarians closely monitored their recovery. Postoperative analgesia was managed by a 0.02 mg/Kg subcutaneous injection of buprenorphine twice a day for two days. See Figure 1.

TABLE 1: A global functional score was calculated based on lameness at walk and trot and normalized (score of lameness at walk + score of lameness at trot)/2.

Score of lameness—walk and trot [26]	
0	Normal (without lameness)
1	Discrete lameness (lameness barely visible and intermittent)
2	Obvious lameness (visible lameness)
3	Severe lameness (evident lameness)
4	Lameness with intermittent support removal
5	Constant support removal

2.3. Clinical Followup

2.3.1. Pain Assessment. Pain threshold was defined as the minimum pressure applied through the 1 cm^2 tip that induced pain, as described by Rompe et al. [24, 25], at the level of zone 2 with an algometer (Dolormeter, EMS, Nyons Suisse). The essence of pressure algometry is that increasing pressure applied to the part of the body to be investigated, and the outcome is the patient's reaction to the pressure. The algometer was calibrated to give an integer between 0 and 5 (5: no pain, 0: maximal pain).

Lameness at walk and trot was evaluated semi-quantitatively according to Millis [26], Table 1.

A global functional score was calculated based on lameness at walk and trot and normalized (score of lameness at walk + score of lameness at trot)/2.

External width (distance between the skin and the plantar edge of the metatarsus) and thickness (distance skin to skin from medial to lateral) of the region of tendons were measured at the level of the surgery to follow up oedema and inflammation. The same person performed all the

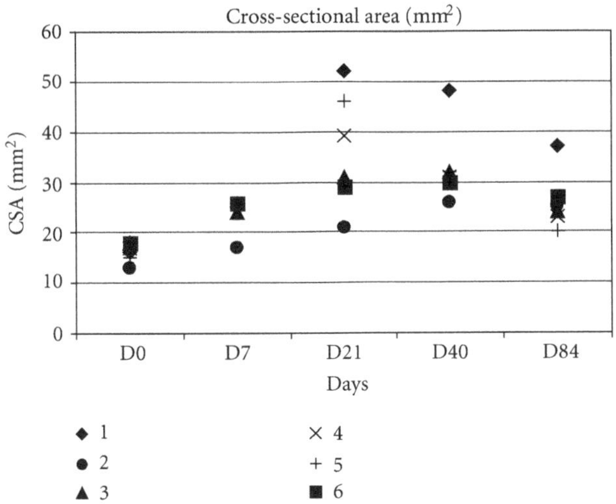

Figure 6: Change in CSA.

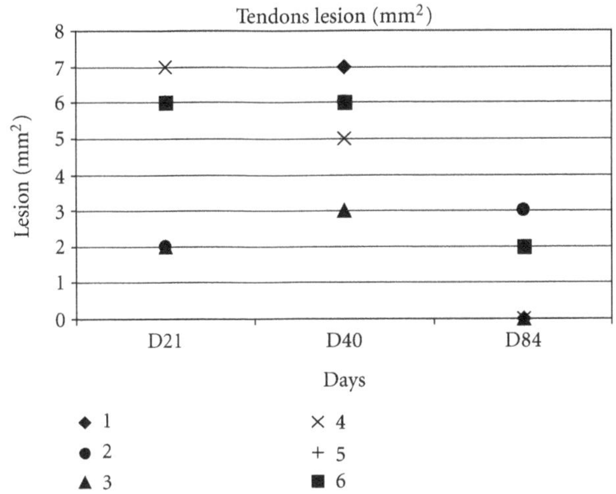

Figure 7: Change in measurements of tendon's lesion.

measurements with a digital calliper ("Casto" 0–150 mm, Castorama, 59175 Templemars, France).

2.4. *In Vivo Ultrasonography (US)*

2.4.1. US Protocol. Ultrasonography of the operated limb was performed *in vivo* without sedation prior to the surgery at days 0 and then 7, 21, 42, and 84 days after the surgery. A protocol for US of the goat metatarsal region was created and standardised, based on the routine US examination protocol used for horse metatarsal region at VetAgro Sup. US examinations were performed with a MyLab70 X-Vision (Esaote) with a linear probe (6 to 18 MHz—Diasus Dynamic Imaging Ltd). Left metatarsal region was clipped; isopropyl alcohol and ultrasound coupling gel were applied to ensure good contact between the skin and the transducer. Examinations were performed with the goats weight-bearing on all four limbs.

Each metatarsal region was divided into three main zones of equal size from the tarsometatarsal joint to the bifurcation of the DDFT, that is, above the ergots. Zone 1 covered the proximal third of the metatarsal region; Zone 3 covered the distal third; Zone 2 was in between and corresponded to the splitting and to the examined zone. US exam was performed before surgery for each animal to record a control image.

2.4.2. US Measurement of the DDFT Lesion. In Zone 2, quantitative measurements of the cross-sectional areas (CSA) of DDFT were done. The measurement was performed when the image showed the smallest CSA (i.e., when the ultrasound probe was perpendicular to the tendon thus preventing from the anisotropic artefact). The lesion areas were measured and the ratio lesion/tendon cross-sectional areas were recorded for each tendon. Measurements and ratio were calculated directly on the US machine's software.

Examinations were carried out by the same operator to avoid interobserver error. The lesion was tagged on the images to help for the next examination and to assure repeatability.

2.5. Statistics. The data were statistically analysed with Excel (Microsoft Office) and R 2.11 for Windows. The effect of time was assessed by comparison of values between the different time points using paired t-test when distribution was normal and Wilcoxon test when it was abnormal.

3. Results

All animals were operated on under the same conditions. Their waking was calm and uneventful. No wounds complications were observed after surgery. All the goats completed the study. The operated area of tendon could be identified and followed up by the same methods for all animals.

3.1. Clinical Examination. The results of local pain assessment are displayed in (Figure 2).

No animal showed local pain before surgery. At day 7, the highest value of pain was obtained with a significant difference compared to day 0 ($P < 0.05$). Between days 7 and 21, the scores stayed high and then decreased progressively until the end of the study when they returned to zero.

The global functional scores are displayed in (Figure 3).

All goats presented the highest score of lameness at day 7 with a significant difference compared to day 0 ($P < 0.05$). Between day 7 and 84, they presented a diminution of their scores. And at day 84, there was no difference compared to day 0.

Measurements of external width and thickness are represented in (Figures 4 and 5).

At day 0, the external width of zone 2 was 14.59 ± 2.26 mm, increased until day 21 (18.13 ± 2.58 mm), and then decreased until the end of the study (17.09 ± 3.46 mm at day 42 and 15.11 ± 2.33 mm at day 84). The difference was significant between day 7 and day 0 ($P = 0.03$) but not significant between days 7 and 42 ($P > 0.3$ between days 42

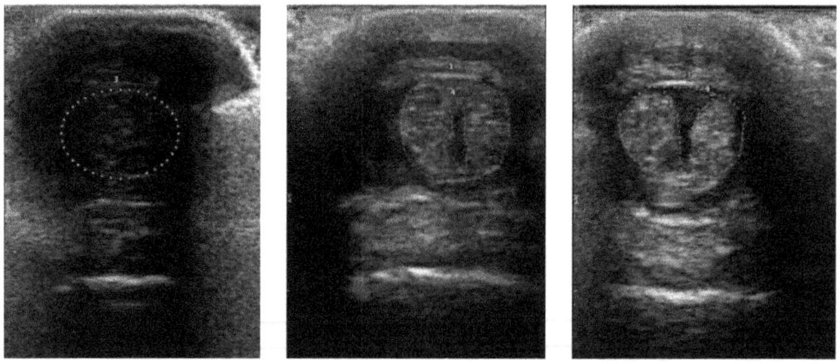

(a) (b) (c)

FIGURE 8: Transversal image at day 7 (a), day 21 (b), and day 42 (c), when the lesion is bigger than at day 21.

and 7 and $P > 0.06$ between days 42 and 21). At day 84, the external width was not significantly different from its initial size.

At day 0, the thickness of zone 2 was 16.71 ± 1.19 mm, increased until day 42 (18.69 ± 1.74 mm) and decreased until day 84. At day 84, the size of zone 2 was not significantly different from its initial size.

3.2. In Vivo Ultrasonography (US). All tendons presented similar images at day 0 (Figure 8). At day 7, on the longitudinal view, the operated tendons appeared to be increased in volume, and a discontinuity of the parallel aspect of the margins was noticed. On this view, we could not detect/visualize the lesions. On the transverse view, a convex deformation of the tendon was apparent around the operated area. At day 7 and at day 21, focal lesions were observed and quantified.

Measurements of CSA and lesion areas are presented in (Figures 6 and 7).

At day 7, all tendons presented an increased CSA (24 ± 3 mm^2) compared to day 0 (16 ± 2 mm^2) with a significant difference ($P < 0.001$). Peritendinous oedemas (anechoic image around the tendon) were observed in all the operated hindlimbs without visible intratendinous lesions (Figure 8). At day 21, the CSA (36 ± 12 mm^2) was at its largest size with a significant difference compared to the day 0 ($P < 0.05$). Lesions were identified and measured in all tendons at day 21 (4.8 ± 2.2 mm^2 or 13.2 ± 5.3% of CSA) (Figure 8). At day 42, CSA was still increased (33 ± 8 mm^2) compared to day 0 ($P < 0.005$) and day 7 ($P < 0.05$) but was lower than at day 21 ($P > 0.5$) (Figure 8).

Lesions appeared hypo to anechoic at day 42 with a larger area than at day 21 (5.5 ± 1.4 mm^2 or 17 ± 4.8%). At day 84 two of six tendons still presented an increased CSA (26 ± 6 mm^2) compared to day 0 ($P > 0.01$).

The highest values of the operated zone external width, thickness and CSA were at day 21. The highest value of the global functional score was at day 7.

No correlation was observed between the global functional score and the external size of the operated zone or its US area.

4. Discussion

This study presents a standardized experimental model of surgically induced tendinopathy: lesions were performed by the same operator, the same technique, and the same material. All the operated tendons presented the same gross changes, and lesions were seen ultrasonographically in all animals at day 21 demonstrating the homogeneity of the lesions.

As in other species, US is a relevant, reliable, and inexpensive examination. It allowed *in vivo*, noninvasive, and longitudinal monitoring of the lesions of tendons and to work in sedation-free conditions, as described by other authors [17, 27]. However, we could not use the longitudinal images to quantify the lesion. We supposed that the elasticity of the tendon did not allow us to observe the lesion itself, but we could observe its consequences.

In human and veterinary medicine, it is described that almost all tendons have an identical echostructure. Here, we noticed the longitudinal and axial US aspects of the goat tendon were similar to the description of Sans et al. [18]. In longitudinal view, they present a broadly hyperechoic, fibrillar structure parallel to the major axis of the tendon, corresponding to bundles of collagen fibres that are surrounded by a structure of middle echogenicity. In axial/transverse view, the tendon is an oval structure, limited by a hyperechoic border, and presenting paint strokes of regular echoes, with a synovial sheath which appears like a hypoechoic fine band [18]. In goats, the DDFT appears less homogeneous than horses DDFT making the US assessment of the fibre's alignment difficult.

Another difficulty of tendon US imaging is the artefact of anisotropy that occurs when the incident ultrasound wave is not perpendicular to the axis of the tendon or parallel to him in the longitudinal plane, so an aspect hypoechoic of the tendons is observed [12, 18]. To prevent anisotropic artefact, we performed measurement of CSA on the image where it appeared the smallest and with the highest signal intensity (i.e., US probe perpendicular to the tendon long axis).

In horses, the literature shows a slight tendency for tall horses to have a higher tendon width and thickness [19, 23]. No correlation was observed between the weight and size of the animals and their tendon's CSA or external size. Variations in the CSA of tendons and ligaments of clinically normal horses have been described in a number of breeds [21, 28–30]. The variation of the CSA observed could be expressed by the individual variation of CSA of the healthy tendon. No published references for the echogenicity or the CSA of goat's tendons were found. Interestingly, we observed that goat's DDFT was more heterogeneous than in horses making the qualitative evaluation of its echogenicity difficult and not reliable. While peritendinous oedemas (anechoic image around the tendon) were observed in all operated legs, no intratendinous lesions could be recognized at day 7 by US. An increase in the tendon mass and CSA appears to occur during the modelling stage of a tendinopathy [31]. This was also found at day 84. In horses, after flexor tendons injuries, at least 6 weeks are required for the tendon to gain sufficient strength to bear weight [6]. Indeed, different authors mention a recovery time of three to six months [1, 2]. However, tendon US morphology does not necessarily correlate with clinical symptoms [32].

The goat is relevant as an experimental model in the study of tendinopathy as they are easy to house and to handle and are cheaper than horse or dog models. In addition, their size allows for performing similar examination to be performed on humans, horses, or dogs (clinical and imaging exams).

Clinical examination and ultrasonography were easy to perform *in vivo* with gentle handling only and provided complementary information on the goat's tendon healing process. The normal US images and tendon CSA presented here could be used as a reference for following studies such as the evaluation of different therapies.

Conflict of Interests

The authors declare that they have no conflict of interests.

Authors' Contribution

All the authors participated in the design of the experiment. A. K. De Grandis, C. Boulocher, S. Sawaya participated in the acquisition, analysis, and interpretation of the data. A. K. De Grandis and C. Boulocher wrote the paper. All authors read and approved the final paper.

Acknowledgment

The authors wish to acknowledge the Claude Bourgelat Institute (ICl-B).

References

[1] S. J. Warden, "Animal models for the study of tendinopathy," *British Journal of Sports Medicine*, vol. 41, no. 4, pp. 232–240, 2007.

[2] P. Sharma and N. Maffulli, "Tendon injury and tendinopathy: healing and repair," *Journal of Bone and Joint Surgery Series A*, vol. 87, no. 1, pp. 187–202, 2005.

[3] S. Boehart, G. Arndt, and B. Carstanjen, "Ultrasonographic morphometric measurements of digital flexor tendons and ligaments of the palmar metacarpal region in haflinger horses," *Journal of Veterinary Medicine Series C*, vol. 39, no. 4, pp. 366–375, 2010.

[4] C. T. Thorpe, P. D. Clegg, and H. L. Birch, "A review of tendon injury: why is the equine superficial digital flexor tendon most at risk?" *Equine Veterinary Journal*, vol. 42, no. 2, pp. 174–180, 2010.

[5] R. B. Williams, L. S. Harkins, C. J. Hammond, and J. L. Wood, "Racehorse injuries, clinical problems and fatalities recorded on British racecourses from flat racing and National Hunt racing during 1996, 1997 and 1998," *Equine Veterinary Journal*, vol. 33, no. 5, pp. 478–486, 2001.

[6] M. Jordana, H. Wilderjans, J. Boswell, J. Dewulf, R. K. W. Smith, and A. Martens, "Outcome after lacerations of the superficial and deep digital flexor tendons, suspensory ligaments and/or distal sesamoidean ligaments in 106 horses," *Veterinary Surgery*, vol. 40, no. 3, pp. 277–283, 2011.

[7] R. C. Dirks and S. J. Warden, "Models for the study of tendinopathy," *Journal of Musculoskeletal Neuronal Interactions*, vol. 11, no. 2, pp. 141–149, 2011.

[8] D. Marsolais, C. H. Côté, and J. Frenette, "Neutrophils and macrophages accumulate sequentially following Achilles tendon injury," *Journal of Orthopaedic Research*, vol. 19, no. 6, pp. 1203–1209, 2001.

[9] R. W. W. Hsu, W. H. Hsu, C. L. Tai, and K. F. Lee, "Effect of shock-wave therapy on patellar tendinopathy in a rabbit model," *Journal of Orthopaedic Research*, vol. 22, no. 1, pp. 221–227, 2004.

[10] S. K. Maiti, N. Kumar, G. R. Singh, M. Hoque, and R. Singh, "Ultrasound therapy in tendinous injury healing in goats," *Journal of Veterinary Medicine Series A*, vol. 53, no. 5, pp. 249–258, 2006.

[11] K. Vanderperren and J. H. Saunders, "Diagnostic imaging of the equine fetlock region using radiography and ultrasonography—part 1: soft tissues," *Veterinary Journal*, vol. 181, no. 2, pp. 111–122, 2009.

[12] W. M. Karlin, A. A. Stewart, S. S. Durgam, J. F. Naughton, K. J. O'dell-Anderson, and M. C. Stewart, "Evaluation of experimentally induced injury to the superficial digital flexor tendon in horses by use of low-field magnetic resonance imaging and ultrasonography," *American Journal of Veterinary Research*, vol. 72, no. 6, pp. 791–798, 2011.

[13] A. Agut, M. L. Martínez, M. A. Sánchez-Valverde, M. Soler, and M. J. Rodríguez, "Ultrasonographic characteristics (cross-sectional area and relative echogenicity) of the digital flexor tendons and ligaments of the metacarpal region in Purebred Spanish horses," *Veterinary Journal*, vol. 180, no. 3, pp. 377–383, 2009.

[14] C. S. Avella, E. R. Ely, K. L. P. Verheyen, J. S. Price, J. L. N. Wood, and R. K. W. Smith, "Ultrasonographic assessment of the superficial digital flexor tendons of National Hunt racehorses in training over two racing seasons," *Equine Veterinary Journal*, vol. 41, no. 5, pp. 449–454, 2009.

[15] M. Kramer, M. Gerwing, V. Hach, and E. Schimke, "Sonography of the musculoskeletal system in dogs and cats," *Veterinary Radiology and Ultrasound*, vol. 38, no. 2, pp. 139–149, 1997.

[16] H. T. M. Van Schie and E. M. Bakker, "Structure-related echoes in ultrasonographic images of equine superficial digital flexor tendons," *American Journal of Veterinary Research*, vol. 61, no. 2, pp. 202–209, 2000.

[17] F. Arnault, E. Cauvin, E. Viguier, E. Kraft, J. Sonet, and C. Carozzo, "Diagnostic value of ultrasonography to assess stifle

lesions in dogs after cranial cruciate ligament rupture: 13 cases," *Veterinary and Comparative Orthopaedics and Traumatology*, vol. 22, no. 6, pp. 479–485, 2009.
[18] N. Sans, N. Boutry, X. Demondion, and S. Lagarde, "Tendons: inflammatory and degenerative pathology," *Journal de Radiologie*, vol. 86, no. 12, pp. 1834–1844, 2005.
[19] R. K. Smith, R. Jones, and P. M. Webbon, "The cross-sectional areas of normal equine digital flexor tendons determined ultrasonographically," *Equine Veterinary Journal*, vol. 26, no. 6, pp. 460–465, 1994.
[20] C. H. Pickersgill, C. M. Marr, and S. W. J. Reid, "Repeatability of diagnostic ultrasonography in the assessment of the equine superficial digital flexor tendon," *Equine Veterinary Journal*, vol. 33, no. 1, pp. 33–37, 2001.
[21] J. M. Vilar, A. Santana, J. Espinosa, and G. Spinella, "Cross-sectional area of the tendons of the tarsal region in Standardbred trotter horses," *Equine Veterinary Journal*, vol. 43, no. 2, pp. 235–239, 2011.
[22] V. B. Reef, *Equine Diagnostic Ultrasound*, W. B. Saunders, Philadelphia, Pa, USA, 1998.
[23] F. Kainberger, F. Mittermaier, G. Seidl, E. Parth, and R. Weinstabl, "Imaging of tendons—adaptation, degeneration, rupture," *European Journal of Radiology*, vol. 25, no. 3, pp. 209–222, 1997.
[24] J. D. Rompe, B. Nafe, J. P. Furia, and N. Maffulli, "Eccentric loading, shock-wave treatment, or a wait- and-see policy for tendinopathy of the main body of tendo Achillis: a randomized controlled trial," *American Journal of Sports Medicine*, vol. 35, no. 3, pp. 374–383, 2007.
[25] J. D. Rompe, J. Furia, and N. Maffulli, "Eccentric loading compared with shock wave treatment for chronic insertional achilles tendinopathy: a randomized, controlled trial," *Journal of Bone and Joint Surgery Series A*, vol. 90, no. 1, pp. 52–61, 2008.
[26] D. L. Millis, "Assessing and measuring outcomes," in *Canine Rehabilitation and Physical Therapy*, D. L. Millis, D. Levine, and R. A. Taylor, Eds., pp. 211–227, Saunders, Elesvier, 2004.
[27] M. L. Esterline, L. Armbrust, and J. K. Roush, "A comparison of palpation guided and ultrasound guided percutaneous biceps brachii tenotomy in dogs," *Veterinary and Comparative Orthopaedics and Traumatology*, vol. 18, no. 3, pp. 135–139, 2005.
[28] G. M. Constantinescu, *Guide to Regional Ruminant Anatomy Based on the Dissection of the Goat*, Iowa State University Press, Ames, Iowa, USA, 2001.
[29] C. Gillis, N. Sharkey, S. M. Stover, R. R. Pool, D. M. Meagher, and N. Willits, "Effect of maturation and aging on material and ultrasonographic properties of equine superficial digital flexor tendon," *American Journal of Veterinary Research*, vol. 56, no. 10, pp. 1345–1350, 1995.
[30] C. Gillis, R. R. Pool, D. M. Meagher, S. M. Stover, K. Reiser, and N. Willits, "Effect of maturation and aging on the histomorphometric and biochemical characteristics of equine superficial digital flexor tendon," *American Journal of Veterinary Research*, vol. 58, no. 4, pp. 425–430, 1997.
[31] P. Sharma and N. Maffulli, "Biology of tendon injury: healing, modeling and remodeling," *Journal of Musculoskeletal Neuronal Interactions*, vol. 6, no. 2, pp. 181–190, 2006.
[32] J. J. Wilson and T. M. Best, "Common overuse tendon problems: a review and recommendations for treatment," *American Family Physician*, vol. 72, no. 5, pp. 811–818, 2005.

A Simple Method for Enema Administration in One-Day-Old Broiler Chicks

Guilherme Augusto Marietto-Gonçalves,[1] Fabrizio Grandi,[2,3] and Raphael Lucio Andreatti Filho[1]

[1] *Laboratory of Avian Pathology, School of Veterinary Medicine and Animal Science, Universidade Estadual Paulista (UNESP), 18618-970 Botucatu, SP, Brazil*
[2] *Department of Pathology, Botucatu Medical School, Universidade Estadual Paulista (UNESP), 18618-970 Botucatu, SP, Brazil*
[3] *Laboratory of Investigative and Comparative Pathology, School of Veterinary Medicine and Animal Science, Universidade Estadual Paulista (UNESP), 18618-970 Botucatu, SP, Brazil*

Correspondence should be addressed to Guilherme Augusto Marietto-Gonçalves, gmarietto_ornito@fmvz.unesp.br

Academic Editor: Takaaki Arigami

The present study aimed to describe a simple technique for enema administration in one-day-old broiler chicks. For this purpose we used 455 unsexed health birds divided into four groups submitted to three different experimental protocols: in the first one, we measured the total length of the large intestine in order to establish a secure distance for probe introduction; in the second, we evaluated maximum compliance of large intestine and diffusion range; finally, based on results obtained we tested the hypothesis in 400 birds in order to standardize the method. Enema solutions applied in an intrarectal manner with a stainless steel gavage BD-10 probe into one-day-old broiler chicks at 0.2 mL at a distance of 1.5 cm proved to be a reliable method.

1. Introduction

Enema is a technical procedure that consists in rectal or colonic administration of several drugs that require rapid systemic absorption such as anticonvulsants, analgesics, antiemetics, anesthetic, and antibacterial agents [1]. Plus, it can be used to remove local toxins by flushing or by increasing the volume of liquid which in turn causes rapid expansion of the lower intestinal tract and evacuation [2, 3].

In veterinary medicine, the technique is used both in clinical and experimental settings [4]. In broiler chicks enemas had been used in a diverse set of experiments including toxicological, nutritional, and immunological assays. Despite this, there is no standardized protocol for enema administration in these animals, the majority being empirical.

The objective of this study is to describe a simple method for enema administration that can be applied to one-day-old broiler chickens in order to better standardize further experiments involving this administration route.

2. Materials and Methods

2.1. Animals. Four hundred fifty-five, one-day-old, unsexed, healthy Cobb Avian Farm broiler chicks (average weight = 42.2 g ± 1.8) were acquired from a commercial incubatory (Céu Azul Alimentos, Pereiras, SP, Brazil) and kept in galvanized wire cages (0,90 × 0,60 × 0,33) in the experimental aviary of the Avian Pathology Laboratory, School of Veterinary Medicine and Animal Science, Universidade Estadual Paulista, UNESP, Botucatu, SP, Brazil. The animals were kept in a controlled environment at a temperature of 27 ± 2°C, a relative humidity of 70 ± 10%, on a 24 h light cycle with a continuous air exchange, and water *ad libitum*. The experiment was approved by the Institutional Ethics Committee of School of Veterinary Medicine and Animal Science, Universidade Estadual Paulista, Botucatu, SP, Brazil.

2.2. Animal Experimental Design. The study was divided into three experiments in order to reduce the total number of birds used. The euthanasia procedure used was cervical dislocation, conforming that recommended by Federal Council of Veterinary Medicine, Brazil [5], and Close et al. [6]. All euthanized birds were submitted to necropsy evaluation by a pathologist. Only those birds with no gross signs of disease were considered in the results.

Experiment 1. Twenty-five birds were randomly selected and euthanized by cervical displacement technique in order to measure the total length of the large intestine. The last was defined as the distance between cloaca and the ileum-cecum-colon junction at the level of caecal tonsils. Measurement was carried out with an analog caliper (Mitutoyo Sul Americana, Santo Amaro, Brazil). The average length was tabulated and used in the standardization of the second experiment.

Experiment 2. Based on the results obtained in the first experiment, thirty animals were randomly selected and divided into two groups ($n = 15$ for each group). Methylene blue dye was administered intrarectally with a stainless steel gavage BD-10 probe (Insight Equipamentos, Ribeirão Preto, SP, Brazil) into broiler chicks at 0.2 or 0.4 mL/animal in order to evaluate the maximum compliance of the large intestine and diffusion range. Signs of dye leakage or rectal evacuation were evaluated up to ten seconds after each enema, after which animals were euthanized and submitted to necropsy.

Experiment 3. This final experiment was conducted in accordance with the values obtained in the first two experiments. To this end, four hundred birds were randomly selected and submitted to a saline enema. Signs of solution leakage or rectal evacuation were evaluated up to ten seconds after each enema. Twenty-four hours after instillation, animals were clinically evaluated and euthanized in order to detect gross abnormalities in large intestine.

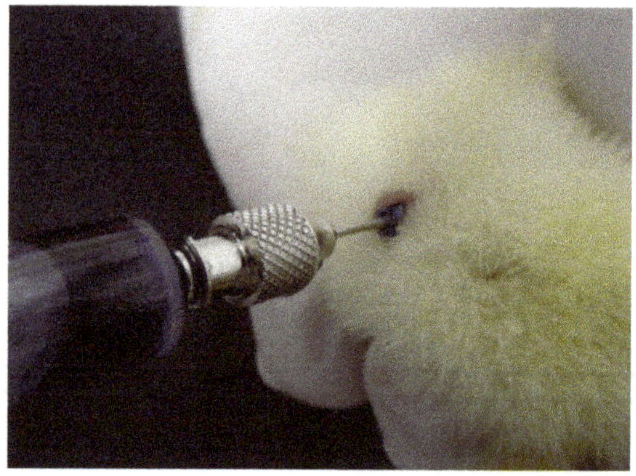

Figure 1: Note leakage of enema in a bird submitted to 0.4 mL methylene blue dye.

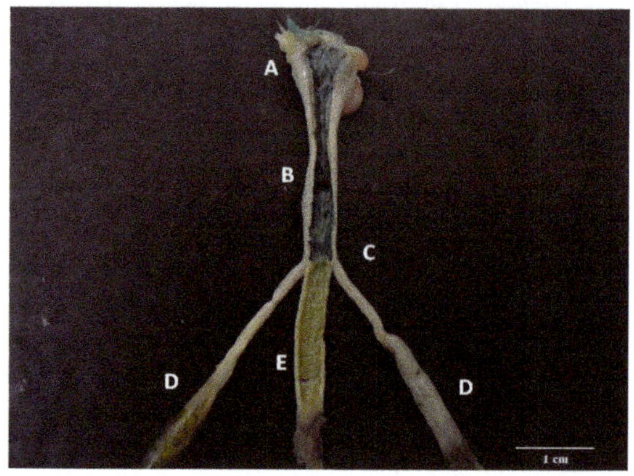

Figure 2: Diffusion range limited to caecal tonsils as evidenced by labeling with the methylene blue dye. A: cloaca; B: rectum; C: caecal tonsils; E: ileum.

3. Results and Discussion

The average length obtained in Experiment 1 was 1.9 cm (±0.2). Based on this, a standard distance of 1.5 cm was established for the next two experiments.

In methylene blue dye enema groups (Experiment 2) there were two different results. The group submitted to a 0.2 mL/bird enema did not show signs of leakage or rectal evacuation during or after the procedure. However, those birds submitted to 0.4 mL/bird enema show signs of leakage (Figure 1) and evacuation reflex in 40% and 100%, respectively. All birds ($n = 30$) displayed a diffusion range limited to caecal tonsils as evidenced by labeling with the dye (Figure 2) and no gross abnormalities on necropsy evaluation. The results are summarized on Table 1.

In saline-enema-treated group (Experiment 3), four hundred birds were submitted to 0.2 mL saline enema at an intrarectal distance of 1.5 cm with no signs of leakage and rectal evacuation up to ten seconds after the procedure. There were no clinical signs or gross abnormalities during or after a period of 24 hours, respectively.

Enema administration for routine use in one-day-broiler chicks involves a series of methodological aspects as seen in this study. The total volume of solution administered should not exceed the maximum capacity retention (compliance) of the lower segments of large intestine, that is, rectum and colon, and therefore was determined in 0.2 mL/bird. The administration of dye at 0.4 mL/bird induces retrograde cloacal reflux and rectal evacuation reflex in some animals which can compromise the total absorbed drug dose in a clinical setting or experimental assay. Additionally, the interval between defecation and enema administration plays a central role in the maintenance of drugs in lower intestinal portions and consequently their absorption [4].

Table 1: Total number of birds showing cloacal reflux, rectal evacuation, or gross abnormalities following methylene blue dye instillation.

Sign	Volumes	
	0.2 mL	0.4 mL
Cloacal reflux	0% [0/15]*	40% [6/15]
Rectal evacuation	0% [0/15]	100% [15/15]
Gross abnormalities	0% [0/15]	0% [0/15]

* Positive number of animals/total number of birds.

The distance for the introduction of the probe was inferior (1.5 cm) compared to the average distance between cloaca and ileum-cecum-colon junction (1.8 cm ±0.2). The former was adopted as the standard distance for Experiments 2 and 3 in order to avoid anatomical limits and therefore lesions to intestinal tract as could be confirmed by necropsy which reveal no gross lesions in all birds evaluated (n = 430).

Clinical applicability of the technique described here includes the administration of drugs and experimental inoculums (e.g., biological agents), radiological contrasts for large intestine analysis, collection of fecal samples for microbiological, immunological (e.g., IgA), and/or parasitological assays.

In conclusion, enema solutions administered with a stainless steel gavage BD-10 probe into one-day-old broiler chicks at 0.2 mL/bird at an intrarectal distance of 1.5 cm proved to be a reliable method. Technical data generated by this study can be applied safely for experimental assays involving young broiler chicks.

Acknowledgment

This research was supported by Fundação de Amparo à Pesquisa do Estado de São Paulo (FAPESP) (Grants nos. 07/54012-9 and 08/51034-4).

References

[1] E. J. Van Hoogdalem, A. G. De Boer, and D. D. Breimer, "Pharmacokinetics of rectal drug administration—part I. General considerations and clinical applications of centrally acting drugs," *Clinical Pharmacokinetics*, vol. 21, no. 1, pp. 11–26, 1991.

[2] R. W. Nelson and C. G. Couto, *Medzicina Interna de Pequenos Animais*, Elsevier, Rio de Janeiro, Brazil, 4th edition, 2010.

[3] M. Sakate, R. M. B. Nogueira, and S. F. Andrade, "Terapêutica das intoxicações," in *Manual de Terapêutica Veterinária*, S. F. Andrade, Ed., pp. 611–645, Roca, São Paulo, Brazil, 2008.

[4] T. Smith, A. Smith, and J. Kelly, "The practical aspects of repeated administration of an enema to beagle dogs," *Toxicology Letters*, vol. 95, p. 200, 1998.

[5] Brasil, Resolução no. 714, de 20 de junho de 2002. Conselho Federal de Medicina Veterinária. Disponível em, http://www.furb.br/site/arquivos/357080-486559/Resolucao%20714_%202002.htm.

[6] B. Close, K. Banister, V. Baumans et al., "Recommendations for euthanasia of experimental animals—part 1," *Laboratory Animals*, vol. 30, no. 4, pp. 293–316, 1996.

Effect of Isosporiasis Prevention with Toltrazuril on Long-Term Pig Performance

K. Rypula,[1] M. Porowski,[1] J. Kaba,[2] M. Gorczykowski,[3] and A. Deniz[4]

[1] *Division of Infectious Diseases and Veterinary Administration, Department of Epizootiology with Clinic of Birds and Exotic Animals, Faculty of Veterinary Medicine, Wrocław University of Environmental and Life Sciences, Grunwaldzki Square 45, 50-366 Wrocław, Poland*
[2] *Division of Infectious Diseases and Epidemiology, Department of Large Animal Diseases, Faculty of Veterinary Medicine, Warsaw University of Life Sciences—SGGW, Nowoursynowska 159c, 02-776 Warsaw, Poland*
[3] *Divison of Parasitology, Department of Internal Diseases with Clinic of Horses, Dogs and Cats, Faculty of Veterinary Medicine, Agricultural University of Wrocław, Poland*
[4] *Bayer HealthCare Animal Health, Leverkusen, Germany*

Correspondence should be addressed to K. Rypula, krzysztof.rypula@up.wroc.pl

Academic Editor: Kunio Ohmiya

The efficacy of toltrazuril treatment was assessed in two experiments in Polish swine herds. Experiment 1 included a toltrazuril treatment group, Group A ($n = 410$), and untreated control, Group B ($n = 386$). Time to sale in Group A was 108 days versus 120 days for Group B, with average body weights at sale of 114.2 kg and 108.8 kg, respectively ($P < 0.05$). In experiment 2, the health status and body weight gain of 238 piglets treated with toltrazuril (Group D) were compared to 235 untreated piglets (Group K). A similar difference was observed in average body weights of slaughtered animals, being on average 104 kg in Group D and 101 kg in Group K ($P < 0.01$). Animals from Group D were slaughtered 5 days earlier than animals from Group K (day 166 versus day 171). Data from clinical trials suggest treatment of coccidiosis with toltrazuril offering potential for improved animal welfare and yields, however this has remained unproven in field conditions in large swine production facilities. The present study confirms the efficacy of toltrazuril treatment when used in the field and the subsequent positive impact on time to weaning, time to market, and on weight gain at all time points.

1. Introduction

Diarrhoea remains a significant, though often underappreciated, issue in both economic and welfare terms on many swine farms worldwide. The most common cause of severe diarrhoea in pigs aged 5–20 days is coccidiosis, caused by infection by the near ubiquitous Eimeriidae coccidium *Isospora suis* [1–3], which has been found in over 75% of farms examined in Ireland, Germany, the Netherlands, Greece, Austria, and Switzerland [4, 5]. A recent study into *I. suis* prevalence in Poland found that 90% of farms tested positive [4].

The *I. suis* parasite lifecycle has prepatent and patent phases; the prepatent usually lasts 5–7 days, and the patent lasts 5–16 days. Along with the characteristic 5–8 days of creamy yellow diarrhoea, serious damage to the mucosal crypts and villi of suckling piglets due to *I. suis* has previously been reported [1, 3]. The rupture of cells of the villi of gut mucosa during infection causes fibrinous enteritis and long-term damage to the gut, leaving piglets more susceptible to other infections, such as *E. coli and Clostridium perfringens* [7, 8]. Maturity of mucosa villous at weaning is of special importance in terms of postweaning feeding performance [9, 10]. Damage to the gut can also have a significant impact on the long-term growth and wellbeing of the piglet, causing decreases in weight at weaning of as much as 1 kg [6], even in asymptomatic pigs [11].

As *I. suis* infection is spread through faecal matter, hygiene is a key component of coccidiosis prevention. In theory, clearing farrowing pens and a programme of thorough, ongoing cleansing with an effective oocysticide may to some extent control the reappearance of coccidiosis, but not totally [12]. However, as *I. suis* infection is so prevalent, this is, in practice, not effective strategy.

Treatment with sulphonamides and diclazuril in experimental studies has not proven effective in managing coccidiosis, but treatment simplicity and efficacy were recently significantly improved by the approval of toltrazuril (Baycox 5%, Bayer Animal Health) for the treatment of coccidiosis in swine. Individual treatment of piglets around day 4 of life with 0.4 mL/kg toltrazuril has proven to be the most effective treatment option available [5, 6].

A number of studies have reported that treatment with toltrazuril can improve the health of the gut and increased weight gain [6, 8, 11], reduce use of antibiotics [13] and rate of diarrhoea in early life [8], and improve postweaning feed conversion ratios [9, 10].

The present study sets out to investigate the efficacy of toltrazuril treatment in swine herds in field conditions in Poland to ascertain whether the efficacy reported in clinical studies can be replicated in the field, particularly in relation to increased weight gain, reduced need for veterinary intervention and faster time to market.

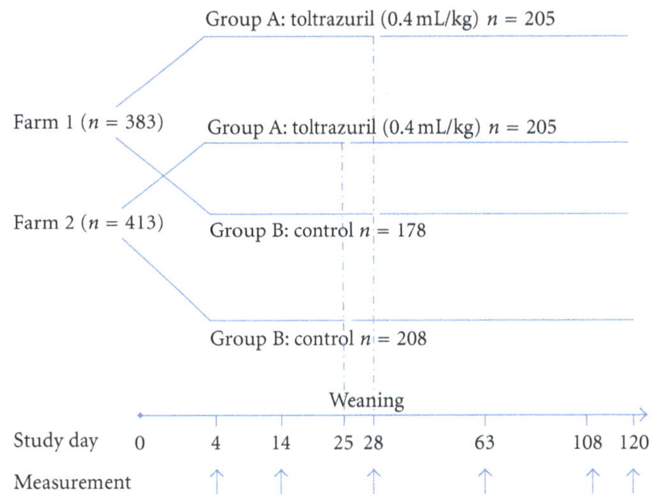

FIGURE 1: Experiment 1: Study design.

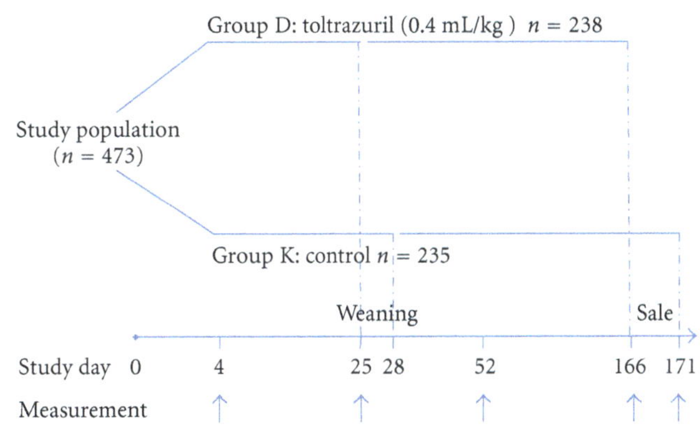

FIGURE 2: Experiment 2: Study design.

2. Materials and Methods

2.1. Experiment 1. The therapeutic efficacy of a single oral treatment with toltrazuril (Baycox 5%, Bayer Animal Health) (0.4 mL/kg BW, equivalent to 20 mg toltrazuril/kg BW) was examined on two pig farms in Lower Silesia and Mazowia voividships, Poland.

Farm 1 operated a closed, continuous flow with all-in-all-out (AIAO) system of production cycle with a basic herd of 130 hybrid Polish Landrace x Polish Large White sows. Study groups comprising 10 sows were created twice a week during the study period. All welfare conditions in the labour sections as well as in the breeding and fattening sections were satisfactory. A history of *I. suis* infection was confirmed on Farm 1.

Farm 2 also operated a closed, continuous flow with AIAO system of production cycle, with a basic herd of 450 hybrid PIC sows. Study groups of 20 sows were created once a week during the study period. All welfare conditions in the labour sections as well as in the breeding and fattening sections were satisfactory. All weaning piglets were sold on. A history of *I. Suis* infection was confirmed on Farm 2.

The study was conducted on 383 pigs from Farm 1 and on 413 pigs from Farm 2 based on simple randomisation. On both farms, the group treated with toltrazuril was labelled Group A (Farm 1, $n = 205$; Farm 2, $n = 205$) and the nontreated control group as Group B (Farm 1, $n = 178$; Farm 2, $n = 208$) (Figure 1). Selection criteria were based on the age of piglets and number of piglets in the litter.

Treatment efficacy assessment was based on weight gain from day 4 (first day of toltrazuril administration) through to day 14—defined as the first stage preweaning period—and from day 14 to the day of weaning—the second stage preweaning period. Piglets were weaned when 28 and 25 days old on farm 1 and 2, respectively. In addition, the frequency of medical interventions (mainly antibiotic injections) required for diarrhoea control was measured. Prior to treatment with toltrazuril, the presence of *I. suis* infection was confirmed by parasitological examination of 10% of piglet faeces in all experimental groups. Oocysts were confirmed in all collected samples.

2.2. Experiment 2. The second experiment was carried out on a production facility in Mazovia viovodship, Poland with a closed, AIAO production cycle and a basic herd of 1,700 hybrid PIC sows and 10 hybrid Polish Landrace x Polish Large White boars. Study groups comprising 90 sows were created once a week during the production cycle. All welfare conditions in the labour sections as well as in the breeding and fattening sections were satisfactory.

The study evaluated the health status and body weight gain of 238 piglets treated with a single dose of toltrazuril (0.4 mL/kg BW, equivalent to 20 mg toltrazuril/kg BW) (Group D) at day 4 of life compared to 235 untreated piglets in the control group (Group K) (Figure 2). The choice of the piglets was conducted as in experiment 1.

TABLE 1: Experiment 1: Mean piglet body weight.

		Piglet body weight					
		Day 4	Day 14	Day 28	Day 63	Day 108	Day 120
Farm 1	Group A	2093 g ± 390	4163 g* ± 854	7745 g ± 1843	21300 g* ±1351	114200 g* ± 3856	—
	Group B	2125 g ± 420	3602 g ± 571	6333 g ± 933	20500 g ± 1381	—	108800 g ± 3036
Farm 2	Group A	2065 g ± 413	3910 g* ± 879	6490 g* ± 1337	—	—	—
	Group B	2062 g ± 374	3040 g ± 440	5385 g ± 1118	—	—	—

*$P < 0.05$.

TABLE 2: Experiment 2: Mean piglet body weight.

	Piglet body weight				
	Day 4	Day 25[a]/28[b]	Day 52	Day 166	Day 171
Group D	1530 g ± 103	6180 g* ± 271	31000 g* ± 1068	104000 g* ± 7026	—
Group K	1540 g ± 97	5830 g ± 245	27900 g ± 1407	—	101000 g ± 7251

*$P < 0.01$.
[a]Day of weaned piglets in group D.
[b]Day of weaned piglets in group K.

Assessments of health status and body weight gain were made on the 4th day of life (start of treatment), on the day of weaning, when moving from the breeding sector to the fattening sector, and finally on the day of sale.

Statistical calculations in both experiments were carried out with Mann-Whitney U test and χ^2 (chi-squared) test with the use of Statistica v. 6.1 software.

3. Results

3.1. Experiment 1. Body weight gain of the piglets in Group A (treatment group), between day 4 and day 14, was 2070 g and 1845 g in Farms 1 and 2, respectively. Additional body weight gain in Farms 1 and 2 in the second phase of weaning (day 14 to weaning) was 3582 g and 2580 g, respectively.

Piglets in Group B (control group) gained 1477 g on Farm 1 and 978 g on Farm 2 between day 4 and 14, and additional 2737 g and 2345 g, respectively, between day 14 and weaning.

In the time to weaning, piglets in Group A required 6 medical interventions in both Farms 1 and 2, compared to 13 and 18 in Farms 1 and 2, respectively, for those in Group B.

Piglets on Farm 1 were also followed through to sale to ascertain the impact of treatment on long-term growth. At transfer from weaning to a feeding group at day 63, average body weight was 21300 g for Group A versus 20500 g in Group B. Time to sale in Group A was 108 days for Group A versus 120 days for Group B, with average body weights at sale of 114200 g and 108800 g ($P < 0.05$), respectively (Table 1).

3.2. Experiment 2. Piglets in experiment 2 of the study were assessed at days 4, 25, 52, 166, and 171. Those piglets in treatment group D ($n = 238$ at birth, $n = 210$ at weaning) weaned on average at 25.6 days, while those in the control group K ($n = 235$ at birth, $n = 194$ at weaning) weaned on average at 28 days.

There was a statistically significant difference ($P = 0.03$) in relation to average daily weight gain between Group D (221 g) and Group K (204 g) at day 25, and a statistically significant difference was also observed between Groups D and K in relation to reports of diarrhoea prior to weaning—4 versus 22 cases, respectively ($P < 0.01$). Body weight at weaning and cases of digestive disorders or death showed no statistical difference between groups.

After moving animals to the breeding sector on day 25, average body weight of the animals in the group receiving the toltrazuril was 6180 g and was greater than the body weight of the piglets in Group K ($P < 0.01$). After weaning, animals were kept in their groups for fattening until day 52. Average body weight of animals transferred to the fattening sector was 31000 g and 27900 g, respectively, for Groups D and K. A similar difference was observed in average body weights of slaughtered animals, being on average 104000 g in Group D and 101000 g in Group K (Table 2). Animals from Group D were slaughtered 5 days earlier than animals from Group K (day 166 versus day 171).

4. Discussion

Alongside the obvious short-term impact of diarrhoeal disease, coccidiosis infection is responsible for significant damage to the gut of piglets, regardless of whether or not they are symptomatic. This damage can have serious long-term effects on their health and growth, leading to significant losses for the pig producer.

A number of experimental trials have demonstrated the impact of toltrazuril on key production criteria including daily weight gain, where treatment-related increases in weight gain have been recorded at 37 g/day to day 28 [6], 25 g/day to weaning [11], and 14 g/day between days 21 and 105 [9], and toltrazuril treatment-related feed conversion rates in weaner-finisher herds of 2.41 versus 2.63 [10] and 1.6 versus 1.77 [9]. Treatment with toltrazuril has also been shown to increase body weight at weaning by 670 g ($P < 0.05$) [6] and 326.6 g ($P = 0.044$) [8] compared to placebo.

While not directly investigating daily weight gains or feed conversion rates, the present study has confirmed the significant improvements in yield suggested by trial results are indeed replicable in the "real world", with treatment-related weight gain of 1412 g and 350 g at weaning and 5400 g and 3000 g, respectively, for experiments 1 and 2 at time to market. It was also notable that all treatment groups reached weaning (3 days) and market weight (between 5 and 12 days) substantially earlier than the untreated controls.

Cases of diarrhoea were also significantly reduced in treated groups, reflecting the previously reported findings of McOrist and others [9] and Westphal and others [8]. The absence of significant reductions in cases of digestive disorders and death among groups in this study is likely to reflect the already low mortality associated with coccidiosis infection along with the multiplicity of infections (Porcine Respiratory Disease Complex) affecting piglets during the weaning phase in a commercial swine production facility.

The results of this study, performed in field conditions, suggest that the use of a single application of toltrazuril is likely to produce results similar to those noted in experimental trials. These results support the view that, in real-world conditions, metaphylaxis with toltrazuril is extremely effective at managing the impact of *I. suis* infection on the health and growth of piglets, leading to substantial improvements in weight gain that continue over the lifetime of the pig, bringing pigs to market weight substantially faster and at a greater weight.

Acknowledgment

The authors thank gratefully Bayer and Ketchum Pleon Limited.

References

[1] B. P. Stuart, D. S. Lindsay, J. V. Ernst, and H. S. Gosser, "Isospora suis enteritis in piglets," *Veterinary Pathology*, vol. 17, no. 1, pp. 84–93, 1980.

[2] Y. Robinson, M. Morin, C. Girard, and R. Higgins, "Experimental transmission of intestinal coccidiosis to piglets: clinical, parasitological and pathological findings," *Canadian Journal of Comparative Medicine*, vol. 47, no. 4, pp. 401–407, 1983.

[3] H. C. Mundt, A. Joachim, M. Becka, and A. Daugschies, "*Isospora suis*: an experimental model for mammalian intestinal coccidiosis," *Parasitology Research*, vol. 98, no. 2, pp. 167–175, 2006.

[4] A. Torres, "Prevalence study of Isospora suis in Europe," in *Proceedings of the 18th IPVS Congress*, Hamburg, Germany, 2004.

[5] H. C. Mundt, A. Cohnen, A. Daugschies et al., "Occurrence of Isospora suis in Germany, Switzerland and Austria," *Journal of Veterinary Medicine Series B*, vol. 52, no. 2, pp. 93–97, 2005.

[6] A. Scala, F. Demontis, A. Varcasia et al., "Toltrazuril and sulphonamide treatment against naturally Isospora suis infected suckling piglets: is there an actual profit?" *Veterinary Parasitology*, vol. 163, no. 4, pp. 362–365, 2009.

[7] C. Chae, D. Kwon, O. Kim et al., "Diarrhoea in nursing piglets associated with coccidiosis: prevalence, microscopic lesions and coexisting microorganisms," *Veterinary Record*, vol. 143, no. 15, pp. 417–420, 1998.

[8] B. Westphal, U. Bernemann, and L. Kathmann, "Mixed *Isospora suis* and Clostridium perfringens infections in suckling pigs immediately post partum?" *Tierarztliche Umschau*, vol. 62, no. 12, pp. 682–689, 2007.

[9] S. McOrist, A. Blunt, H. El-Sheikha, A. Morillo-Alujas, M. Ocak, and A. Deniz, "Evaluation of efficacy of oral toltrazuril (Baycox 5%) for the improvement of post-weaning gut health in pigs," *The Pig Journal*, vol. 63, pp. 73–79, 2010.

[10] S. McOrist, D. Spiru, M. Ocak, and A. Deniz, "Evaluation of efficacy of oral toltrazueril (Baycox 5%) for the improvement of post-weaning gut health in pigs in Romania," in *Proceedings of the 21st IPVS Congress*, Vancouver, Canada, July 2010.

[11] D. Maes, P. Vyt, P. Rabaeys, and D. Gevaert, "Effects of toltrazuril on the growth of piglets in herds without clinical isosporosis," *Veterinary Journal*, vol. 173, no. 1, pp. 197–199, 2007.

[12] E. Straberg and A. Daugschies, "Control of piglet coccidiosis by chemical disinfection with a cresol-based product (Neopredisan 135-1)," *Parasitology Research*, vol. 101, no. 3, pp. 599–604, 2007.

[13] S. J. Driesen, V. A. Fahy, and P. G. Carland, "The use of toltrazuril for the prevention of coccidiosis in piglets before weaning," *Australian Veterinary Journal*, vol. 72, no. 4, pp. 139–141, 1995.

A Survey on Prevalence and Pathological Findings of Gallstones in Lori-Bakhtiari Sheep in Iran

Afshin Raoofi,[1] Alireza Rahmani Shahraki,[2] Abdolrasool Namjoo,[3] and Hasan Momtaz[4]

[1] *Department of Clinical Sciences, Faculty of Veterinary Medicine, University of Tehran, P.O. Box 14155-6453, Tehran, Iran*
[2] *Club of Young Researchers, Islamic Azad University, Shahrekord Branch, P.O. Box 166, Shahrekord, Iran*
[3] *Department of Clinical Sciences, Faculty of Veterinary Medicine, Islamic Azad University, Shahrekord Branch, P.O. Box 166, Shahrekord, Iran*
[4] *Department of Microbiology, Faculty of Veterinary Medicine, Islamic Azad University, Shahrekord Branch, P.O. Box 166, Shahrekord, Iran*

Correspondence should be addressed to Afshin Raoofi, raoofi@ut.ac.ir

Academic Editor: Udeni B. R. Balasuriya

In a survey of 430 Lori-Bakhtiari sheep at a slaughterhouse in Iran, gallstones were found in the gallbladder of 7 sheep (1.6%). Biliary calculi were more frequent in adult and female sheep ($P < 0.05$). Chemical analysis of the gallstones revealed 6 sheep with pigment (bilirubin) stones and 1 sheep with cholesterol stones. Chemical composition of bile in these sheep was evaluated. Bacteriologic analysis of the bile in the affected sheep revealed bacteria (*Streptococcus* spp., *Klebsiella* spp., *Escherichia coli*, and *Salmonella* spp.) in 5 sheep. Microscopic examination of gallbladders revealed focal calcification, cystic glands, necrosis and atrophy of mucosal layer, edema, diffuse and focal infiltration of lymphocytes in submucosal layer, and hypertrophy of smooth muscles in sheep with gallstones. It was concluded that the prevalence of both types of gallstones in Lori-Bakhtiari sheep is low. Cholelithiasis can cause chronic inflammation of the gallbladder, but it is not likely to become clinically significant.

1. Introduction

The Lori-Bakhtiari sheep is one of the most common native breeds in the southwestern part of Iran, with more than 1.7 million head population, and the largest fat-tail size among all the breeds in Iran. Majority of the sheep population, are managed under a migratory system, utilizing the ranges as the major source of feed [1, 2]. Choleliths or gallstones are concretions of normally soluble components of bile. They occur infrequently in all the domestic species, but they are especially well described in ruminants [3]. There are two major types of gallstones (pigment and cholesterol), which seem to form due to distinctly different pathogenic mechanisms. Pigment stones are composed of large quantity of bile pigments, along with less amounts of cholesterol and calcium salts. Cholesterol stones can be almost pure cholesterol or mixtures of cholesterol and substances such as mucin [4]. Biliary stone formation begins with the precipitation or aggregation of normally soluble components of bile. Other mechanisms involved in the pathogenesis include ascariasis, ascending biliary infection or inflammation, biliary stasis, changes in bile composition, and presence of a foreign body [5]. Choleliths in the gallbladder usually do not become clinically significant unless they migrate and obstruct the extrahepatic bile ducts [3]. The pigment gallstones are more frequently detected in sheep (8.6%), and they are associated with high total bilirubin concentration in the bile [6]. Amazingly, the foetal sheep gallbladder is capable of containing concentrated bile that can produce gallstones. These stones are composed of calcium palmitate and pigment [7].

The clinical signs associated with cholelithiasis in the large animals are anorexia, weight loss, low milk yield, chronic intermittent diarrhea, recurrent attacks of sever abdominal pain, alimentary tract stasis, pain on percussion over the liver, pyrexia, jaundice, recumbency, depression, and coma. [8–10]. Hyperammonemic hepatic encephalopathy and photosensitization are other less common features of cholelithiasis. A subclinical presentation, caused by partial

Table 1: Characteristics of the sheep and their gallstones.

Sheep number	Gender	Age (year)	Gallstone Number	Diameter (mm)	Total weight (g)	Color	Consistency
1	Female	3	5	4	0.02	Green	Soft
2	Female	4	9	2	0.01	Brown	Semi hard
3	Female	4	10	1	0.03	Green	Soft
4	Male	3	6	1	0.05	Green	Soft
5	Male	4	2	4	0.02	Dark green	Soft
6	Female	1	8	1	0.01	Dark green	Soft
7	Female	1	9	1	0.02	Dark green	Soft

Table 2: Chemical composition of gallstones in the sheep.

Sheep number	Gallstone Bilirubin (%)	Cholesterol (%)	Oxalate (%)	Calcium (%)	Phosphorous (%)
1	12	38	20	25	5
2	9	41	30	20	—
3	—	18	—	72	10
4	3	5	—	81	11
5	—	80	—	15	5
6	4	7	—	76	13
7	80	3	—	16	1

obstruction of the biliary tree, may be recognized only on postmortem examination [5]. Choleliths may be associated with chronic cholecystitis [3]. The lack of observational models for noninduced cholelithiasis in animals had contributed to the absence of epidemiologic studies, which have been done in human beings [6]. In view of the paucity of information on cholelithiasis in sheep, this paper reports the prevalence and composition of choleliths in a main breed of Iranian sheep. Bacteriologic analysis and histopathological findings were reviewed.

2. Materials and Methods

The study was carried out on 430 Lori-Bakhtiari sheep (279 males and 151 females) at Juneghan abattoir in Chaharmahal-Bakhtiari province of Iran from November 2009 to June 2010. Before slaughter, an antemortem examination was done on all sheep during which their age and gender were evaluated. A division of young ($\leq$2 years, n = 297) and adult (>2 years, n = 133) sheep were done after inspection of their teeth. After slaughtering the sheep, the gallbladder was removed and the surface and some sections of the liver were examined macroscopically. A short incision was made in the gallbladder by use of a scissors. In sterile conditions, a sample of bile was collected by a swab for bacterial culture. Then, the gallbladder was opened and its contents passed through a filter (fourfold gauze) to collect the gallstones. A sample of bile was also collected from the sheep with gallstones for chemical analysis. Number, diameter, weight, color, consistency, and chemical composition of gallstones were determined. Gallstones were analyzed for the determination of cholesterol (CHOD-PAP), bilirubin (DCA), calcium (arsenazo), and phosphorous (phosphometric UV) concentrations. Measurements were performed by commercial kits (Pars Azmoon, Tehran, Iran) using an automated biochemical analyzer (Biotecnica, Roma, Italy) in accordance with the instructions by the manufacturers. Oxalate was determined (enzymatic method) with a commercial kit (Darman Kav, Tehran, Iran) using a spectrophotometer (Clima, Madrid, Spain). Bile samples were analyzed by the same methods using Hitachi 704 autoanalyzer (Tokyo, Japan). Tissue specimens from gallbladders with gallstones were fixed in neutral buffered 10% formalin, processed, and sectioned. Tissue sections were stained with hematoxylin-eosin and prepared for histopathological examination.

The SPSS version 16 statistical package was used for data analysis. The chi-square and Fisher's exact tests were used for comparing the groups, and $P < 0.05$ was considered to be significant.

3. Results

Seven of the 430 sheep (1.6%) had 2 to 10 gallstones in their gallbladders. The clinical sings associated with cholelithiasis were not observed in the affected sheep. Necropsy examination revealed no visible findings in the liver of sheep with gallstones. Number, diameter, weight, color, consistency, and chemical composition of gallstones are shown in Tables 1 and 2. Chemical analysis of the gallstones revealed 6 sheep with pigment (bilirubin) stones and 1 sheep with cholesterol stones. Bacteriologic analysis of the bile in 7 sheep with gallstones revealed bacteria

TABLE 3: Chemical composition of bile in the sheep with gallstones.

	Bile				
Sheep Number	Total bilirubin (mg/dL)	Direct bilirubin (mg/dL)	Cholesterol (mg/dL)	Calcium (mg/dL)	Phosphorous (mg/dL)
1	13.2	7.5	120	22	24
2	8.2	6	82	22	20
3	12	4.5	40	17	14
4	4	3	39	14	10
5	3	0.5	73	10	20
6	8.8	4	55	10	20
7	14	5	66	19	22

(*Streptococcus* spp., *Klebsiella* spp., *Escherichia coli,* and *Salmonella* spp.) in 5 sheep. Concentrations of total and direct bilirubin, cholesterol, calcium and phosphorous in the bile of the sheep with gallstones are shown in Table 3. The gallstones were more frequently found in adult than in young sheep ($P < 0.05$) and in female, rather than male ($P < 0.05$). Microscopic examination of gallbladders revealed focal calcification, cystic glands, necrosis and atrophy of mucosal layer, edema, diffuse and focal infiltration of lymphocytes in submucosal layer, and hypertrophy of smooth muscles in sheep with gallstones.

4. Discussion

The prevalence of gallstones in surveyed sheep was 1.6%, which was less than the prevalence in sheep (8.6%) reported by Cavallini et al. [6]. A study on prevalence of cholelithiasis in sheep indicated that 11.7% of sheep had gallstones [11]. Khaki [12] reported that the prevalence of gallstones in sheep and cattle slaughtered in Tehran abattoirs in Iran were 4.75% and 5.6%, respectively. A study on the gallbladders of 36 fetal sheep of gestational age 102–147 days revealed a 50% incidence of gallstones [7].

In the present investigation, the gallstones were more frequently found in adult than young sheep. The risk of gallstones increases with age in human beings. An increase in age may be directly proportional with an increase in cholesterol secretion and saturation [13].

The current study shows that the biliary calculi are more frequent in females compared with males. This is in agreement with what was reported by Cavallini et al. [6]. Female sex hormones are the obvious basis for this gender difference [13]. Progesterone and also probably estrogen impair gallbladder emptying and are associated with hypersecretion of cholesterol into bile. In addition, estrogen treatment reduces synthesis of bile acids. These proprecipitation factors peak during late pregnancy when the levels of these steroids hormones are at the highest [4]. However, the results of one study indicated higher frequency of gallstones in male sheep [11].

In this study, most of the gallstones found in the sheep were pigment stones. This is in agreement with the results reported by Petruzzi et al. [11], Cavallini et al. [6], and Khaki [12]. All gallstones that they found in sheep and cattle were pigment type. These findings indicate that pigment cholelithiasis is more common in ruminants.

Bacteriologic analysis of the bile in 5 of the 7 sheep with gallstones revealed bacteria (*Streptococcus* spp., *Klebsiella* spp., *Escherichia coli,* and *Salmonella* spp.). Isolation of bacteria from bile is common. In one study, bacteriologic analysis of the bile in 10 sheep with gallstones and 10 controls (without gallstones) revealed bacteria in 50% of the first group and 75% of the second group [6].

Microscopic examination of gallbladders revealed focal calcification, cystic glands, necrosis and atrophy of mucosal layer, edema, diffuse and focal infiltration of lymphocytes in submucosal layer, and hypertrophy of smooth muscles. These findings indicate chronic cholecystitis which is most likely to be due to the mechanical irritation of the gallbladder by biliary calculi. Cholecystitis may occur as a result of bacterial infections such as salmonellosis. Other bacteria, either derived from the blood or ascended from the intestine, can cause acute or chronic cholecystitis. Chronic cholecystitis typically accompanies prolonged bacterial infection of the biliary tree or ongoing irritation from choleliths or parasites of the gallbladder [3].

Based on the results of this study, the prevalence of both types of gallstones in Lori-Bakhtiari sheep is low. Although cholelithiasis can cause chronic inflammation of the gallbladder, it is not likely to become clinically significant.

Acknowledgments

The authors wish to thank Dr. A. Khodabakhsh Sarbandi, Dr. H. Shojaei, Dr. A. Badakhsh, and Dr. S. Baradaran for their contributions and support.

References

[1] G. H. Shadnoush, G. R. Ghorbani, and M. A. Edris, "Effect of different energy levels in feed and slaughter weights on carcass and chemical composition of Lori-Bakhtiari ram lambs," *Small Ruminant Research*, vol. 51, no. 3, pp. 243–249, 2004.

[2] M. Vatankhah and F. Zamani, "Phenotypic and genetic characteristics of longevity in Lori-Bakhtiari sheep," *Biotechnology in Animal Husbandry*, vol. 23, pp. 323–329, 2007.

[3] J. M. Cullen, "Diseases of the gallbladder," in *Pathologic Basis of Veterinary Diseases*, M. D. Mc Gavin and J. F. Zachary, Eds.,

pp. 453–455, Mosby Elsevier, St. Louis, Mo, USA, 4th edition, 2007.

[4] D. E. Johnston and M. M. Kaplan, "Medical progress: pathogenesis and treatment of gallstones," *New England Journal of Medicine*, vol. 328, no. 6, pp. 412–421, 1993.

[5] T. C. Gerros, "Gallbladder and biliary tract disease," in *Large Animal Internal Medicine*, B. P. Smith, Ed., pp. 920–921, Mosby Elsevier, St. Louis, Mo, USA, 4th edition, 2009.

[6] A. Cavallini, C. Messa, V. Mangini et al., "Prevalence of pigment gallstones in sheep," *American Journal of Veterinary Research*, vol. 52, no. 12, pp. 2043–2045, 1991.

[7] J. R. Wood, V. M. France, and D. J. Sutor, "Occurrence of gallstones in foetal sheep," *Laboratory Animals*, vol. 8, no. 2, pp. 155–159, 1974.

[8] H. J. West and R. Hogg, "Biliary calculi in a herd of shorthorn cattle in Lancashire," *Veterinary Record*, vol. 122, no. 11, pp. 251–256, 1988.

[9] J. K. Johnston, T. J. Divers, V. B. Reef, and H. Acland, "Cholelithiasis in horses: ten cases (1982–1986)," *Journal of the American Veterinary Medical Association*, vol. 194, no. 3, pp. 405–409, 1989.

[10] O. M. Radostits, C. C. Gay, K. W. Hinchcliff, and P. B. Constable, *Veterinary Medicine*, Saunders, Edinburgh, UK, 10th edition, 2007.

[11] J. Petruzzi, V. Mangini, C. Messa, and G. Misciagna, "Spontaneous cholelithiasis in sheep: prevalence survey and analysis of gallstones and bile," *Journal of Comparative Pathology*, vol. 98, no. 3, pp. 367–369, 1988.

[12] Z. Khaki, "Gallstones in sheep and cows slaughtered at Tehran abattoir," *Journal of the Faculty of Veterinary Medicine, University of Tehran*, vol. 60, pp. 401–403, 2005.

[13] E. A. Shaffer, "Epidemiology of gallbladder stone disease," *Best Practice and Research*, vol. 20, no. 6, pp. 981–996, 2006.

22

Effects of Feeding of Two Potentially Probiotic Preparations from Lactic Acid Bacteria on the Performance and Faecal Microflora of Broiler Chickens

Paula Fajardo,[1] Lorenzo Pastrana,[1] Jesús Méndez,[2]
Isabel Rodríguez,[1] Clara Fuciños,[1] and Nelson P. Guerra[1]

[1] *Departamento de Química Analítica y Alimentaria, Facultade de Ciencias de Ourense, Universidade de Vigo, As Lagoas s/n, 32004 Ourense, Spain*
[2] *Cooperativas Orensanas Sociedad Cooperativa Ltda (COREN), Polígono San Ciprián de Viñas, 32901 Ourense, Spain*

Correspondence should be addressed to Nelson P. Guerra, nelsonpg@uvigo.es

Academic Editors: G. Tellez and I. Valpotic

The aim of this study was to evaluate the potential of two probiotic preparations, containing live lactic acid bacteria (*Lactococcus lactis* CECT 539 and *Lactobacillus casei* CECT 4043) and their products of fermentation (organic acids and bacteriocins), as a replacement for antibiotics in stimulating health and growth of broiler chickens. The effects of the supplementation of both preparations (with proven probiotic effect in weaned piglets) and an antibiotic (avilamycin) on body weight gain (BWG), feed intake (FI), feed consumption efficiency (FCE), relative intestinal weight, and intestinal microbiota counts were studied in 1-day posthatch chickens. The experiments were conducted with medium-growth Sasso X44 chickens housed in cages and with nutritional stressed Ross 308 broiler distributed in pens. Consumption of the different diets did not affect significantly the final coliform counts in Sasso X44 chickens. However, counts of lactic acid bacteria and mesophilic microorganisms were higher in the animals receiving the two probiotic preparations ($P < 0.05$). In the second experiment, although no differences in BWG were observed between treatments, Ross 308 broilers receiving the probiotic *Lactobacillus* preparation exhibited the lowest FCE values and were considered the most efficient at converting feed into live weight.

1. Introduction

Antibiotics have been extensively used in animal feed to improve production in poultry and piglet industries [1]. However, the use of these substances as growth promoters can lead to the development of antibiotic resistances. Such resistances can occur not only in pathogenic bacteria [2, 3], which can be transferred from poultry products to human population [4], but also in commensal bacteria [5], constituting a reservoir of resistance genes for pathogenic bacteria [6]. In recent years, the interest in finding alternatives to the use of antibiotics in animal feed has been increased due to the ban of subtherapeutic antibiotic usage in Europe. The research is mostly focused on incorporating into animal feeds, substances derived from plants, animals, bacteria and fungi, as well as organic acid, essential oils, and bacteriocins, that could interfere in colonisation of pathogens [7–9].

Due to their potential to reduce enteric disease in poultry, probiotics are considered to be a good alternative to the use of antibiotics [10]. The production of antimicrobial compounds (mainly organic acids and bacteriocins) by many lactic acid bacteria (LAB) into the intestine has provided these organisms with a competitive advantage over other microorganisms to be used as probiotics [11, 12]. Moreover, the presence of some *Lactobacillus* in the chicken gastrointestinal tract (GIT) has been described to be of great importance for regulating the composition of the intestinal microflora, developing immunity of the intestine, and promoting the health of chickens [13].

The administration of highly concentrated bacterial cultures, containing both the live cells and their products of fermentation, was an effective way to promote body weight gain (BWG) and improve feed conversion efficiency (FCE) in chickens [6, 14–16]. In fact, probiotics are used nowadays by compound feed industry to improve the poultry production [17, 18].

In a previous work [1], two potentially probiotic preparations, containing the live cells of *Lactococcus lactis* CECT 539 or *Lactobacillus casei* CECT 4043, as well as their fermentation products, were evaluated as probiotic additives to replace antibiotics in weaning pig diets. The administration of these potentially probiotic preparations improved BWG and feed intake (FI). In the same study, Guerra et al. [1] observed that the two above-mentioned LAB fulfil many of the probiotic criteria [19], because they are (i) nonpathogenic, (ii) able to survive during processing and storage, (iii) resistant to bile and acid environment, and (iv) producer of inhibitory compounds (organic acids and antibacterial activity).

Since probiotic effects are strain dependent [1] and may also depend on the host and their immunologic state [20], the observed probiotic effects of the *L. lactis* CECT 539 and *Lact. casei* CECT 4043 preparations in piglets might not be observed in other host entities. Therefore, in an attempt for testing the latter hypothesis, the *L. lactis* CECT 539 and *Lact. casei* CECT 4043 preparations (containing both the live cells and their products of fermentation) were evaluated as a replacement for antibiotics in stimulating health and growth of broilers.

2. Materials and Methods

2.1. Bacterial Strains. Lactobacillus casei subsp. *casei* CECT 4043 (a high lactic acid-producing strain) and *Lactococcus lactis* subsp. *lactis* CECT 539 (a nisin-producing strain) were obtained from the Spanish Type Culture Collection (CECT). Stock cultures of both LAB strains were maintained at −40°C in nutrient broth supplemented with 15% glycerol. Working cultures, maintained at 4°C on de Man, Rogosa, and Sharpe (MRS, Cultimed) agar, were prepared monthly from frozen stock cultures.

2.2. Production of the Potentially Probiotic Preparations of the Two LAB. The potentially probiotic preparations of the strains CECT 4043 and CECT 539 were obtained by using a fed-batch fermentation technique based on successive realkalizations of the culture media, which were prepared with cheese whey from a local dairy plant [21]. The fermentation medium was a diluted whey (DW: concentrated whey (CW) mixed with wash water), which contained (in g/L): total sugars, 20.54; total nitrogen, 0.45; total phosphorus, 0.25, and soluble proteins, 2.04 [1]. The substrates used as feeding media were a concentrated lactose solution (400 g/L) and CW medium. The latter substrate contained (in g/L): total sugars, 48.11; total nitrogen, 1.05; total phosphorus, 0.43, and soluble proteins, 5.02 [1].

The realkalized fed-batch cultures with each LAB strain were carried out at a controlled temperature of 30°C in a 10 L bench top bioreactor tailored at an agitation speed of 200 rpm and continuous record of pH as described before [1, 21, 22].

Table 1: Mean composition of the probiotic preparations obtained from realkalized fed-batch cultures of *Lact. casei* CECT 4043 and *L. lactis* CECT 539.

Composition	CECT 4043	CECT 539
Total sugars (g/L)	16.16	19.71
Nitrogen (g/L)	1.37	1.59
Phosphorous (g/L)	0.07	0.36
Protein (g/L)	6.09	9.15
pH	7.00	7.00
Viable cells (CFU/mL)[1]	3.69×10^9	3.34×10^9
Antibacterial activity (AU/mL)[2]	28.85	164.49
Lactic acid (g/L)	33.47	17.54
Formic acid (g/L)	0.10	0.85

[1] CFU: colony-forming units.
[2] AU: activity units.

At the end of each realkalized fed-batch culture, the media were adjusted to pH 7.0 to facilitate the adsorption of the bacteriocin onto the producer strains [23]. Subsequently, the cultures (cells plus the fermentation products) were preserved at −20°C with skim milk powder (300 g/L of fermented medium) until further use, as indicated by Guerra et al. [1].

2.3. Preparation of the Experimental Feeds. The potentially probiotic preparations of the two LAB (composition in Table 1) were defrosted and mixed with the commercial mash broiler feed (named basal diet which composition is showed in Table 2) using an end-over-end mixer in a ratio of 20 mL probiotic preparation/kg feed. No pellet was made with the experimental feeds. This can contribute to increase feed wastage and, so, to increase feed conversion values; however for comparative purposes between treatments it is worth keeping high probiotic counts. The probiotic preparations were added weekly to the basal diets as recommended by Guerra et al. [1]. In the group receiving the antibiotic, the basal diet was supplemented with 10 mg of avilamycin per kg of feed.

2.4. Analytical Determinations. The concentrations of total sugars, phosphorous, nitrogen, protein, lactic acid, formic acid and antibacterial activity in the probiotic preparations were determined by methods previously described [23, 24].

2.5. Experimental Animals and Management. The two experiments were carried out in the experimental farm of COREN, S.C.L. (Ourense, Spain). One-day-old males were used in both experiments and fed *ad libitum*. Four experimental groups were assayed: a control group fed with unsupplemented basal diet, a second group fed with the probiotic *Lactobacillus casei* preparation, a third group fed with the probiotic *Lactococcus lactis* preparation, and an antibiotic (avilamycin) supplemented fed group.

2.5.1. Experiment 1. A total of 120 medium-growth Sasso X44 chickens were distributed into 12 replicates of 10 birds

TABLE 2: Composition of the basal diets of both experiments.

Composition (g/Kg of diet)	Experiment 1	Experiment 2
Barley	20.0	70.0
Wheat	300.0	500.0
Maize	300.0	0.0
Animal fat	15.0	48.2
Full fat soybean	35.0	28.6
Soybean meal 440	272.0	20.0
Gluten feed	20.0	0.0
Soybean meal 470	0.0	287.4
Sodium bicarbonate	0.3	0.5
Calcium carbonate	14.0	11.2
Monocalcium phosphate	13.5	19.6
Sodium chloride	3.9	3.5
L-Choline 75	0.9	0.9
DL(+)-Methionine	1.9	3.4
L-Threonine	0.0	0.6
L-Lysine	0.7	3.3
Coccidiostate[a]	0.6	0.6
Mineral premix[b]	1.1	1.1
Vitamin premix[c]	1.1	1.1

[a]C-Maxiban G150.
[b]Premix contained per kg of diet: Co 0.15 g, Cu 8 g, Fe 40 g, I 1.9 g, Mn 80 g, Se 0.25 g, Zn 65 g.
[c]Premix contained per kg of diet: Vitamin A 12000 IU, Vitamin D_3 4000 IU, Vitamin E 50 IU, Vitamin K 3.5 mg, Vitamin B_1 2.5 mg, Vitamin B_2 7 mg, pantothenic acid 14 mg, Vitamin B_6 3 mg, Vitamin B_{12} 15 mg, nicotinic acid 55 mg, folic acid 1 mg, biotin 0.17 mg.

each (three replicates per treatment) during an experimental period of 42 days. Each replicate was housed separately in individual metal cages (75 × 40 × 105 cm), situated at 80 cm from the floor to limit the consumption of faeces. The cycle of light was natural environment (12 h of daylight) and the temperature during the treatment, maintained with propane heating, was the following: first week, 32°C, second week, 30°C, and third week, 26°C. From day 21, the temperature was maintained between 20 and 24°C. The BWG, FI, and FCE were calculated at 7, 14, 21, and 42 days after the animals received the experimental diets.

2.5.2. Experiment 2. A total of 1200 commercial Ross 308 broiler chicks were distributed into 24 pens (12.7 animals/m^2) of 50 birds (six replicates per treatment) during an experimental period of 31 days on wood shaving floor to simulate farm conditions. According to the good manufacturing practices of Coren S.C.L., the light program consisted in 24 h for the first 12 days, one hour alternating light and dark from day 15 to day 21, and 2 h alternating light and dark from day 21 until the end of the experiment. The temperature program was similar to that of experiment 1. BWG, FI, and FCE were determined at 16 and 31 days.

2.6. Sample Collection. At 7, 14, 21, and 42 days (in case of experiment 1) and at 7, 16, and 31 days (in case of experiment 2), 24 chickens (2 per replicate, so 6 per treatment) in experiment 1 and 48 chickens (2 per replicate, so 12 per treatment) in experiment 2 were chosen randomly and sacrificed. Animal management followed the animal care and welfare guidelines of COREN S.C.L. The abdominal cavity was opened and the gastrointestinal tract was excised to determine the number of bacterial counts. In experiment 1 the whole gastrointestinal tract, from crop to caeca, was used. In experiment 2 only the caeca were excised.

2.7. Bacterial Counts in Gastrointestinal Samples. All gastrointestinal samples emptied of faeces were weighed and placed in a sterile bag with sterile phosphate buffered saline (PBS, pH 7, 100 mM NaCl) in proportion 1 : 10 (w/v) and pummelled for 2 min in a Stomacher. Tenfold serial dilutions in sterile PBS were performed up to 10^7 and aliquots (0.1 mL) of each dilution were pour-plated in MRS agar (Cultimed), eosin methylene blue agar (EMB, Levine Formulation, Cultimed), and Tryptone Soy Agar (TSA, Cultimed) to determine the main representative cultivable LAB microbiota, coliforms, and total mesophilic counts, respectively. The plates were incubated at 37 ± 1°C for 24 h for coliform counts and at 30 ± 1°C for 24 h and 48 h for mesophilic bacteria and LAB counts, respectively. The results were expressed as the number of colony-forming units per gram (wet weight) of intestinal content (CFU/g).

2.8. Statistical Analysis. Data on growth performance, bacterial counts, and relative intestine weight were statistically analyzed using the software package SPSS 13.0 for Windows (Release 13.0.1; SPSS Inc., Chicago, IL, 2004). Viable counts in the intestinal content were transformed by logarithm ($\log_{10}$) before statistical analysis. Normal distribution of data as well as the independence and homogeneity of variances among treatment groups was verified by looking at the distribution of the data and the Fisher F-test (which is included in the t-test output), respectively. A one-way analysis of variance (ANOVA) with the step-down multiple-stage F post hoc test (Ryan-Einot-Gabriel-Welsch multiple F-test (P = 0.05) was used to distinguish treatment mean differences [1].

3. Results

3.1. Probiotic Preparations. The mean compositions of the two probiotic preparations obtained from the realkalized fed-batch fermentations with *Lact. casei* and *L. lactis* on whey are shown in Table 1. As it can be observed, both probiotic preparations contained relatively high concentrations of inhibitory products (lactic acid and antibacterial activity) and relatively low concentrations of formic acid, which were accumulated at different concentrations in the culture media during the realkalized fed-batch fermentations.

In addition, both preparations were characterized with high concentrations of viable cells (3.69 × 10^9 CFU/mL in case of *Lact. casei* and 3.34 × 10^9 CFU/mL in case of *L. lactis*). Therefore, addition of the two potential probiotic preparations at the dose of 20 mL/kg of feed offered the possibility of preparing feeds with viable cells concentrations of 7.38 × 10^7 CFU of *Lact. casei* or 6.68 × 10^7 CFU of *L. lactis*

Table 3: Effect of dietary probiotic preparations (CECT 4043, CECT 539) or antibiotic (avilamycin) on growth performance parameters of medium-growth Sasso X44 chickens during 42 days (experiment 1).

Treatment[1]	BWG (g per chicken)	FI (g per chicken)	FCE (g of FI/g of BWG)	Relative intestine weight (g of organ/g of BW)
		Chicken performance (days 1–21)		
Control	436 ± 21[a]	749 ± 16[a]	1.72 ± 0.05	0.066 ± 0.006
CECT 4043	425 ± 5[ab]	754 ± 9[a]	1.78 ± 0.01	0.064 ± 0.003
CECT 539	395 ± 13[b]	654 ± 80[b]	1.65 ± 0.15	0.067 ± 0.007
Avilamycin	440 ± 17[a]	766 ± 15[a]	1.74 ± 0.05	0.060 ± 0.009
F	5.477	4.630	1.179	0.965
d.f. (N)[2]	3 (12)	3 (12)	3 (12)	3 (24)
		Chicken performance (days 1–42)		
Control	1336 ± 33	2864 ± 140	2.14 ± 0.07	0.046 ± 0.004[a]
CECT 4043	1348 ± 33	2858 ± 97	2.12 ± 0.05	0.045 ± 0.002[a]
CECT 539	1314 ± 16	2800 ± 120	2.13 ± 0.07	0.048 ± 0.006[a]
Avilamycin	1503 ± 16	3084 ± 84	2.06 ± 0.14	0.040 ± 0.004[b]
F	3.935	3.741	0.584	4.242
d.f. (N)	3 (12)	3 (12)	3 (12)	3 (24)

[a–c]Means within columns followed by different letters are significantly different ($P < 0.05$).
[1]The chickens from the control group were not given probiotic preparations or antibiotic. The chickens in the CECT 4043, CECT 539, and avilamycin groups were fed with *Lactobacillus casei* CECT 4043 (7.38×10^{10} CFU/Kg diet), *Lactococcus lactis* CECT 539 (6.68×10^{10} CFU/Kg diet) preparations, and avilamycin (10 mg/Kg diet), respectively. BWG: body weight gain, FI: feed intake, FCE: feed conversion efficiency.
[2]d.f.: degree of freedom. N: number of samples.

per g of feed. Both concentrations are higher than that of the recommended dose of viable probiotic cells (10^6 CFU per g or mL) necessary to observe beneficial effects [25, 26].

3.2. Performance of Medium-Growth Sasso X44 Chickens in Cages (Experiment 1). The BWG, FI, and FCE values of medium-growth Sasso X44 chickens fed with the different diets during the experimental period are shown in Table 3. Broilers fed the *L. lactis* CECT 539 preparation showed the lowest values of BWG and FI during the first 21 d of treatment ($P < 0.05$), but no differences were found for FCE among groups. In addition, for the entire experimental period, diets did not affect any of the growth performance parameters studied.

Interestingly, at the end of the experiment (42 d), avilamycin feeding resulted in a reduction ($P < 0.05$) in the mean relative intestinal weight (0.040 g of organ/g of BW) in comparison to the control group (0.046 g of organ/g of BW) and the groups receiving *Lact. casei* (0.045 g of organ/g of BW) and *L. lactis* (0.048 g of organ/g of BW). However, no significant differences in the relative intestine weight were observed between the two groups receiving the two probiotic preparations and the control group (Table 3).

3.3. Effect of the Feeding with Probiotic Preparations on the Intestinal Microbiota of Medium-Growth Sasso X44 Chickens in Cages (Experiment 1). The viable counts of the different groups of bacteria analyzed in this trial are shown in Figure 1. With regard to the coliforms (upper part of Figure 1), no significant differences were found in total counts among diets, probably because birds were placed in cages elevated 80 cm above the barn floor, where no reconsume of faeces occurred.

However, in broilers fed the probiotic preparations, the final average LAB counts (8.16 $\log_{10}$ CFU/g in case of strain CECT 4043 and 8.18 $\log_{10}$ CFU/g in case of strain CECT 539) were higher ($P < 0.10$) than that (7.64 $\log_{10}$ CFU/g) of the control group (middle part of Figure 1). In chickens fed avilamycin, the average LAB counts decreased progressively until reaching a final value at the end of the experiment (6.35 $\log_{10}$ CFU/g) significantly lower ($P < 0.05$) than those final levels obtained in the other three groups (middle part of Figure 1).

As expected, the final average mesophilic counts in the groups fed the probiotic preparations (7.66 $\log_{10}$ CFU/g in case of strain CECT 4043 and 7.65 $\log_{10}$ CFU/g in case of strain CECT 539) by day 42 were significantly higher ($P < 0.05$) than that (7.21 $\log_{10}$ CFU/g) of the avilamycin group (lower part of Figure 1).

3.4. Performance of Broiler Chickens in Pens with Wood Shaving Litter and Subjected to Nutritional Stress (Experiment 2). Table 4 summarizes the effect of dietary probiotic preparations or avilamycin on growth performance parameters in stressed chickens. With regard to the final BWG, no significant differences were observed among treatments during the whole experimental period. However, broilers fed avilamycin had higher FCE values ($P < 0.05$) than the other three groups. At 16 days of treatment, the FCE values in the groups fed the probiotic preparations (1.86 ± 0.08 in case of strain CECT 4043 and 1.82 ± 0.08 in case of strain CECT 539) were lower than those of the avilamycin (2.15 ± 0.18, $P < 0.05$) and control (2.04 ± 0.20) groups. Although the FCE values increased in the four groups at the end of the experimental period, broilers fed *Lact. casei* CECT 4043 preparation were more efficient than those fed avilamycin ($P < 0.05$) or

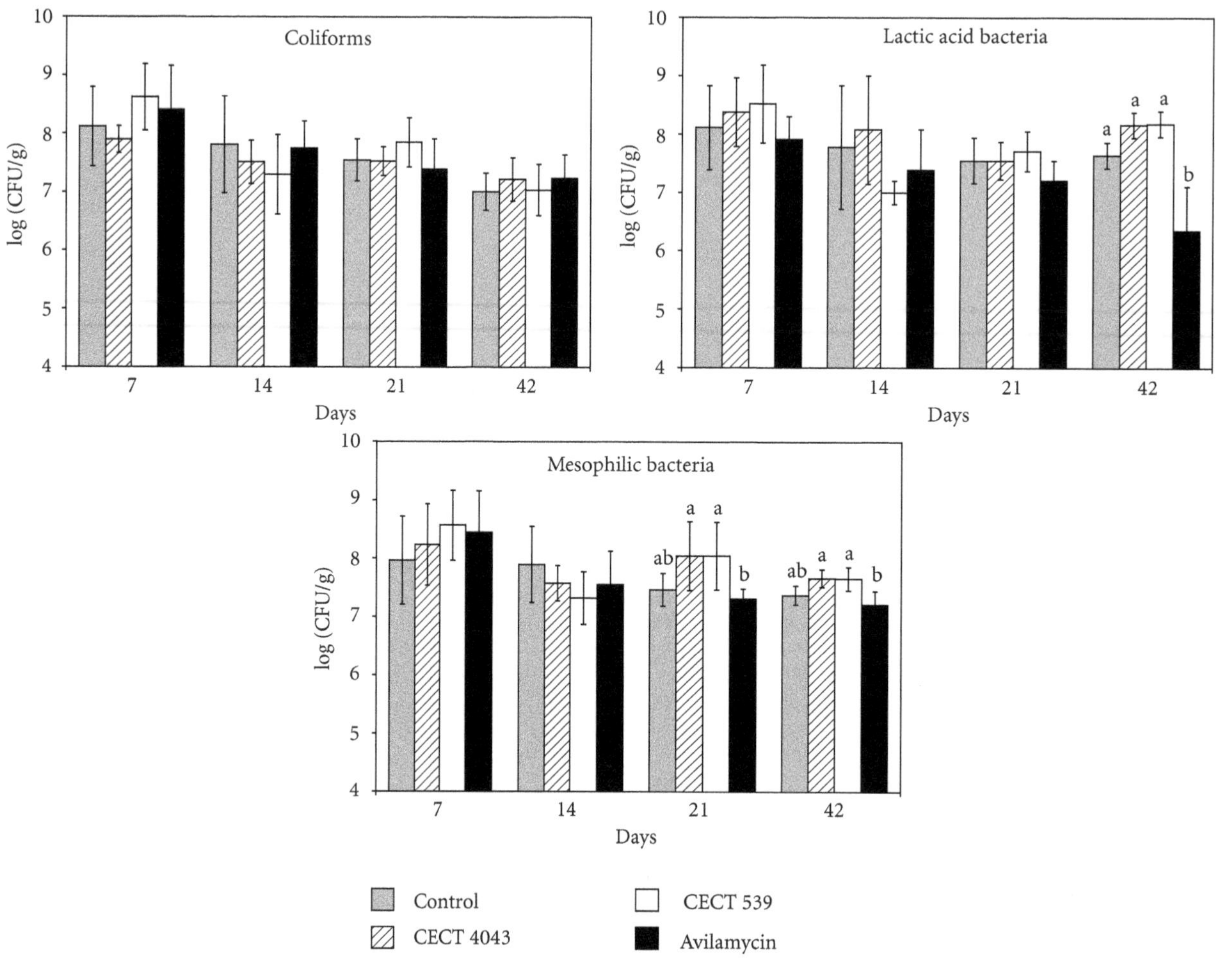

FIGURE 1: Viable plate counts (means ± standard deviations) of coliforms, lactic acid bacteria and mesophilic bacteria in the intestinal content of medium-growth Sasso X44 chickens fed with a non supplemented diet (control), or diets supplemented with the probiotic *Lact. casei* CECT 4043 or *L. lactis* CECT 539 preparations or avilamycin. [a–c]Means within columns followed by different letters are significantly ($P < 0.05$).

unsupplemented feed ($P < 0.10$). In the present study, mortality was not significantly ($P < 0.05$) affected by probiotic treatment over the experimental period (data not shown).

Although, at the end of the experiment, the relative weight of caeca values in all the groups were approximately 1% of the animal weight, as described by Redig [27], no significant differences were found between broilers fed with the different diets.

3.5. Total Coliform Counts in the Caeca of Ross 308 Broiler Chickens (Experiment 2). Coliform counts in the caeca were highly variable throughout the assay, with large variance of values within individual treatment groups and variations observed in counts at different time points (Figure 2). Consequently, no significant difference in fecal coliform counts ($P < 0.05$) was observed in the four groups during the experimental period.

4. Discussion

The results obtained in experiment 1 showed that, at the end of the experimental period (42 days), consumption of the different diets did not affect any of the growth performance parameters of medium-growth Sasso X44 chickens. However, a significant decrease in the relative intestinal weight ($P < 0.05$) was observed in the group receiving avilamycin as compared with the nontreated control group and the groups fed diets with the probiotic preparations. A similar result was observed when bacitracin and virginiamycin, two antibiotic growth promoters, were assayed as additives in corn-soybean meal diets for Ross × Ross broiler chicks [28]. This decrease in the intestinal weight because of consumption of antibiotics has been documented by other authors [29, 30] before knowing their positive effect as growth promoters in chicks. Reduction in intestinal weight has been associated to a thinning of the gastrointestinal walls tract probably due to an inhibition of the microbial production of polyamines and volatile fatty acids [31].

Interestingly, in the present study, the groups receiving the two probiotic preparations had similar relative intestine weights than the group fed control diet (Table 3), suggesting that the mechanism of action of avilamycin and the probiotic preparations was different.

TABLE 4: Effect of dietary probiotic preparations (CECT 4043, CECT 539) or antibiotic (avilamycin) on growth performance parameters of Ross 308 broiler chickens subjected to nutritional stress (experiment 2).

Treatment[1]	BWG (g per chicken)	FI (g per chicken)	FCE (g of FI/g of BWG)	Relative caeca weight (g of organ/g of BW)
		Chicken performance (days 1–16)		
Control	397 ± 34	805 ± 42^{a}	2.04 ± 0.20^{ba}	0.012 ± 0.003
CECT 4043	387 ± 13	721 ± 9^{b}	1.86 ± 0.08^{cb}	0.011 ± 0.003
CECT 539	388 ± 15	706 ± 18^{b}	1.82 ± 0.08^{c}	0.011 ± 0.002
Avilamycin	369 ± 39	789 ± 47^{a}	2.15 ± 0.18^{a}	0.012 ± 0.003
F	1.025	13.042	6.810	1.669
d.f (N)[2]	3 (24)	3 (24)	3 (24)	3 (48)
		Chicken performance (days 1–31)		
Control	1377 ± 82	2909 ± 154	2.11 ± 0.10^{ab}	0.009 ± 0.003
CECT 4043	1388 ± 42	2802 ± 34	2.02 ± 0.05^{b}	0.009 ± 0.003
CECT 539	1364 ± 46	2812 ± 56	2.06 ± 0.07^{ab}	0.008 ± 0.003
Avilamycin	1319 ± 87	2872 ± 33	2.18 ± 0.12^{a}	0.007 ± 0.003
F	1.221	2.135	3.689	3.446
d.f (N)	3 (24)	3 (24)	3 (24)	3 (44)

$^{a-c}$Means within columns followed by different letters are significantly different ($P < 0.05$).
[1]The chickens from the control group were not given probiotic preparations or antibiotic. The chickens in the CECT 4043, CECT 539, and avilamycin groups were fed with *Lactobacillus casei* CECT 4043 (7.38×10^{10} CFU/Kg diet), *Lactococcus lactis* CECT 539 (6.68×10^{10} CFU/Kg diet) preparations, and avilamycin (10 mg/Kg diet), respectively. BWG: body weight gain, FI: feed intake, FCE: feed conversion efficiency.
[2]d.f.: degree of freedom. N : number of samples.

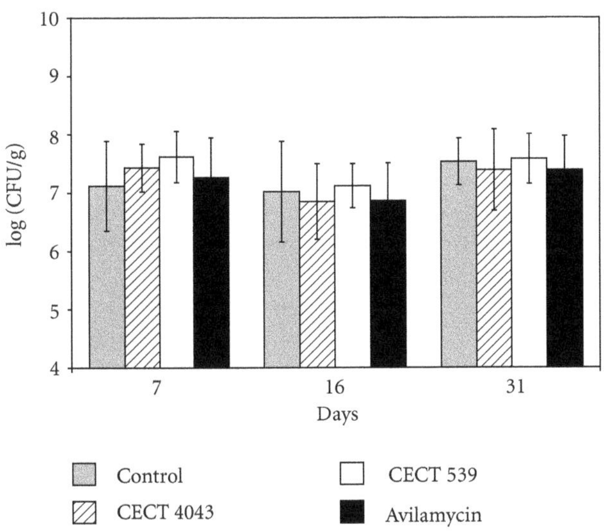

FIGURE 2: Viable plate counts (means ± standard deviations) of coliforms in the caeca of Ross 308 broilers fed with a non supplemented diet (control) or diets supplemented with the probiotic *Lact. casei* CECT 4043 or *L. lactis* CECT 539 preparations or avilamycin.

In the first experiment, no significant differences were found in total coliform counts among groups (Figure 1). In this way, when a pathogen colonizes the intestine, infection in the other chickens happens by horizontal transmission through faeces [32], but, in this assay, chickens had a minimum contact with their faeces and, consequently, the growth of enteric bacterial contamination was avoided.

At the end of the experimental period, LAB counts in the probiotic fed groups were higher than that of the control group. The strains CECT 4043 and CECT 539 used in this experiment have proven to be resistant to acid and bile salts *in vitro* under conditions that mimic the animal GIT environment [1]. Therefore, the higher LAB counts found in chickens fed probiotics could be due to the presence of the *Lact. casei* CECT 4043 and *L. lactis* CECT 539 in the GIT, permanently as a result of the colonization of the intestinal mucus, or temporarily and dependent on the diet consumed by the birds. Another possible reason to explain the increase in LAB counts could be the growth of other epiphytic LAB due to the probiotic cells supplemented in the diet. Contrarily, chickens fed with avilamycin showed a continuous decrease in LAB counts, which were at the end of the experiment (42 days), significantly lower than those of the groups receiving the two probiotic preparations. These results suggest that the feeding with avilamycin inhibits the development of LAB. Also the highest counts of mesophilic bacteria were found in chicks fed the two probiotic preparations. As mesophilic bacteria also include LAB, the increase in mesophilic counts observed in the probiotic groups could be due to the same reasons previously discussed for LAB counts. Yu et al. [33] also reported that Arbor Acres broiler fed a *Lactobacillus reuteri* Pg4 transformant in pens showed higher total aerobic and *Lactobacillus* spp. counts in the ileum and caecum than unsupplemented control birds. In conclusion, the experimental system chosen in this first trial for the handling of animals, which reduces their contact with faeces, could mask a potential protective effect of probiotic or antibiotic. These results suggested the need of choosing other handling conditions.

Then, in experiment 2, the effect of the probiotic preparations containing *Lact. casei* CECT 4043 and *L. lactis* CECT 539 cultures was evaluated in wood shaving floor, using the similar conditions of temperature, cycle of light, and handling as the farm conditions. With this approach, the transmission of microorganisms between animals could be facilitated. The medium-growth Sasso X44 chickens previously used in the first trial were replaced by Ross 308 broilers in the second trial. In order to obtain a more accurate analysis, both the number of animals per treatment and the number of replicates were increased. Additionally, a feed based on barley and wheat was used to promote intestinal adverse conditions that could be reversed or improved by using a probiotic treatment. These cereals contain high amounts of nonstarch polysaccharides (NSPs), which have "anti-nutritive effects" and increase the viscosity of the intestinal content [34]. The use of barley can deteriorate the intestinal structure, causing decrease of length and width of villi and their atrophy [35, 36]. Otherwise, Hofshagen and Kaldhusdal [37] observed that the counts of *Lactobacillus* and *Streptococcus* strains were higher in chickens fed with diets based on corn than chickens fed diets with barley. Moreover, Dalloul et al. [38] observed an increase in resistance to coccidiosis in chickens fed with a *Lactobacillus*-based probiotic diet. These results support the hypothesis that these bacteria could control the necrotic enteritis and it could be expected that the probiotic feed used in this trial would protect against this infection.

In this second experiment the FCE values of broilers fed with *Lact. casei* CECT 4043 preparation were lower ($P < 0.10$) than that of the broilers fed with the control diet at 16 and 31 days. With respect to avilamycin, the decrease of FCE was statistically significant ($P < 0.05$) in both periods. This positive effect of *Lactobacillus*-supplemented diets on FCE has been previously reported. Thus, laying hens, that received *L. acidophilus* supplemented diets for a 48-week period [39], had significantly better FCE than control birds. In the same way, the addition of either the single *L. acidophilus* or a mixture of 12 *Lactobacillus* cultures significantly improved FCE in broilers [14].

The use of the wheat and barley diet did not increase mortality in any of the treatments. Thus, in the second experiment, slighter and subclinic necrotic enteritis could occur, as this type of enteritidis is asymptomatic [40]. Consequently, it is probable that the nutritional stress induced in this trial was not enough to see the growth-stimulating effects of the probiotic bacteria in animal exposed to stress reported by other authors [41, 42].

In experiment 1, no significant differences were found between treatments in total coliform counts in the whole intestinal tract (Figure 1). However, it has been reported that bacterial distribution along the gastrointestinal tract is not uniform [33]. The high acidity in the stomach as well as the concentration of bile components in the proximal intestine determines a strain selection [43] and reduces the bacteria counts in the proximal segments of intestine, crop, and ileum, in comparison with the caecum. But the homogenization of the contents of the whole intestine could minimize differences among the different segments. In this manner, Jin et al. [14] did not observe significant differences in the coliform population in the small intestine of broilers fed diets supplemented with *Lactobacillus* during the experimental period, although the number of coliforms was significantly reduced in the caeca. For these reasons, and considering that the caecum is a distal part where more favourable conditions for bacterial development exist, in experiment 2, this part was used to analyze the number of total coliform counts. However, no significant differences ($P < 0.05$) were found in total coliform counts between the treatments (Figure 2).

Probiotics inhibit the adhesion of certain pathogenic bacteria such as *E. coli* and *Salmonella enterica* to the epithelial cells *in vitro* [44]. Competitive binding to receptors or the stimulation of host factors such as the production of mucin has been proposed as possible reasons to explain this inhibition [45]. However, not always inhibitory effects of probiotic strains on the growth of coliforms are observed in *in vivo* trials because host-dependent mechanisms are important in reducing the coliform level [46]. Guerra et al. [1], reported that viable coliform counts in pigs fed *L. lactis* CECT 539 and *Lact. casei* CECT 4043 preparations dropped on average for 1.8 and 1.4 log units, respectively mean; while viable coliform counts did not change in the control group. However, in the current experiment, the above discussed coliform counts reduction was not observed. The host-dependent theory suggested by Meimandipour et al. [46] could be used to explain this fact.

On the other hand, when *Lact. casei* CECT 4043 preparation was tested as probiotic in pigs, the mean final BWG and FI values were higher than those observed in the control group [1]. However, these researchers did not observe significant differences in FCE between the two groups receiving probiotic preparations and the control group. In contrast, the results of present study showed that, by day 31, the final BWG values in chickens receiving the different diets were not significantly different (Table 4), but the animals fed *Lact. casei* CECT 4043 preparation improved their final FCE in comparison to chickens fed avilamycin.

However, it is worth highlighting that differences usually found in BWG between chickens fed with antibiotics and chickens fed with diets without growth promoters were not present in this case (Tables 3 and 4). Patterson and Burkholder [10] recommended that studies in which there is no response to the growth promotant antibiotics should not be considered negative for the probiotic treatment. Then, the lack of differences between antibiotic and control groups in both experiments (medium-growth Sasso X44 chickens and Ross 308 broilers) suggests that the probiotic effect of *Lact. casei* CECT 4043 preparation observed in chickens has been of minor magnitude because of the good condition of the animals.

5. Conclusions

The ability of *Lact. casei* CECT 4043 to improve the FCE in chickens, together with its capability to stimulate the growth and to reduce coliform counts in the faeces of postweaning piglets, indicates that the probiotic *Lact. casei* CECT 4043 preparation could be successfully used as a feed additive for the animal feed industry. In addition the different probiotic effect observed in pigs and broilers supports the hypothesis that probiotic mechanisms are host dependent. The results obtained in this study reinforce previous reports on the probiotic effect of *Lactobacillus* sp. on chicken and pig growth.

Acknowledgments

This research was financially supported by the Instituto Nacional de Investigación y Tecnología Agraria y Alimentaria (project CAL01-045-C2-2) and The Xunta de Galicia, Spain (project PGIDIT02PXIC38). The authors thank COREN, S.C.L. (Ourense, Spain) for its collaboration in the elaboration of this work.

References

[1] N. P. Guerra, P. F. Bernárdez, J. Méndez, P. Cachaldora, and L. Pastrana Castro, "Production of four potentially probiotic lactic acid bacteria and their evaluation as feed additives for weaned piglets," *Animal Feed Science and Technology*, vol. 134, no. 1-2, pp. 89–107, 2007.

[2] F. M. Aarestrup, F. Bager, and S. J. Andersen, "Association between the use of avilamycin for growth promotion and the occurrence of resistance among Enterococcus faecium from broilers: epidemiological study and changes over time," *Microbial Drug Resistance*, vol. 6, no. 1, pp. 71–75, 2000.

[3] L. P. Randall, A. M. Ridley, S. W. Cooles et al., "Prevalence of multiple antibiotic resistance in 443 Campylobacter spp. isolated from humans and animals," *Journal of Antimicrobial Chemotherapy*, vol. 52, no. 3, pp. 507–510, 2003.

[4] A. E. van den Bogaard and E. E. Stobberingh, "Epidemiology of resistance to antibiotics: links between animals and humans," *International Journal of Antimicrobial Agents*, vol. 14, no. 4, pp. 327–335, 2000.

[5] J. Lukášová and A. Šustáčková., "Enterococci and antibiotic resistance," *Acta Veterinaria Brno*, vol. 72, pp. 315–323, 2003.

[6] D. F. Apata, "Antibiotic resistance in poultry," *International Journal of Poultry Science*, vol. 8, no. 4, pp. 404–408, 2009.

[7] Y. Yang, P. A. Iji, and M. Choct, "Dietary modulation of gut microflora in broiler chickens: a review of the role of six kinds of alternatives to in-feed antibiotics," *World's Poultry Science Journal*, vol. 65, no. 1, pp. 97–114, 2009.

[8] M. E. Hume, "Historic perspective: prebiotics, probiotics, and other alternatives to antibiotics," *Poultry Science*, vol. 90, no. 11, pp. 2663–2669, 2011.

[9] M. Ganan, J. M. Silván, A. V. Carrascosa, and A. J. Martínez-Rodríguez, "Alternative strategies to use antibiotics or chemical products for controlling Campylobacter in the food chain," *Food Control*, vol. 24, no. 1-2, pp. 6–14, 2012.

[10] J. A. Patterson and K. M. Burkholder, "Application of prebiotics and probiotics in poultry production," *Poultry Science*, vol. 82, no. 4, pp. 627–631, 2003.

[11] P. Marteau, P. Pochart, Y. Bouhnik, and J. C. Rambaud, "The fate and effects of transiting, nonpathogenic microorganisms in the human intestine," *World Review of Nutrition and Dietetics*, vol. 74, pp. 1–21, 1993.

[12] S. Salminen, M. A. Deighton, Y. Benno, and S. L. Gorbach, "Lactic acid bacteria in health and disease," in *The Lactic Acid Bacteria: Microbiology and Functional Aspects*, S. Salminen and Wright A. von, Eds., pp. 211–253, Marcel Dekker, New York, NY, USA, 2nd edition, 1998.

[13] W. I. Muir, W. L. Bryden, and A. J. Husband, "Immunity, vaccination and the avian intestinal tract," *Developmental and Comparative Immunology*, vol. 24, no. 2-3, pp. 325–342, 2000.

[14] L. Z. Jin, Y. W. Ho, N. Abdullah, and S. Jalaludin, "Growth Performance, Intestinal Microbial Populations, and Serum Cholesterol of Broilers Fed Diets Containing Lactobacillus Cultures," *Poultry Science*, vol. 77, no. 9, pp. 1259–1265, 1998.

[15] S. M. L. Kabir, M. M. Rahman, M. B. Rahman, M. M. Rahman, and S. U. Ahmed, "The dynamics of probiotics on growth performance and immune response in broilers," *International Journal of Poultry Sciences*, vol. 3, pp. 361–364, 2004.

[16] W. L. Willis and L. Reid, "Investigating the effects of dietary probiotic feeding regimens on broiler chicken production and Campylobacter jejuni presence," *Poultry Science*, vol. 87, no. 4, pp. 606–611, 2008.

[17] J. P. Griggs and J. P. Jacob, "Alternatives to antibiotics for organic poultry production," *Journal of Applied Poultry Research*, vol. 14, no. 4, pp. 750–756, 2005.

[18] G. M. Nava, L. R. Bielke, T. R. Callaway, and M. P. Castañeda, "Probiotic alternatives to reduce gastrointestinal infections: the poultry experience," *Animal Health Research Reviews*, vol. 6, no. 1, pp. 105–118, 2005.

[19] R. Simmering and M. Blaut, "Pro- and prebiotics—the tasty guardian angels?" *Applied Microbiology and Biotechnology*, vol. 55, no. 1, pp. 19–28, 2001.

[20] V. Delcenserie, D. Martel, M. Lamoureux, J. Amiot, Y. Boutin, and D. Roy, "Immunomodulatory effects of probiotics in the intestinal tract," *Current Issues in Molecular Biology*, vol. 10, no. 1, pp. 37–54, 2008.

[21] N. Pérez Guerra, P. Fajardo Bernárdez, A. Torrado Agrasar, C. López Macías, and L. Pastrana Castro, "Fed-batch pediocin production by *Pediococcus acidilactici* NRRL B-5627 on whey," *Biotechnology and Applied Biochemistry*, vol. 42, no. 1, pp. 17–23, 2005.

[22] P. F. Bernárdez, I. R. Amado, L. P. Castro, and N. P. Guerra, "Production of a potentially probiotic culture of Lactobacillus casei subsp. casei CECT 4043 in whey," *International Dairy Journal*, vol. 18, no. 10-11, pp. 1057–1065, 2008.

[23] N. P. Guerra, M. L. Rua, and L. Pastrana, "Nutritional factors affecting the production of two bacteriocins from lactic acid bacteria on whey," *International Journal of Food Microbiology*, vol. 70, no. 3, pp. 267–281, 2001.

[24] N. Pérez Guerra and L. Pastrana Castro, "Enhancement of nisin production by Lactococcus lactis in periodically re-alkalized cultures," *Biotechnology and Applied Biochemistry*, vol. 38, no. 2, pp. 157–167, 2003.

[25] W. P. Charteris, P. M. Kelly, L. Morelli, and J. K. Collins, "Development and application of an in vitro methodology to determine the transit tolerance of potentially probiotic Lactobacillus and Bifidobacterium species in the upper human gastrointestinal tract," *Journal of Applied Microbiology*, vol. 84, no. 5, pp. 759–768, 1998.

[26] Y. K. Lee, C. Y. Lim, W. L. Teng, A. C. Ouwehand, E. M. Tuomola, and S. Salminen, "Quantitative approach in the study of adhesion of lactic acid bacteria to intestinal cells and their competition with enterobacteria," *Applied and Environmental Microbiology*, vol. 66, no. 9, pp. 3692–3697, 2000.

[27] P. T. Redig, "The avian ceca: obligate combustion chambers or facultative afterburners? The conditioning influence of diet," *Journal of Experimental Zoology*, no. 3, pp. 66–69, 1989.

[28] R. D. Miles, G. D. Butcher, P. R. Henry, and R. C. Littell, "Effect of antibiotic growth promoters on broiler performance, intestinal growth parameters, and quantitative morphology," *Poultry Science*, vol. 85, no. 3, pp. 476–485, 2006.

[29] M. E. Coates, M. K. Davies, and S. K. Kon, "The effect of antibiotics on the intestine of the chick," *British Journal of Nutrition*, vol. 9, pp. 110–119, 1955.

[30] C. H. Hill, A. D. Keeling, and J. W. Kelly., "Studies on the effect of antibiotics on the intestinal weights of chicks," *Journal of Nutrition*, vol. 62, pp. 255–267, 1957.

[31] M. Bedford, "Removal of antibiotic growth promoters from poultry diets: implications and strategies to minimise subsequent problems," *World's Poultry Science Journal*, vol. 56, no. 4, pp. 362–365, 2000.

[32] R. K. Gast and P. S. Holt, "Experimental horizontal transmission of *Salmonella enteritidis* strains (phage types 4, 8, and 13a) in chicks," *Avian Diseases*, vol. 43, no. 4, pp. 774–778, 1999.

[33] B. Yu, J. R. Liu, F. S. Hsiao, and P. W. S. Chiou, "Evaluation of *Lactobacillus reuteri* Pg4 strain expressing heterologous β-glucanase as a probiotic in poultry diets based on barley," *Animal Feed Science and Technology*, vol. 141, no. 1-2, pp. 82–91, 2008.

[34] X. Meng, B. A. Slominski, and W. Guenter, "The effect of fat type, carbohydrase, and lipase addition on growth performance and nutrient utilization of young broilers fed wheat-based diets," *Poultry Science*, vol. 83, no. 10, pp. 1718–1727, 2004.

[35] A. Viveros, A. Brenes, M. Pizarro, and M. Castaño, "Effect of enzyme supplementation of a diet based on barley, and autoclave treatment, on apparent digestibility, growth performance and gut morphology of broilers," *Animal Feed Science and Technology*, vol. 48, no. 3-4, pp. 237–251, 1994.

[36] E. Teirlynck, L. Bjerrum, V. Eeckhaut et al., "The cereal type in feed influences gut wall morphology and intestinal immune cell infiltration in broiler chickens," *British Journal of Nutrition*, vol. 102, no. 10, pp. 1453–1461, 2009.

[37] M. Hofshagen and M. Kaldhusdal, "Barley inclusion and avoparcin supplementation in broiler diets. 1. Effect on small intestinal bacterial flora and performance," *Poultry Science*, vol. 71, no. 6, pp. 959–969, 1992.

[38] R. A. Dalloul, H. S. Lillehoj, T. A. Shellem, and J. A. Doerr, "Enhanced mucosal immunity against *Eimeria acervulina* in broilers fed a *Lactobacillus*-based probiotic," *Poultry Science*, vol. 82, no. 1, pp. 62–66, 2003.

[39] M. S. Y. Haddadin, S. M. Abdulrahim, E. A. R. Hashlamoun, and R. K. Robinson, "The effect of Lactobacillus acidophilus on the production and chemical composition of hen's eggs," *Poultry Science*, vol. 75, no. 4, pp. 491–494, 1996.

[40] M. Kaldhusdal and M. Hofshagen, "Barley inclusion and avoparcin supplementation in broiler diets. 2. Clinical, pathological, and bacteriological findings in a mild form of necrotic enteritis," *Poultry Science*, vol. 71, no. 7, pp. 1145–1153, 1992.

[41] F. Abe, N. Ishibashi, and S. Shimamura, "Effect of administration of bifidobacteria and lactic acid bacteria to newborn calves and piglets," *Journal of Dairy Science*, vol. 78, no. 12, pp. 2838–2846, 1995.

[42] B. Bogovic Matijasic, S. Stojković, J. Salobir, Š. Malovrh, and I. Rogelj, "Evaluation of the *Lactobacillus gasseri* K7 and LF221 strains in weaned piglets for their possible probiotic use and their detection in the faeces," *Animal Research*, vol. 53, no. 1, pp. 35–44, 2004.

[43] B. Hyronimus, C. Le Marrec, A. Hadj Sassi, and A. Deschamps, "Acid and bile tolerance of spore-forming lactic acid bacteria," *International Journal of Food Microbiology*, vol. 61, no. 2-3, pp. 193–197, 2000.

[44] H. S. Gill, "Probiotics to enhance anti-infective defences in the gastrointestinal tract," *Bailliere's Best Practice and Research in Clinical Gastroenterology*, vol. 17, no. 5, pp. 755–773, 2003.

[45] Y. K. Lee and K. Y. Puong, "Competition for adhesion between probiotics and human gastrointestinal pathogens in the presence of carbohydrate," *British Journal of Nutrition*, vol. 88, no. 1, pp. S101–S108, 2002.

[46] A. Meimandipour, M. Shuhaimi, M. Hair-Bejo et al., "In vitro fermentation of broiler cecal content: the role of *Lactobacilli* and pH value on the composition of microbiota and end products fermentation," *Letters in Applied Microbiology*, vol. 49, no. 4, pp. 415–420, 2009.

Subcutaneous Administration of Tramadol after Elective Surgery Is as Effective as Intravenous Administration in Relieving Acute Pain and Inflammation in Dogs

Salisu Buhari,[1,2] Kalthum Hashim,[1] Goh Yong Meng,[3]
Noordin Mohamed Mustapha,[4] and Siew Hua Gan[5]

[1] *Department of Veterinary Clinical Studies, Faculty of Veterinary Medicine, Universiti Putra Malaysia, 43400 Serdang, Selangor, Malaysia*
[2] *Department of Veterinary Surgery & Radiology, Faculty of Veterinary Medicine, Usmanu Danfodiyo University Sokoto, PMB 2346, Sokoto, Nigeria*
[3] *Department of Veterinary Preclinical Studies, Faculty of Veterinary Medicine, Universiti Putra Malaysia, 43400 Serdang, Selangor, Malaysia*
[4] *Department of Veterinary Pathology and Microbiology, Faculty of Veterinary Medicine, Universiti Putra Malaysia, 43400 Serdang, Selangor, Malaysia*
[5] *Human Genome Centre, School of Medical Sciences, Universiti Sains Malaysia, Kelantan, 16150 Kubang Kerian, Malaysia*

Correspondence should be addressed to Kalthum Hashim, kalthum@vet.upm.edu.my

Academic Editors: G. T. Pharr, J. L. Romalde, and B. I. Yoon

Subcutaneous (SC) administration of tramadol was compared with intravenous (IV) administration to evaluate analgesia following canine ovariohysterectomy (OHE). Healthy female dogs ($n = 12$) between 1 and 3 years of age (1.95 ± 0.65 years), weighing between 10.5 and 17.1 kg (13.12 ± 1.95 kg), were used. Pain was assessed at baseline before surgery and then hourly for 8 hr after surgery. Tramadol was administered both SC and IV at a dose of 3 mg/kg and provided significant postoperative analgesia, as indicated by analgesiometry, β-endorphin levels, and interleukin 6 (IL-6) levels. The respiratory rates and rectal temperatures remained normal and were not significantly different between or within the groups. A significant increase in heart rate was observed at 4 hr for dogs in both groups relative to the baseline, but there was no significant difference in heart rates between the groups at any time point. A significant decrease in mechanical pain threshold was observed within each group after surgery, but both groups responded similarly, suggesting that SC administration of tramadol is as effective as IV administration. Increased serum levels of both IL-6 and β-endorphin 3 hr postoperatively further indicate that both routes of administration achieve similar pain control. Thus, the relative analgesic efficacy of SC tramadol is comparable to that of IV administration and can be used to achieve similar effects for postsurgical pain management in dogs undergoing OHE.

1. Introduction

Inflammatory pain is characterized by an increased sensitivity to mechanical or heat stimuli in the affected tissue [1]. Following tissue injury, an inflammatory response is generated by local macrophages and then amplified by migrating blood cells. Various inflammatory mediators, as well as tissue acidification, act synergistically to induce and maintain pain and hyperalgesia [2]. Regardless of the nature of the event initiating tissue damage, pain usually progresses in a predictable manner and eventually leads to multiple organ failure [3].

Pain recognition in humans is subjective, and pain in animals can be challenging to identify because many species have evolved to mask signs of illness and distress [4]. However, it is the consensus among veterinarians and researchers that predictable alterations in animals' behavior are likely to accompany pain. It is therefore accepted that pain or distress in animals, including those used for biomedical research, should be prevented or minimized as much as possible [5].

In veterinary practice, the clinical application of most nonsteroidal anti-inflammatory drugs for pain management is limited due to their potentially harmful side effects, which include gastrointestinal discomfort, cardiopulmonary depression [6], and decreased antibody production [7]. The use of opioids in the management of both acute and chronic pain is therefore a useful alternative. Opioids are considered the most reliable and effective analgesic, although they can produce reversible behavioral [8] and physiological [9] side effects in dogs.

Tramadol is an analgesic with a dual mechanism of action. It both binds to the μ_1 opioid receptor [10, 11] and inhibits the monoaminergic pathway, which is responsible for noradrenaline (NA) and serotonin (5HT) reuptake [12, 13]. For this reason, tramadol is considered an "atypical opioid" and is only partially inhibited by naloxone, an opioid antagonist [13]. Preemptive administration of tramadol has been shown to significantly reduce the amount of inhalant anesthetic required for procedures in humans [14] and dogs [15].

Several studies have described the efficacy of tramadol following intravenous (IV) [11, 13], oral [11, 16], intramuscular [17] and epidural administration [18]. The subcutaneous (SC) administration of analgesic drugs has been advocated to reduce the risk of overdose and to sustain effective plasma levels for longer durations [19]. Despite the wide use of SC drugs in dogs, the efficacy of SC tramadol for pain control after surgery is not well documented. Although previous studies have investigated the SC administration of tramadol in red-eared sliders [20], chicks [21], and cats [22], none have assessed its efficacy in dogs. This study aimed to compare tramadol's efficacy when administered SC versus IV as a postoperative analgesic agent in dogs undergoing routine ovariohysterectomy (OHE).

2. Materials and Methods

Female dogs ($n = 12$) ranging in age from 1 to 3 years old (1.95 ± 0.65) and weighing between 10.5 and 17.1 kg (13.12 ± 1.95) were obtained from a local animal shelter where they were available for adoption (Progressive Animal Welfare Society, PAWS, Subang Airport road, Malaysia). All dogs were determined to be clinically healthy based on a physical examination by a qualified veterinarian prior to surgery. The dogs were familiarized with the handler prior to the study and individually housed in a kennel that was kept quiet and clean. The study was ethically approved by the Universiti Putra Malaysia Animal Care and Utility Committee (UPM/FPV/PS/3.2.1.551/AUP-R86) and adhered to the Declaration of Helsinki.

3. Experimental Procedures

Dogs were fasted for 12 hr prior to surgery but had water ad libitum until two hours before premedication. On the morning of surgery, a 20-gauge, 1.25-inch sterile catheter (Terumo, Somerset NJ, USA) was placed and secured in one of the cephalic veins. A baseline venous blood sample (2 mL) was collected from each dog prior to the administration of tramadol. The dogs were randomly divided into 2 groups ($n = 6$ for each group) depending on the route of tramadol administration. At the time of premedication, group 1 received 3 mg/kg tramadol SC, while group 2 received the same dose of tramadol IV.

4. Anesthesia and Surgery

The dogs were premedicated with atropine (0.04 mg/kg) (Troy laboratory PTY Ltd, Australia) and xylazine (0.5 mg/kg) (Troy laboratory PTY Ltd, Australia). Anesthesia was induced with ketamine hydrochloride (Narketan, Vetoquinol SA, 70204 Lure, Cedex, France) at 10 mg/kg (IV) given to effect. Following jaw relaxation, the dogs were quickly intubated, and the lungs were ventilated by an assistant using an Ambu bag. The dogs were then prepared for surgery aseptically, and OHE was performed through a ventral midline approach. The same veterinarian performed every surgery, and the mean duration of the procedure was approximately 23 min (22.5 ± 4.6 min).

5. Pain Assessment

Pain was assessed both subjectively and objectively. Physiologic parameters, such as cardiopulmonary rates and rectal temperature before and after the surgery, were measured based on criteria defined by the University of Melbourne [23]. In addition, serum levels of interleukin-6 (IL-6) and β-endorphin, as well as mechanical pressure thresholds, were measured for the unrestrained dogs before and after surgery.

Pain was evaluated before the surgery as a baseline (0 h) and at 1, 2, 3, 4, 5, 6, 7, and 8 h after recovery from anesthesia. Pain assessments were made by an observer who was blinded with respect to the route of administration. Rectal temperatures and cardiopulmonary rates were recorded for each dog prior to palpation of the surgical site. The mechanical nociceptive thresholds were then measured using a clinical algometer (FPX 25, Wagner instrument, Greenwich CT, USA), which records sensitivity to pressure. Pain was first assessed 2 hr before drug administration and then hourly until 8 hr after anesthetic recovery.

Constant pressure was applied 2 cm from the incision site cranially, caudally, and laterally to the left and right. The pressure threshold was read at the point of a positive reaction, with an average of four readings per site. A positive reaction was considered to be a leg shake, a head turned toward the site, snapping or biting at the instrument, barking, or vocalizing. The instrument was calibrated with a progressively increasing force, and a cut-off point of 15 N was used to prevent mechanical damage to the tissue. Ascending values with an increase in pressure indicated less pain, while descending values with minimal pressure indicated pain in that area.

6. Measurement of Serum β-Endorphin and IL-6 Levels

Serum β-endorphin and IL-6 concentrations were determined before premedication, during surgery (1 hr after

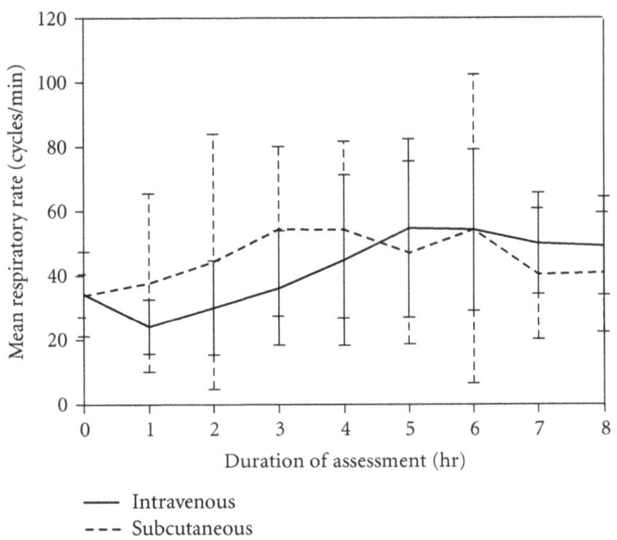

FIGURE 1: Mean respiratory rates over time for the IV and SC groups (IV group, $P = 0.069$; SC group, $P = 0.904$).

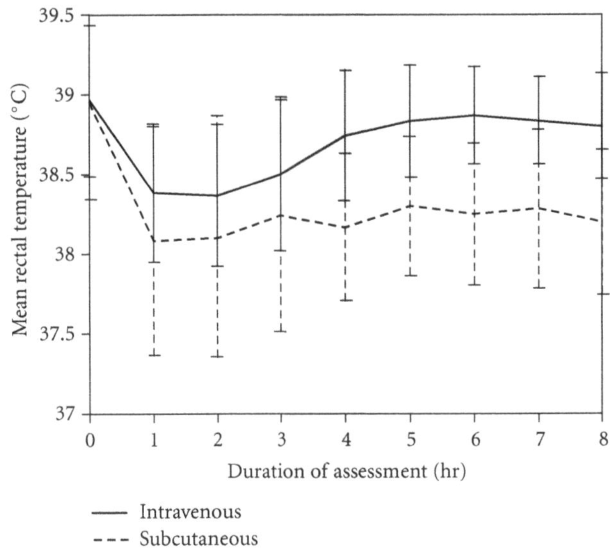

FIGURE 2: Mean rectal temperatures over time for the IV and SC groups (IV group, $P = 0.082$; SC group, $P = 0.331$).

tramadol administration), and after surgery at 2, 3, 6, and 9 hr following tramadol administration. Blood samples (2 mL) were collected from a jugular catheter and centrifuged at 1000 ×g for 10 min. The serum was separated and kept frozen at −80°C until analysis with commercially available enzyme-linked immunosorbent assay (ELISA) kits (Cusabio Biotech Co., Ltd, Wuhan China) specific for canine β-endorphin and IL-6. A wavelength of 450 nm was selected for optical density measurements on an ELISA microplate reader (Bio-Rad model 680, Bio-Rad Laboratories Inc., Tokyo, Japan).

7. Statistical Analysis

Physiological parameters, mechanical pain threshold values, and serum levels of β-endorphin and IL-6 were analyzed using parametric statistical methods. Heart rates, respiratory rates, and rectal temperatures were analyzed using repeated measures ANOVA. One-way ANOVA was used to compare differences within treatment groups, and two-way repeated measures ANOVA was used to compare differences between the two treatments over time. Fisher's Least Significant Difference (LSD) multiple comparison test was used to compare differences at each time point. Multiple linear regression analysis was used to test the relationship between objective parameters and the mechanical pain threshold values generated with the analgesiometer. A value of $P < 0.05$ was considered to be significant. The data were reported as the mean ± SD.

8. Results

8.1. Physiological Parameters. During the study period, respiratory rate (Figure 1) and rectal temperature (Figure 2) remained within normal range and were not significantly different between or within the two groups, indicating that comparable pain control was achieved. Dogs in both groups had increased heart rates compared to the baseline at 4, 5, 6, 7, and 8 hr (Figure 3), indicating that the dogs recovered at similar rates from anesthesia.

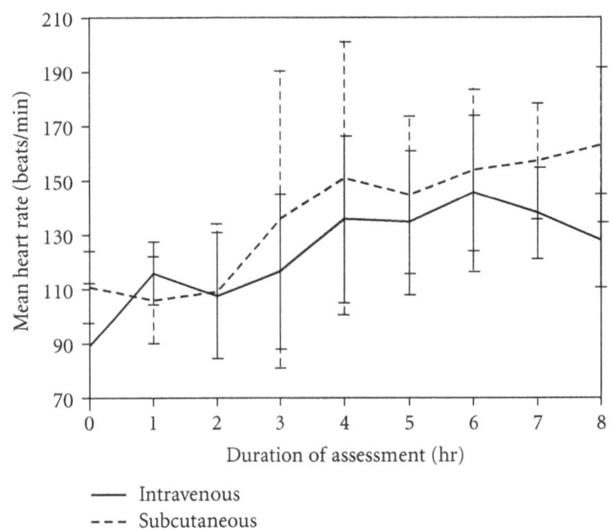

FIGURE 3: Mean heart rates over time are not significantly different between the IV and SC groups. Values within the IV group are significantly different from the baseline measurements at 4 hr ($P = 0.02$), 5 hr ($P = 0.02$), 6 hr ($P = 0.00$), 7 hr ($P = 0.001$), and 8 hr ($P = 0.009$). Values within the SC group are significantly different from the baseline measurements at 4 hr ($P = 0.042$), 6 hr ($P = 0.029$), 7 hr ($P = 0.019$), and 8 hr ($P = 0.009$).

8.2. Pain Assessment. No significant differences were observed between the SC and IV groups when they were evaluated for mechanical pain thresholds, indicating similar analgesic effects of tramadol via both routes (Table 1). A

TABLE 1: Reaction times in the analgesiometer test demonstrate a progressive decrease in the mechanical pain threshold for dogs that received tramadol via both routes, indicating comparable increases in pain perception over time. The results are listed as the mean ± SD.

Time (hr) before (0) tramadol administration and after recovery from anesthesia	Mechanical pain threshold assessment score (Newton) IV group ($n = 6$)	SC group ($n = 6$)
0	14.92 ± 0.1	14.76 ± 0.5
1	15.00 ± 1.8	14.94 ± 1.6
2	14.90 ± 1.6	15.00 ± 0.1
3	7.99 ± 2.7	7.77 ± 2.0
4	5.96 ± 2.8	6.66 ± 2.1
5	4.94 ± 2.2	5.00 ± 1.0
6	4.34 ± 2.1	3.68 ± 0.4
7	3.41 ± 2.0	3.20 ± 0.4
8	2.76 ± 1.8	2.61 ± 0.7

TABLE 2: The relationship between the subjective parameters and mechanical pain threshold was assessed using multiple linear regression.

Model	IV route		Confidence interval		SC route		Confidence interval	
Constants independent variables	Beta	P value ($P < 0.05$)	Lower bound	Upper bound	Beta	P value ($P < 0.05$)	Lower bound	Upper bound
Respiratory rate (cycles/min)	−0.472	0.001	−0.19	−0.053	−0.319	0.008	−0.101	−0.016
Rectal temperature (°C)	0.004	0.972	−3.029	3.139	0.13	0.244	−0.779	2.996
Heart rate (beats/min)	−0.16	0.233	−0.08	0.20	−0.652	0.00	−0.121	−0.059

Dependent variable: mechanical pain threshold (N).

significant decrease in the mechanical pain threshold was observed for both groups over time, further indicating that pain perception was similar for the two groups. Respiratory and heart rates were significantly associated with the mechanical pain scores in dogs receiving IV tramadol, but only respiratory rates are significantly associated with the mechanical pain threshold for dogs in the SC group (Table 2).

8.3. Serum IL-6 and β-Endorphin Levels. There were no significant differences in serum levels of IL-6 ($P = 0.701$) or β-endorphin ($P = 0.806$) between the two groups, suggesting that dogs from both groups had similar perception and responses to painful stimulation (Figures 4 and 5).

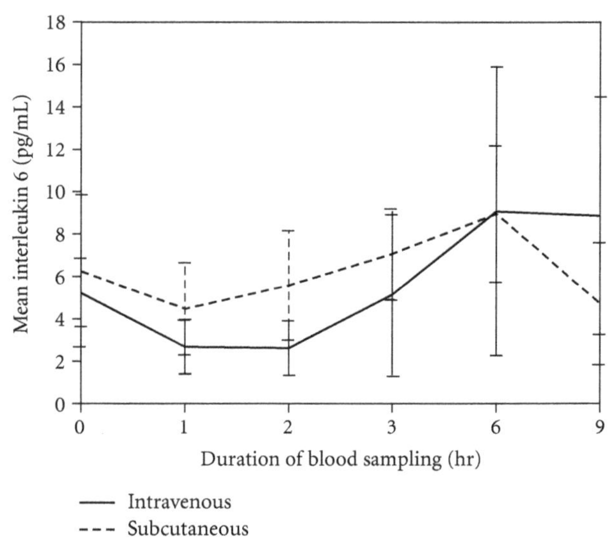

FIGURE 4: Mean serum IL-6 concentrations for the IV and SC groups at different sampling times after tramadol administration ($P = 0.701$).

9. Discussion

In humans, SC administration of analgesics is widely used because it achieves relatively similar pain control compared to the intramuscular and IV routes [24]. Information on SC tramadol administration in dogs, however, is limited. Our study is the first to demonstrate that SC administration of tramadol is a reliable and effective method for controlling pain with limited side effects in dogs after OHE.

Although tramadol has a rapid onset of effect when given to dogs IV or intramuscularly, it can also produce unwanted side effects such as nausea, salivation, increased swallowing, and retching [11, 13]. Another effective analgesic strategy, epidural analgesia, carries the risk of nerve injury and side effects that include pruritus, urinary retention, hypoventilation and hypotension, [10, 18, 25]. In contrast, better patient compliance with minimal restraint was achieved in the SC group. In this study, none of the dogs suffered from adverse effects of tramadol, regardless of the route of administration. According to Hendrix et al. [26], marked respiratory depression is not observed in dogs, even with morphine administration. In addition, although vomiting is

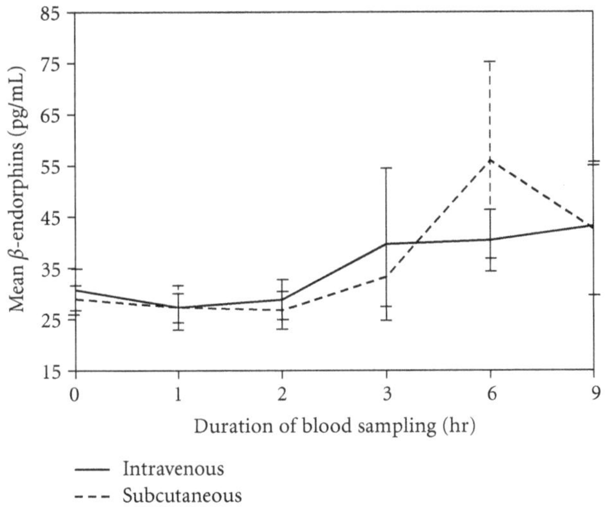

FIGURE 5: Mean serum β-endorphin concentrations for the IV and SC groups at different sampling times after tramadol administration ($P = 0.806$).

reported to occur within 5–10 min of SC administration of morphine, this effect is not reported with other opioids [27].

Physiologic indicators of acute pain in animals include increased heart rate, increased blood pressure, peripheral vasoconstriction, cardiac dysrhythmias, sweating, hyperventilation, and reduced peristalsis [27]. In our study, other than the slightly decreased rectal temperatures observed in the SC group two hours after recovery, heart rates, respiratory rates, and rectal temperatures did not vary significantly from the baseline or between the groups. Similar observations were made following epidural administration of tramadol in dogs undergoing stifle surgery [10]. In horses that received epidural tramadol, good analgesia was achieved without significantly influencing the horses' behavioral and physiological parameters [28]. The parameters evaluated here demonstrated that the severity of pain had no detectable physiologic influence on the patients as judged by an observer, and the variability among these parameters was consistent for all tests between the groups. It is important to note that the anesthetic agents used in this study may have resulted in residual central nervous system depression, making pain assessment a challenge postoperatively.

Based on consistently decreasing algometer values for the nociceptive thresholds beginning 2 hours after recovery, increased pain was suspected around the incision site and thus warranted an additional dose of tramadol to maintain analgesia in dogs from both groups. These results suggest that the increased pressure thresholds until 3 hr after tramadol administration are associated with adequate analgesia, although tramadol dosed at 3 mg/kg results in no more than 3 hours of postsurgical analgesia in dogs [11]. The general lack of effect on the pressure threshold after 3 hours may be due to the complexity of pain neurophysiology, the different receptors involved [22], and the rapid clearance of tramadol in dogs [11]. In veterinary medicine, tramadol is typically used in dogs and cats at doses that do not exceed 4.0 mg/kg [29].

In the present study, the subjective pain scales combined with the mechanical nociceptive thresholds indicated that SC tramadol is similar in efficacy to IV in controlling pain after OHE. The effectiveness of the SC route for postsurgical pain management was previously demonstrated in a study comparing the analgesic effects of butorphanol and meloxicam in dogs [30] and tramadol in cats [31] after elective OHE. Progressive increases in the pain scores 3 hours after recovery correspond to the decreasing values observed for the mechanical pain thresholds, suggesting that pain sensation around the incision area increased over time. Due to the rapid elimination of tramadol, a dosing frequency of every four hours is necessary to maintain plasma concentrations sufficient for analgesia in dogs [11, 13]. In humans, the elimination half-life of 6 to 7 hours provides prolonged analgesia and a less frequent dosing schedule [32, 33]. Both subjective and objective indicators for pain were negatively correlated with respiratory and heart rates to mechanical pain thresholds but were positively correlated with rectal temperatures in both groups. Similar relationships were observed in a study that established interval level measurements for a prototype composite measure pain scale assessing acute pain in dogs and in a prospective study that investigated experimental orthopedic pain in beagle dogs [34, 35].

The IL-6 and β-endorphin levels may be useful objective indicators of pain in animals [2, 36]. Over the years, numerous studies on the role of cytokines in pain control have been conducted. During pathologic situations associated with increased pain and hyperalgesia, the pleiotropic cytokine IL-6 is markedly upregulated. Elevated serum IL-6 levels were detected in patients with neurological disorders, musculoskeletal injuries, and autoimmune and inflammatory conditions [2]. In the current study, serum IL-6 levels decreased gradually after tramadol administration and remained low throughout the surgery.

A significant increase in IL-6 over the baseline was observed at 3, 6, and 9 hours following administration ($P = 0.028$) via both routes. This observation is similar to that in previous reports, in which gradual increases in IL-6 were observed after both laparoscopic and open surgeries [37]. Similar increases in IL-6 plasma concentrations have been noted in response to cardiopulmonary bypass [38]. Proinflammatory and pronociceptive roles for IL-6 have been described in rats receiving intraplantar and intrathecal injections of IL-6 to induce hyperalgesia or allodynia [39]. In a human study, low synovial fluid concentrations of IL-6 and reduced joint pain were reported following tramadol administration [40], demonstrating its analgesic efficacy and cytokine modulating effects.

β-endorphin plays a significant role as biomarker [36] and modulator in acute traumatic conditions such as surgery [41]. Measurements of plasma concentrations of β-endorphin have been used extensively in the assessment of pain following castration and tail docking [42]. In our study, serum β-endorphin levels at 1 and 2 hours after tramadol administration were significantly lower than levels between 3 and 9 hours after administration. The sharp rise of plasma β-endorphin beginning at 3 hours after surgery may be related to the rapid metabolism and clearance of tramadol in dogs [11, 13] and can be correlated with postsurgical pain stimulation. Both groups exhibited similar pain responses as indicated by β-endorphin levels. A previous study indicated that serum β-endorphin levels over time in severely injured dogs exceeded the levels in moderately traumatized dogs [43]. The increases in serum concentrations due to painful stimuli remained elevated much longer than those due to nonpainful stimuli such as stress from handling [36].

A future crossover study in which dogs receive medication via both routes of administration may help to confirm these findings. In addition, it will be useful to investigate the effects of tramadol administered SC at multiple doses and establish the pharmacokinetic profile of the drug given by this route.

10. Conclusion

Postsurgical pain management strategies are improving with the incorporation of SC administration of drugs. The identification of less painful and more reliable routes of drug administration is very important for effectively controlling pain in small animals. We conclude that the relative analgesic efficacy of SC tramadol is comparable to IV administration and can be used independently for postsurgical pain management in dogs. One significant difference between the two routes of administration is the faster time of onset for IV tramadol, which must be considered in emergency situations when a more rapid onset and distribution of analgesia is required.

Acknowledgments

The author acknowledge the financial support from Research University Grant Scheme (RUGS) ((UPM/TNCPI/RMC/91465) and (USM/1001/PPSP/815058)). They are also grateful to Muhammad Saed Ibrahim from Institute of Bioscience for technical support.

References

[1] T. Foulkes and J. N. Wood, "Pain genes," *PLoS Genetics*, vol. 4, no. 7, Article ID e1000086, 2008.

[2] C. Sommer and M. Kress, "Recent findings on how proinflammatory cytokines cause pain: peripheral mechanisms in inflammatory and neuropathic hyperalgesia," *Neuroscience Letters*, vol. 361, no. 1-3, pp. 184–187, 2004.

[3] G. Moalem and D. J. Tracey, "Immune and inflammatory mechanisms in neuropathic pain," *Brain Research Reviews*, vol. 51, no. 2, pp. 240–264, 2006.

[4] A. B. de Sousa, A. C. D. dos Santos, J. C. Florio, and H. S. Spinosa, "Pharmacokinetics of tramadol administered by intravenous and intramuscular routes to female dogs submitted to ovariohysterectomy," *Brazilian Journal of Veterinary Research and Animal Science*, vol. 45, no. 3, pp. 239–247, 2008.

[5] J. V. Roughan and P. A. Flecknell, "Evaluation of a short duration behaviour-based post-operative pain scoring system in rats," *European Journal of Pain*, vol. 7, no. 5, pp. 397–406, 2003.

[6] M. Elghazali, I. M. Barezaik, A. A. Abdel Hadi, F. M. Eltayeb, J. Al Masri, and I. A. Wasfi, "The pharmacokinetics, metabolism and urinary detection time of tramadol in camels," *Veterinary Journal*, vol. 178, no. 2, pp. 272–277, 2008.

[7] S. Bancos, M. P. Bernard, D. J. Topham, and R. P. Phipps, "Ibuprofen and other widely used non-steroidal anti-inflammatory drugs inhibit antibody production in human cells," *Cellular Immunology*, vol. 258, no. 1, pp. 18–28, 2009.

[8] B. KuKanich, B. K. Hogan, L. A. Krugner-Higby, and L. J. Smith, "Pharmacokinetics of hydromorphone hydrochloride in healthy dogs," *Veterinary Anaesthesia and Analgesia*, vol. 35, no. 3, pp. 256–264, 2008.

[9] A. E. Wagner, *Opioids*, Mosby, St. Louis, Mo, USA, 2002.

[10] A. G. P. Guedes, C. C. Natalini, E. P. Robinson, S. D. L. Alves, and S. T. Oliveira, "Epidural administration of tramadol as an analgesic technique in dogs submitted to stifle surgery," *The International Journal of Applied Research in Veterinary Medicine*, vol. 3, no. 4, pp. 352–359, 2005.

[11] B. Kukanich and M. G. Papich, "Pharmacokinetics of tramadol and the metabolite O-desmethyltramadol in dogs," *Journal of Veterinary Pharmacology and Therapeutics*, vol. 27, no. 4, pp. 239–246, 2004.

[12] R. Kubota, T. Komiyama, Y. Miwa et al., "Pharmacokinetics and postoperative analgesia of epidural tramadol: a prospective, pilot study," *Current Therapeutic Research*, vol. 69, no. 1, pp. 49–55, 2008.

[13] C. J. McMillan, A. Livingston, C. R. Clark et al., "Pharmacokinetics of intravenous tramadol in dogs," *Canadian Journal of Veterinary Research*, vol. 72, no. 4, pp. 325–331, 2008.

[14] J. Wordliczek, M. Banach, J. Garlicki, J. Jakowicka-Wordliczek, and J. Dobrogowski, "Influence of pre- or intraoperational use of tramadol (preemptive or preventive analgesia) on tramadol requirement in the early postoperative period," *Polish Journal of Pharmacology*, vol. 54, no. 6, pp. 693–697, 2002.

[15] M. R. Seddighi, C. M. Egger, B. W. Rohrbach, S. K. Cox, and T. J. Doherty, "Effects of tramadol on the minimum alveolar concentration of sevoflurane in dogs," *Veterinary Anaesthesia and Analgesia*, vol. 36, no. 4, pp. 334–340, 2009.

[16] M. Giorgi, G. Saccomanni, B. Łebkowska-Wieruszewska, and C. Kowalski, "Pharmacokinetic evaluation of tramadol and its major metabolites after single oral sustained tablet administration in the dog: a pilot study," *Veterinary Journal*, vol. 180, no. 2, pp. 253–255, 2009.

[17] A. B. de Sousa, A. C. D. dos Santos, J. C. Florio, and H. S. Spinosa, "Pharmacokinetics of tramadol administered by intravenous and intramuscular routes to female dogs submitted to ovariohysterectomy," *Brazilian Journal of Veterinary Research and Animal Science*, vol. 45, no. 3, pp. 239–247, 2008.

[18] E. Vettorato, A. Zonca, M. Isola et al., "Pharmacokinetics and efficacy of intravenous and extradural tramadol in dogs," *Veterinary Journal*, vol. 183, no. 3, pp. 310–315, 2010.

[19] A. Waterman and W. Kalthum, "The absorption and distribution of subcutaneously administered pethidine in the dog," *Journal of Association of Veterinary Anaesthesia*, vol. 16, pp. 51–52, 1989.

[20] B. B. Baker, K. K. Sladky, and S. M. Johnson, "Evaluation of the analgesic effects of oral and subcutaneous tramadol administration in red-eared slider turtles," *Journal of the American Veterinary Medical Association*, vol. 238, no. 2, pp. 220–227, 2011.

[21] N. O. Tawfik, G. A. Taqa, and T. A. Alsandook, "Evaluation of antinocicpetive effect of tramadol in chicks," *Iraqi Journal of Veterinary Sciences*, vol. 23, no. 1, pp. 19–22, 2009.

[22] P. V. Steagall, P. M. Taylor, J. T. Brondani, S. P. Luna, M. J. Dixon, and T. H. Ferreira, "Effects of buprenorphine, carprofen and saline on thermal and mechanical nociceptive

thresholds in cats," *Veterinary Anaesthesia and Analgesia*, vol. 34, no. 5, pp. 344–350, 2007.

[23] A. M. Firth and S. L. Haldane, "Development of a scale to evaluate postoperative pain in dogs," *Journal of the American Veterinary Medical Association*, vol. 214, no. 5, pp. 651–659, 1999.

[24] S. Negro, A. Martín, M. L. Azuara, Y. Sánchez, and E. Barcia, "Stability of tramadol and haloperidol for continuous subcutaneous infusion at home," *Journal of Pain and Symptom Management*, vol. 30, no. 2, pp. 192–199, 2005.

[25] A. S. Bigham, S. Habibian, F. Ghasemian, and S. Layeghi, "Caudal epidural injection of lidocaine, tramadol, and lidocaine-tramadol for epidural anesthesia in cattle," *Journal of Veterinary Pharmacology and Therapeutics*, vol. 33, no. 5, pp. 439–443, 2010.

[26] P. K. Hendrix, M. R. Raffe, E. P. Robinson, L. J. Felice, and D. A. Randall, "Epidural administration of bupivacaine, morphine, or their combination for postoperative analgesia in dogs," *Journal of the American Veterinary Medical Association*, vol. 209, no. 3, pp. 598–607, 1996.

[27] M. Pearson, "Practical pain management in animals," in *Proceedings of the Australian Animal Welfare Strategy Science Summit on Pain and Pain Management*, pp. 1–9, May 2007.

[28] C. C. Natalini and E. P. Robinson, "Evaluation of the analgesic effects of epidurally administered morphine, alfentanil, butorphanol, tramadol, and U50488H in horses," *American Journal of Veterinary Research*, vol. 61, no. 12, pp. 1579–1586, 2000.

[29] D. C. Plumb, "Tramadol HCl," in *Veterinary Drug Handbook*, pp. 1113–1114, Blackwell, Ames, Iowa, USA, 5th edition, 2005.

[30] N. Caulkett, M. Read, D. Fowler, and C. Waldner, "A comparison of the analgesic effects of butorphanol with those of meloxicam after elective ovariohysterectomy in dogs," *Canadian Veterinary Journal*, vol. 44, no. 7, pp. 565–570, 2003.

[31] J. T. Brondani, S. P. Loureiro Luna, S. L. Beier, B. W. Minto, and C. R. Padovani, "Analgesic efficacy of perioperative use of vedaprofen, tramadol or their combination in cats undergoing ovariohysterectomy," *Journal of Feline Medicine and Surgery*, vol. 11, no. 6, pp. 420–429, 2009.

[32] S. H. Gan, R. Ismail, W. A. Wan Adnan, and Z. Wan, "Method development and validation of a high-performance liquid chromatographic method for tramadol in human plasma using liquid-liquid extraction," *Journal of Chromatography B*, vol. 772, no. 1, pp. 123–129, 2002.

[33] L. J. Scott and C. M. Perry, "Tramadol: a review of its use in perioperative pain," *Drugs*, vol. 60, no. 1, pp. 139–176, 2000.

[34] C. M. Morton, J. Reid, E. M. Scott, L. L. Holton, and A. M. Nolan, "Application of a scaling model to establish and validate an interval level pain scale for assessment of acute pain in dogs," *American Journal of Veterinary Research*, vol. 66, no. 12, pp. 2154–2166, 2005.

[35] P. Rialland, S. Authier, D. Gauvin et al., "Physiologic responses and pain-related behaviors in beagle dogs undergoing trochleoplasty surgery," *Journal of Veterinary Behavior*, vol. 5, no. 3, p. 156, 2010.

[36] N. A. Rasmussen and L. A. Farr, "Beta-endorphin response to an acute pain stimulus," *Journal of Neuroscience Methods*, vol. 177, no. 2, pp. 285–288, 2009.

[37] M. Kristiansson, L. Saraste, M. Soop, K. G. Sundqvist, and A. Thörne, "Diminished interleukin-6 and C-reactive protein responses to laparoscopic versus open cholecystectomy," *Acta Anaesthesiologica Scandinavica*, vol. 43, no. 2, pp. 146–152, 1999.

[38] W. J. Dreyer, S. C. Phillips, M. L. Lindsey et al., "Interleukin 6 induction in the canine myocardium after cardiopulmonary bypass," *Journal of Thoracic and Cardiovascular Surgery*, vol. 120, no. 2, pp. 256–263, 2000.

[39] R. F. De Jongh, K. C. Vissers, T. F. Meert, L. H. D. J. Booij, C. S. De Deyne, and R. J. Heylen, "The role of interleukin-6 in nociception and pain," *Anesthesia and Analgesia*, vol. 96, no. 4, pp. 1096–1103, 2003.

[40] M. Bianchi, M. Broggini, P. Balzarini et al., "Effects of tramadol on synovial fluid concentrations of substance P and interleukin-6 in patients with knee osteoarthritis: comparison with paracetamol," *International Immunopharmacology*, vol. 3, no. 13-14, pp. 1901–1908, 2003.

[41] A. R. Shahed and D. A. Shoskes, "Correlation of β-endorphin and prostaglandin E2 levels in prostatic fluid of patients with chronic prostatitis with diagnosis and treatment response," *Journal of Urology*, vol. 166, no. 5, pp. 1738–1741, 2001.

[42] R. K. Tume and F. D. Shaw, "Beta-endorphin and cortisol concentrations in plasma of blood samples collected during exsanguination of cattle," *Meat Science*, vol. 31, no. 2, pp. 211–217, 1992.

[43] P. L. De Riu, V. Petruzzi, G. Palmieri et al., "β-Endorphin in experimental canine spinal ischemia," *Stroke*, vol. 20, no. 2, pp. 253–258, 1989.

Effects of Zearalenone on IL-2, IL-6, and IFN-γ mRNA Levels in the Splenic Lymphocytes of Chickens

Y. C. Wang,[1] J. L. Deng,[1] S. W. Xu,[2] X. Peng,[3] Z. C. Zuo,[4] H. M. Cui,[3] Y. Wang,[4] and Z. H. Ren[4]

[1] *College of Veterinary Medicine, Sichuan Agricultural University, Yaan, Sichuan 625014, China*
[2] *Department of Veterinary Medicine, Northeast Agricultural University, Harbin 150030, China*
[3] *Sichuan Key Laboratory of Animal Disease and Human Health, Yaan, Sichuan 625014, China*
[4] *Sichuan Key Laboratory of Environmental Hazards Disease, Yaan, Sichuan 625014, China*

Correspondence should be addressed to J. L. Deng, dengjl213@126.com

Academic Editors: R. Pohjanvirta and A. Tsatsakis

Zearalenone (ZEN) is an estrogenic mycotoxin produced by several *Fusarium* species, which can contaminate food and feed. These compounds elicit a wide spectrum of toxic effects, including the capacity to alter normal immune function. In this study, the in vitro effects of the treatment of ConA-stimulated splenic lymphocytes with ZEN (0–25 μg/mL) were examined. ZEN modulates the expression of IL-2, IL-6, and IFN-γ. The IL-2 levels were up to fourfold higher ($P < 0.05$) compared with the levels in the control at toxin concentrations of 25 μg/mL after 48 h of treatment. The IL-6 levels were critically suppressed at this concentration; these changes were very statistically significant ($P < 0.05$). At lower ZEN concentrations (0.1, 0.4 and 1.6 μg/mL), the IFN-γ levels changed slightly; however at 6.25 and 25 μg/mL, the IFN-γ results reached statistical significance compared with the control levels ($P < 0.05$). These data suggest that ZEN has potent effects on the expression of chicken splenic lymphocytes cytokines at the mRNA level.

1. Introduction

Zearalenone (ZEN) is a mycotoxin produced by several field fungi, including *Fusarium graminearum* (Gibberella zeae), *F. culmorum*, *F. cerealis*, *F. equiseti*, and *F. semitectum* [1, 2]. It exists widely in many cereal crops such as corn, barley, wheat, oats, sorghum, and sesame seeds, as well as in hay and corn silage. These are all ingredients in many food products for human or animal nutrition [3–5].

ZEN is a macrocyclic lactone with a high binding affinity for estrogen receptors. It is biologically potent, but it is hardly toxic. Rather, it has an estrogenic effect that causes alterations in the reproductive tract of laboratory animals (mice, rats, and guinea pigs) and farm animals [6, 7]. The mechanism of the estrogenic effects of ZEN appears to be mediated via binding of this mycotoxin or its metabolites to the cytoplasmic estrogen receptor [8–10]. This increases cell proliferation [11], resulting in uterine hyperplasia as well as cervical and vaginal metaplasia [12, 13].

The immune system is a potential target for estrogenic endocrine disruptors because various cells of the immune system have estrogen receptors [14]. However, only few studies have been carried out regarding the effects of ZEN on spleen immunity in chickens, specifically on lymphocytes. In the present study, we investigated the in vitro effects of ZEN at different concentrations on IL-2, IL-6, and IFN-γ mRNA expression levels in poultry spleen lymphocytes.

2. Materials and Methods

2.1. Reagents. All chemicals were of the highest grade of purity available. Fetal bovine serum (FBS) was purchased from Sijiqing Biological Engineering Material (Hangzhou, China). Zearalenone, RPMI 1640 medium, and Histopaque 1077 were purchased from Sigma-Aldrich, USA. Trizol reagent was purchased from Invitrogen Biotechnology Co. Ltd. (Shanghai, China). SYBR PremixScript RT-PCR Kit II was purchased from Takara, Shiga, Japan.

TABLE 1: Real-time PCR primer sequences and products.

Gene	Primer	Sequences (5′ → 3′)	Product size (bp)
β-actin	β-Actin Forward	CACCACAGCCGAGAGAGAAAT	135
	β-Actin Reverse	TGACCATCAGGGAGTTCATAGC	
IL-2	IL-2 Forward	GCTAATGACTACAGCTTATGGAGCA	138
	IL-2 Reverse	TGGGTCTCAGTTGGTGTGTAGAG	
IL-6	IL-6 Forward	AAATCCCTCCTCGCCAATCT	106
	IL-6 Reverse	CCCTCACGGTCTTCTCCATAAA	
IFN-γ	IFN-γ Forward	AAGTCATAGCGGCACATCAAAC	132
	IFN-γ Reverse	CTGGAATCTCATGTCGTTCATCG	

2.2. Cell Culture. All chickens used in this experiment were approved by the Institutional Animal Care and Use Committee of Northeast Agricultural University. The spleens of two-month-old *Isa Brown* chicken were teased through a 200-mesh cell strainer into a Petri dish containing phosphate-buffered saline (PBS). The cell suspension was overlaid onto Histopaque 1077 and was centrifuged at 400 ×g for 15 min at room temperature. The lymphocytes at the interface were collected, washed twice with PBS at 250 g for 5 min at room temperature, and suspended in RPMI-1640 medium (without phenol red, a weak estrogen mimic) supplemented with 10% fetal calf serum, 100 U/mL penicillin, 100 U/mL streptomycin. More than 95% of cells were viable based on the trypan blue dye exclusion. The spleen cells were cultured in 6-well tissue culture plates (6×10^6 cell/mL) in triplicate and stimulated with concanavalin A (ConA, 12.5 μg/mL, to induce the proliferation of T cells) at 0, 0.1, 0.4, 1.6, 6.25, and 25 μg/mL ZEN at 41.5°C in a humidified 5% CO_2 environment for 48 h [15]. The mycotoxin concentrations were selected based on preliminary dose-response experiments (data not shown). After 48 h of incubation, cells were collected for RNA isolation, then frozen at −80°C.

2.3. Quantification of IL-2, IL-6, and IFN-γ mRNA. Total RNA was isolated from cells using Trizol reagent according to the instructions of the manufacturer. The RNA concentrations were determined using the GeneQuant 1300.

The 40 μL reverse transcription reaction mixture consisted of the following components: 10 μg of total RNA, 1 μL of Moloney murine leukemia virus reverse transcriptase, 1 μL of RNase inhibitor, 4 μL of deoxynucleoside triphosphate, 2 μL of Oligo dT, 4 μL of dithiothreitol, and 8 mL of 5x reverse transcriptase buffer. The reverse transcription was performed according to the instructions of the manufacturer (Invitrogen). The reverse transcription products (cDNA) were stored at −20°C for PCR.

To design primers, we used the chicken IL-2, IL-6, and IFN-γ mRNA GenBank sequence with accession numbers of NM204153.1, NM204628.1, and DQ470471.1, respectively. Chicken β-actin (GenBank accession number L08165.1), a housekeeping gene, was used as the internal reference. The primers (Table 1) were designed using the Prime 5 Software (Molecular Biology Insights, Cascade, CO) and were synthesized by Invitrogen Biotechnology Co. Ltd., Shanghai, China.

Real-time PCR was performed to detect the expression of IL-2, IL-6, and IFN-γ genes in different cDNA sample using SYBR Premix Ex Taq (Takara, Shiga, Japan). Each sample was assayed in three replicates. The reaction mixtures were incubated in an ABI PRISM 7500 real-time PCR system (Applied Biosystems, Foster City, CA). The program included 1 cycle at 95°C for 30 s, 40 cycles at 95°C for 5 s, and 60°C for 34 s. The dissociation curves were analyzed using Dissociation curve 1.0 Software (Applied Biosystems) for each PCR reaction to detect and eliminate the possible primer dimer and nonspecific amplification. Results (fold changes) are expressed using the Pfaffl method [16, 17] with the following formula:

$$\text{Ratio} = \frac{\left(E_{\text{target}}\right)^{\Delta CT,\ \text{target (calibrator-test)}}}{\left(E_{\text{ref}}\right)^{\Delta CT,\ \text{ref (calibrator-test)}}} \quad (1)$$

where ΔCT, target (calibrator-test) = $(CT_{\text{target}})_{\text{control group}} - (CT_{\text{target}})_{\text{treatment group}}$, ΔCT, ref (calibrator-test) = $(CT_{\text{ref}})_{\text{control group}} - (CT_{\text{ref}})_{\text{treatment group}}$, E_{target} is the real-time PCR efficiency of target gene transcript, and E_{ref} is the real-time PCR efficiency of a reference gene transcript.

2.4. Statistical Analysis. Statistical analysis of all data was performed using SAS procedures (SAS Institute Inc, NC); differences in mean RT-PCR results were compared by one-way ANOVA. All values are expressed as mean ± SD, and $P < 0.05$ were considered as significant difference.

3. Results

To compare the effects of ZEN on cytokine expression in residual living cells among individuals, the results were calculated as mean fold changes in cytokine levels above the control (treated with only ConA) cultures at the same time points. Treatment of the ConA-stimulated cells with ZEN at concentrations ranging from 0 to 25 μg/mL consistently increased the IL-2 levels above those in the ConA-only stimulated cells (Figure 1). These results were statistically significant ($P < 0.05$) with toxin concentrations of 0.1, 0.4, 1.6, 6.25, and 25 μg/mL at 48 h (Figure 1). In contrast, the ZEN treatment moderately inhibited IL-6 levels in these cells; these changes were very statistically significant with toxin

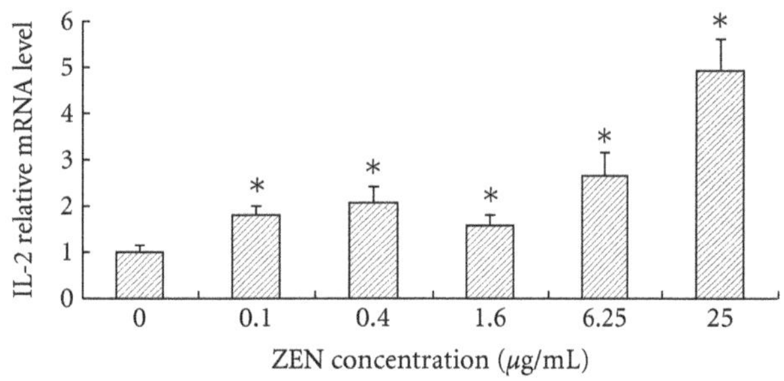

Figure 1: The effect of ZEN on the IL-2 relative mRNA level in ConA-stimulated lymphocytes at toxin concentration of 0, 0.1, 0.4, 1.6, 6.25, and 25 μg/mL at 48 h. The reporter activity in response to ConA alone is expressed as 100%. Values are the means ± SD from three independent experiments. Statistical analysis was performed using one-way ANOVA followed by Dunnett's post hoc test ($^*P < 0.05$ versus ConA treated control).

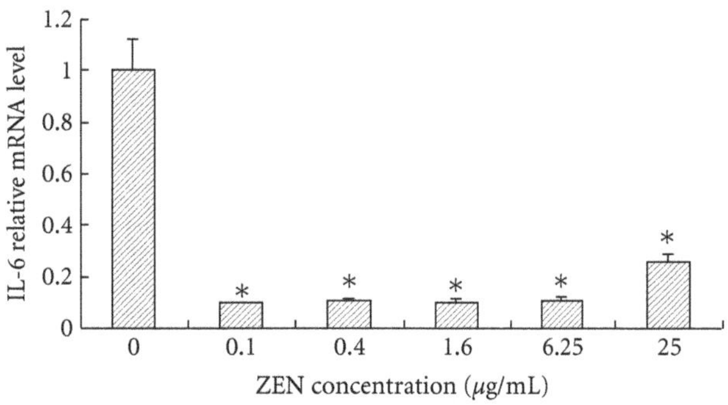

Figure 2: The effect of ZEN on the IL-6 relative mRNA level in ConA-stimulated lymphocytes at toxin concentrations of 0, 0.1, 0.4, 1.6, 6.25, and 25 μg/mL at 48 h. The reporter activity in response to ConA alone is expressed as 100%. Values are the means ± SD from three independent experiments. Statistical analysis was performed using one-way ANOVA followed by Dunnett's post hoc test ($^*P < 0.05$ versus ConA treated control).

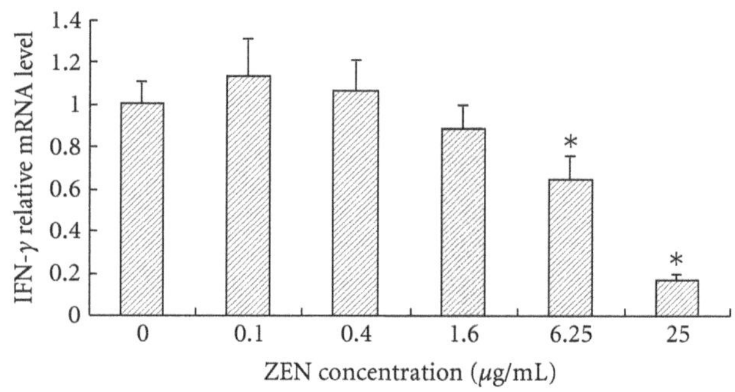

Figure 3: The effect of ZEN on the IFN-γ relative mRNA level in ConA-stimulated lymphocytes at toxin concentrations of 0, 0.1, 0.4, 1.6, 6.25, and 25 μg/mL at 48 h. The reporter activity in response to ConA alone is expressed as 100%. Values are the means ± SD from three independent experiments. Statistical analysis was performed using one-way ANOVA followed by Dunnett's post hoc test ($^*P < 0.05$ versus ConA treated control).

concentration in all treated groups ($P < 0.05$). The IL-6 levels were critically suppressed (Figure 2).

To understand further the specific effects of ZEN on cytokine profiles, a characteristic TH 1 cytokine, IFN-γ, was measured in addition to IL-2 and TH 2, IL-6. A lower dose of ZEN (0.1, 0.4, and 1.6 μg/mL) was selected to eliminate the possibility of cytotoxic effects, which contributes to modulation; however, the two highest doses (6.25 and 25 μg/mL) reached statistical significance compared with the control ($P < 0.05$). The IFN-γ levels were slightly suppressed by the ZEN treatment (Figure 3).

4. Discussion

There is major concern over the potential for mycotoxins to influence poultry negatively. In the present study, the use of cell cultures offers several advantages over other methods, particularly in terms of the quantification of toxic effects and for defining the immune organ specificity related to a preferential action of a particular cell type. We addressed the issue by evaluating the effects of ZEN on the immune function through in vitro assessment of its activity on the splenic lymphocytes of chickens. The splenic lymphocytes of chickens have been a very useful model for different immunologic studies. ConA is a polyclonal T-cell mitogen, and we determined the effects of ZEN on ConA-stimulated lymphocytes on certain T-helper cell (TH), cytokine profiles (IL-2, IL-6, and IFN-γ) were assessed.

To date, there have been no studies regarding the effects of ZEN on the cytokine profiles of chicken splenic lymphocyte. The addition of ZEN in vitro to ConA-stimulated lymphocytes caused a fivefold increase in the expression of IL-2 cytokines at the mRNA level. As the chemical structure of ZEN enables its binding to the estrogenic receptors, our data are not in line with previous results, which indicate that 17-beta-estradiol reduced IL-2 gene transcription in the Jurkat T-cell line [18]. Considering that T-lymphocyte proliferation is essentially mediated by IL-2, the observed inhibition could be considered a primary mechanism of ZEN-induced immunosuppression also acting in vivo. Accordingly, inhibition of the mRNA expression of IL-2 cytokines by α-ZEN remain unclear assuming an estrogen-like activity [18]. Our results on IL-2 are not broadly in agreement with studies on cytokine protein expression in humans [19]. However, several alterations in immunologic parameters have been associated with ZEN concentrations in humans [20]and mice [21] including in vitro inhibition of mitogen-stimulated lymphocyte proliferation, increase of IL-2 and IL-5, and induction of immunosuppressive effects [22, 23]. Alterations in immunologic parameters such as the inhibition of mitogenstimulated lymphocyte proliferation and the increase in IL-2 production were found at high ZEA concentrations in vitro [22]. In addition, populations that are continuously exposed to ZEN may chronically produce IL-2; therefore, IL-6 is decreased. There are only few reports regarding the effects of ZEN on IL-6. Aside from ZEN, *Fusarium* can also produce other mycotoxins such as deoxynivalenol (DON), fumonisin B1 (FB1), and T-2 toxin. The effect of these mycotoxins on IL-6 has been studied. A study [24] quantified IL-6 in the spleen, ileum, and mesenteric lymph nodes of 24 pigs which received either control feeds or feeds naturally contaminated with 2.2–2.5 mg/kg of DON feed for 9 weeks using RT-PCR. FB_1 inhibited the LPS-induced expression of IL-6 in human dendritic cells (DCs) [25], whereas the modulation of FB_1 toxicity in the brain of female BALB/c mice; FB_1 augments the LPS-induced IL-6 expression in the brain [26]. The effects of in vivo exposure to T-2 toxin on the alteration of IL-6 in lipopolysaccharide-stimulated peritoneal macrophages [27]; IL-6 mRNA from activated peritoneal macrophages showed no significant differences between the control and the treatment groups. The effects of different *Fusarium* toxins on IL-6 varied because of differences in toxicities and animal models.

IFN-γ is a master cytokine that affects the functioning of all cells of the immune system and plays a major role in host defense against intracellular infections [28]. This cytokine has also been implicated in autoimmune and inflammatory diseases [29]. Importantly, the IFN-γ levels in ConA-activated splenic lymphocytes that were exposed to zearalenone decreased after 48 h of culture, consistent with previous findings. Studies revealed that zearalenone causes a decrease in IFN-γ in geriatric mice [30], and a slight reduction in both the mitotic index and the cell survival of bovine lymphocytes [31].

To our knowledge, this is the first study that investigates the effects of ZEN on the cellular immune response of chickens. Although the exact mechanism of action of these toxins is still unknown, the results of the current study suggest that ZEN may have divergent effects on chicken lymphocyte cell viability, and production of IL-2, IL-6 and IFN-γ. Further studies are needed to elucidate the specific mechanisms by which ZEN affects immune functions.

Disclosure

All other authors have read the paper and have agreed to submit it in its current form for consideration for publication in The Scientific World Journal.

Acknowledgments

The present work was supported by the National Natural Science Foundation of China Funds (grant no. 31072182) and the Changjing Scholars & Innovative Reasearch Team of Ministry of Education of China Funds (Grant no. IRTO848). The authors gratefully acknowledge the members of the Veterinary Internal Medicine Laboratory in the College of Veterinary Medicine, Sichuan Agricultural University, and in College of Veterinary Medicine, Northeast Agricultural University for their help in feeding the laboratory animals and analyzing the data.

References

[1] J. L. Richard, "Some major mycotoxins and their mycotoxicoses-An overview," *International Journal of Food Microbiology*, vol. 119, no. 1-2, pp. 3–10, 2007.

[2] J. W. Bennett and M. Klich, "Mycotoxins," *Clinical Microbiology Reviews*, vol. 16, no. 3, pp. 497–516, 2003.

[3] S. J. Macdonald, S. Anderson, P. Brereton et al., "Determination of zearalenone in barley, maize and wheat flour, polenta, and maize-based baby food by immunoaffinity column cleanup with liquid chromatography: interlaboratory study," *Journal of AOAC International*, vol. 88, no. 6, pp. 1733–1740, 2005.

[4] G. Engelhardt, J. Barthel, and D. Sparrer, "Fusarium mycotoxins and ochratoxin A in cereals and cereal products: results from the Bavarian Health and Food Safety Authority in 2004," *Molecular Nutrition and Food Research*, vol. 50, no. 4-5, pp. 401–405, 2006.

[5] C. Tabuc, D. Marin, P. Guerre, T. Sesan, and J. D. Bailly, "Molds and mycotoxin content of cereals in southeastern romania," *Journal of Food Protection*, vol. 72, no. 3, pp. 662–665, 2009.

[6] U. Tiemann and S. Dänicke, "In vivo and in vitro effects of the mycotoxins zearalenone and deoxynivalenol on different non-reproductive and reproductive organs in female pigs: a review," *Food Additives and Contaminants*, vol. 24, no. 3, pp. 306–314, 2007.

[7] F. Minervini and M. E. D. Aquila, "Zearalenone and reproductive function in farm animals," *International Journal of Molecular Sciences*, vol. 9, no. 12, pp. 2570–2584, 2008.

[8] B. S. Katzenellenbogen, J. A. Katzenellenbogen, and D. Mordecai, "Zearalenones: characterization of the estrogenic potencies and receptor interactions of a series of fungal β-resorcylic acid lactones," *Endocrinology*, vol. 105, no. 1, pp. 33–40, 1979.

[9] S. O. Mueller, "Overview of in vitro tools to assess the oestrogenic and antioestrogenic activity of phytooestrogens," *Journal of Chromatography B*, vol. 777, no. 1-2, pp. 155–156, 2002.

[10] U. Tiemann, T. Viergutz, L. Jonas, and F. Schneider, "Influence of the mycotoxins α- and β-zearalenol and deoxynivalenol on the cell cycle of cultured porcine endometrial cells," *Reproductive Toxicology*, vol. 17, no. 2, pp. 209–218, 2003.

[11] D. S. Coffey, "Similarities of prostate and breast cancer: evolution, diet, and estrogens," *Urology*, vol. 57, no. 4, supplement 1, pp. 31–38, 2001.

[12] M. Gajecki, "Zearalenone—undesirable substances in feed," *Polish Journal of Veterinary Sciences*, vol. 5, no. 2, pp. 117–122, 2002.

[13] W. Zwierzchowski, M. Przybyłowicz, K. Obremski et al., "Level of zearalenone in blood serum and lesions in ovarian follicles of sexually immature gilts in the course of zearalenone micotoxicosis," *Polish Journal of Veterinary Sciences*, vol. 8, no. 3, pp. 209–218, 2005.

[14] H. Igarashi, T. Kouro, T. Yokota, P. C. Comp, and P. W. Kincade, "Age and stage dependency of estrogen receptor expression by lymphocyte precursors," *Proceedings of the National Academy of Sciences of the United States of America*, vol. 98, no. 26, pp. 15131–15136, 2001.

[15] M. Okamura, H. S. Lillehoj, R. B. Raybourne, U. S. Babu, and R. A. Heckert, "Cell-mediated immune responses to a killed Salmonella enteritidis vaccine: lymphocyte proliferation, T-cell changes and interleukin-6 (IL-6), IL-1, IL-2, and IFN-γ production," *Comparative Immunology, Microbiology and Infectious Diseases*, vol. 27, no. 4, pp. 255–272, 2004.

[16] W. P. Michael, "A new mathematical model for relative quantification in real-time RT-PCR," *Nucleic Acids Research*, vol. 29, no. 900, pp. 2004–2007, 2001.
[17] S. Čikoš, A. Bukovská, and J. Koppel, "Relative quantification of mRNA: comparison of methods currently used for real-time PCR data analysis," *BMC Molecular Biology*, vol. 8, article 113, 2007.
[18] R. W. McMurray, K. Ndebele, K. J. Hardy, and J. K. Jenkins, "17-β-estradiol suppresses IL-2 and IL-2 receptor," *Cytokine*, vol. 14, no. 6, pp. 324–333, 2001.
[19] D. Luongo, L. Severino, P. Bergamo, R. De Luna, A. Lucisano, and M. Rossi, "Interactive effects of fumonisin B1 and α-zearalenol on proliferation and cytokine expression in Jurkat T cells," *Toxicology in Vitro*, vol. 20, no. 8, pp. 1403–1410, 2006.
[20] L. Berek, I. B. Petri, Á. Mesterházy, J. Téren, and J. Molnár, "Effects of mycotoxins on human immune functions in vitro," *Toxicology in Vitro*, vol. 15, no. 1, pp. 25–30, 2001.
[21] M. L. Marin, J. Murtha, W. Dong, and J. J. Pestka, "Effects of mycotoxins on cytokine production and proliferation in EL-4 thymoma cells," *Journal of Toxicology and Environmental Health*, vol. 48, no. 4, pp. 379–396, 1996.
[22] G. S. Eriksen and J. Alexander, Eds., *Fusarium Toxins in Cereals—A Risk Assessment*, vol. 502, Nordic Council of Ministers, Copenhagen, Denmark, 1998.
[23] H. Murata, P. Sultana, N. Shimada, and M. Yoshioka, "Structure-activity relationships among zearalenone and its derivatives based on bovine neutrophil chemiluminescence," *Veterinary and Human Toxicology*, vol. 45, no. 1, pp. 18–20, 2003.
[24] P. Pinton, F. Accensi, E. Beauchamp et al., "Ingestion of deoxynivalenol (DON) contaminated feed alters the pig vaccinal immune responses," *Toxicology Letters*, vol. 177, no. 3, pp. 215–222, 2008.
[25] H. Stockmann-Juvala, H. Alenius, and K. Savolainen, "Effects of fumonisin B1 on the expression of cytokines and chemokines in human dendritic cells," *Food and Chemical Toxicology*, vol. 46, no. 5, pp. 1444–1451, 2008.
[26] M. F. Osuchowski, Q. He, and R. P. Sharma, "Endotoxin exposure alters brain and liver effects of fumonisin B 1 in BALB/c mice: implication of blood brain barrier," *Food and Chemical Toxicology*, vol. 43, no. 9, pp. 1389–1397, 2005.
[27] R. R. Dugyala and R. P. Sharma, "Alteration of major cytokines produced by mitogen-activated peritoneal macrophages and splenocytes in T-2 toxin-treated male CD-1 mice," *Environmental Toxicology and Pharmacology*, vol. 3, no. 1, pp. 73–81, 1997.
[28] J. E. Durbin, T. R. Johnson, R. K. Durbin et al., "The role of IFN in respiratory syncytial virus pathogenesis," *The Journal of Immunology*, vol. 168, no. 6, pp. 2944–2951, 2002.
[29] N. H. R. Hamilton, J. L. Banyer, A. J. Hapel et al., "IFN-γ regulates murine interferon-inducible T cell alpha chemokine (I-TAC) expression in dendritic cell lines and during experimental autoimmune encephalomyelitis (EAE)," *Scandinavian Journal of Immunology*, vol. 55, no. 2, pp. 171–177, 2002.
[30] J. Calemine, J. Zalenka, E. Karpuzoglu-Sahin, D. L. Ward, A. Lengi, and S. A. Ahmed, "The immune system of geriatric mice is modulated by estrogenic endocrine disruptors (diethylstilbestrol, α-zearalanol, and genistein): effects on interferon-γ," *Toxicology*, vol. 194, no. 1-2, pp. 115–128, 2003.
[31] M. B. Lioi, A. Santoro, R. Barbieri, S. Salzano, and M. V. Ursini, "Ochratoxin A and zearalenone: a comparative study on genotoxic effects and cell death induced in bovine lymphocytes," *Mutation Research*, vol. 557, no. 1, pp. 19–27, 2004.

Intrahost Diversity of Feline Coronavirus: A Consensus between the Circulating Virulent/Avirulent Strains and the Internal Mutation Hypotheses?

Aline S. Hora,[1,2] Karen M. Asano,[1,2] Juliana M. Guerra,[3] Ramon G. Mesquita,[3] Paulo Maiorka,[3] Leonardo J. Richtzenhain,[1,2] and Paulo E. Brandão[1,2]

[1] *Department of Preventive Veterinary Medicine and Animal Health, College of Veterinary Medicine, University of São Paulo, Avenida Professor Dr. Orlando Marques de Paiva 87, Cidade Universitária, 05508-270 São Paulo, SP, Brazil*
[2] *Coronavirus Research Group, College of Veterinary Medicine, University of São Paulo, Avenida Professor Dr. Orlando Marques de Paiva 87, Cidade Universitária, 05508-270 São Paulo, SP, Brazil*
[3] *Department of Pathology, College of Veterinary Medicine, University of São Paulo, Avenida Professor Dr. Orlando Marques de Paiva 87, Cidade Universitária, 05508-270 São Paulo, SP, Brazil*

Correspondence should be addressed to Aline S. Hora; alineshora@gmail.com

Academic Editors: G. T. Pharr, J. L. Romalde, and B. I. Yoon

To evaluate the most controversial issue concerning current feline coronavirus (FCoV) virology, the coexisting hypotheses of the intrahost and interhost origins of feline infectious peritonitis virus (FIPV) in regard to the pathogenesis of feline infectious peritonitis (FIP), this study aimed to assess the molecular diversity of the membrane gene FCoVs in 190 samples from 10 cats with signs of FIP and in 5 faecal samples from cats without signs of FIP. All samples from the non-FIP cats and 25.26% of the samples from the FIP cats were positive for the FCoV membrane (M) gene. Mutations in this gene consisted of SNP changes randomly scattered among the sequences; few mutations resulted in amino acid changes. No geographic pattern was observed. Of the cats without FIP that harboured FECoV, the amino acid sequence identities for the M gene were 100% among cats (Cats 1–3) from the same cattery, and the overall sequence identity for the M gene was ≥91%. In one cat, two different lineages of FCoV, one enteric and one systemic, were found that segregated apart in the M gene tree. In conclusion, the in vivo mutation transition hypothesis and the circulating high virulent-low virulent FCoV hypothesis have been found to be plausible according to the results obtained from sequencing the M gene.

1. Introduction

Feline coronavirus (FCoV), a widespread pathogen of domestic cat populations worldwide, is an enveloped single-stranded RNA virus of the order Nidovirales, family Coronaviridae, subfamily Coronavirinae, genus *Alphacoronavirus*, species *alphacoronavirus 1*. Most infections are either asymptomatic or result in a mild, self-limiting gastrointestinal disease, and, in these cases, the causative agent is the feline enteric coronavirus (FECoV) pathotype. In contrast, feline infectious peritonitis (FIP), a possible complication of FCoV infection in a small proportion of cats, is a lethal, systemic immune-mediated disease caused by a second FCoV pathotype, feline infectious peritonitis virus (FIPV) [1, 2].

FIP is characterised by fibrinous/granulomatous serositis, with protein-rich effusions in the body cavities of affected cats, as well as granulomatous-necrotising lesions, periphlebitis, and granulomatous inflammatory lesions in several organs, particularly in the liver, kidney, spleen, leptomeninges, and eyes [3]. The pathogenesis of FIP is not fully understood, but it has been shown that monocyte-triggered vasculitis, in association with systemic monocyte and endothelial cell activation, is an essential event [3], most likely in combination with antibody-mediated enhancement and complement activation [4]. Specific genetic determinants of these clinical outcomes have yet to be discovered in cats. This disease is one of the most serious viral infections in cats, not only because of its fatal nature but also because of the difficulties in diagnosing FIP antemortem and in controlling the spread of FCoV [5].

The key to a deeper understanding of FCoV diseases in cats is the exact nature of the relationship between the two FCoV pathotypes; two important hypotheses have been suggested. The hypothesis known as the "internal mutation theory" is widely accepted [1, 2, 6–9], and it states that FIP occurs when a cat is exposed to variants of FCoV that have mutated within the host and are able to disseminate from the gut (the primary site of infection) by gaining the ability to efficiently replicate within the macrophages [1, 2]. However, any stable genetic differences between FECoV and FIPV that can account for their differing pathogenicities remain to be identified [10].

The alternate "circulating high virulent-low virulent" FCoV hypothesis of viral pathogenesis suggests that both distinctive pathogenic and benign lineages of FECoV might be present in a cat population and that the disease will develop only in those cats infected by the virulent strains already available from other infected cats [5]. The existence of distinct "high virulent-low virulent FCoVs" is an alternate and less popular hypothesis for FIP pathogenesis [5, 10]. As FIP occurs sporadically and outbreaks of FIP in domestic cat populations are rather uncommon, there has been little epidemiologic support for this hypothesis [1].

Most authors have concurred that although a low-level monocyte-associated viraemia is found with FECoV infections, this virus is mainly confined to the gut [10, 11]. This is in contrast to the highly virulent FIPV, which disseminates systemically with high viral titres. Thus, obtaining sequence data from enteric and nonenteric FCoVs found within individual cats with FIP may shed more light on any genetic differences between FECoV and FIPV [10].

To evaluate the most controversial issue concerning current FCoV virology, the coexisting hypotheses of the intrahost and interhost origins of FIPV in regard to FIP pathogenesis and to gain more insight into FCoV evolution, this study aimed to assess the molecular diversity of FCoVs in multiple organs of cats with signs of FIP and in faecal samples from cats without signs of FIP.

2. Materials and Methods

2.1. Animals and Sample Collection. During 2010–2012, tissue samples (eye, cerebrum, cerebellum, lung, heart muscle, thoracic lymph node, thymus, liver, spleen, stomach, mesenteric lymph node, peripancreatic lymph node, kidneys, large and small intestines, and urinary bladder), abdominal, thoracic, and pericardial effusions, aqueous humour, and faecal samples were collected at necropsies from 10 deceased or euthanised unrelated cats with suspected FIP, for a total of 190 samples. Sterile instruments and disposable materials were used for sample collection.

Additionally, faecal samples from five cats without clinical signs of FIP were also collected; none of these had cats developed FIP as of the time of writing this study. These cats came from 3 multiple cat households, one of them with an outbreak of diarrhoea at the time that the 3 samples from the different cats were collected. All samples were flash-frozen in liquid nitrogen and stored at −80 °C until the RNA extraction.

2.2. Total RNA Extraction. Organ samples were prepared as 30% (v/v) suspensions in UltraPure diethyl pyrocarbonate-(DEPC-) treated water (Invitrogen, Carlsbad, CA, USA), submitted to 3 freeze-thaw cycles in liquid nitrogen at 56°C, and clarified at 5,000 ×g for 15 min at 4°C. Effusion and aqueous humour were concentrated at 12,000 ×g for 15 min at 4°C. Faecal samples were prepared as 30% (v/v) suspensions in UltraPure diethyl pyrocarbonate-(DEPC-) treated water (Invitrogen, Carlsbad, CA, USA), clarified at 12,000 ×g for 15 min at 4°C. The total RNA was extracted from the supernatants of organs and faecal suspensions and pellets from effusions with TRIzol reagent (Invitrogen, Carlsbad, CA, USA), according to the manufacturer's instructions. The RNA was eluted in 30 μL of UltraPure DEPC-treated water.

2.3. RT-PCR for the Detection of the FCoV mRNA of the Membrane (M) Gene. All samples were screened for the presence of FCoV M gene mRNA using primers previously described [12], with modifications (2RNAmA TAATRM-CATARACGADCCAGCT, nt 26440–26461, and 2RNAmS GTGCTAGVTTTGTCTTCGGACAMC, nt 60–83, positions regarding strain FIPV 79–1179).

A positive RNA control was prepared from the abdominal effusion of a cat with FIP by an in vitro transcription with a MEGAscript T7 kit (Ambion, Austin, TX, USA) according to the manufacturers' instructions, using the above-mentioned primers. UltraPure DEPC-treated water (Invitrogen, Carlsbad, CA, USA) was used as a negative control.

For the 190 samples, the cDNA was synthesised in 10 μL reactions using 3.5 μL of the RNA solution and 1 μM 2RNAmS of the reverse primer and M-MLV Reverse Transcriptase (Invitrogen, Carlsbad, CA, USA), as per the manufacturer's instructions.

The subgenomic mRNA of the M gene was then amplified using 0.5 μM of each primer and GoTaq Green Master Mix 1X (Promega Corporation, Madison, WI, USA) according to the manufacturer's protocols. The primer annealing temperature was 50°C. The PCR products (295 bp) were visualised by electrophoresis on 1.5% agarose gels stained with SYBR Green I nucleic acid gel stain (Invitrogen, Carlsbad, CA, USA).

2.4. Partial M Gene Amplification and Sequencing. cDNA was synthesised using Random Primers (Invitrogen, Carlsbad, CA, USA) and M-MLV Reverse Transcriptase (Invitrogen, Carlsbad, CA, USA), according to the manufacturer's protocols. The partial M gene (575 bp) was then amplified using 0.5 μM of both reverse (26925–26944 nt positions regarding strain FCoV UU47) and forward primers (26968–26292 nt positions regarding strain FCoV UU47) [5] and GoTaq Green

Master Mix 1X (Promega Corporation, Madison, WI, USA) as per the manufacturer's instructions.

Amplicons were purified from agarose gels with Illustra (GE Healthcare, Buckinghamshire, UK) and submitted to bidirectional DNA sequencing with BigDye 3.1 (Applied Biosystems, Carlsbad, CA, USA), according to the manufacturer's protocols. Products were resolved using a 3500 Genetic Analyzer (Applied Biosystems, Foster City, CA, USA), and the chromatograms were analysed with Phred at http://asparagin.cenargen.embrapa.br/phph/. Positions with a quality score >20 were used to generate contiguous sequences with Cap-contig implemented in the software BioEdit 7.0.9.0 [13]. Those sequences were then submitted to BLAST/n at http://www.ncbi.nlm.nih.gov/BLAST to confirm the Amplicon identities.

The M gene partial sequences and the putative amino acid sequences from each sample were aligned with homologous sequences from both FCoVs pathotypes retrieved from GenBank (Figure 1) with CLUSTAL/W in BioEdit 7.0.9.0 [13], and a phylogenetic tree for the nucleotide sequences was generated with the neighbour-joining distance algorithm and the maximum composite likelihood model with 1,000 bootstrap replicates using MEGA 5.0 [14]. Amino acid alignment was used to search for previously reported pathotype-specific markers [5].

2.5. Histopathologic Analysis. Organ samples were also fixed in 10% buffered formalin and routinely embedded in paraffin. Sections (5 μm) were stained with hematoxylin and eosin (HE). The HE-stained slides of the organ sections were evaluated for evidence of granulomatous and pyogranulomatous lesions.

3. Results

3.1. RT-PCR for the Detection of FCoV mRNA of the Membrane Gene. In all 10 cats with FIP, FCoV mRNA was detected in at least one of the samples. Of the 190 individual samples, 77 (40.53%) were positive for the M gene. The abdominal effusions (5/6), mesenteric lymph nodes (7/10), large intestines (7/10), lungs (6/10), thoracic effusions (4/8), kidneys (10/20), and aqueous humours (8/20) were the most frequent FCoV replication sites. Of the 5 faecal samples from cats without FIP, 3 were positive for FCoV M gene mRNA.

3.2. Partial M Gene Amplification, Sequencing, and Phylogenic Analysis. Of the euthanised or diseased cats, 25.26% samples (48/190) were positive for the FCoV M gene. Multiple samples from each cat were determined to be positive, by RT-PCR, for the FCoV M gene. Of these, the most frequently positive samples were the contents of the large intestine (5/11), spleen (4/10), and lungs (4/10). All faecal samples from the 5 cats without FIP were positive for the FCoV M gene.

The sequences obtained in this study were submitted to the GenBank database under the accession numbers JQ627051-JQ627090.

When compared by phylogenic analysis, the nucleotide sequences of the M gene (positions from 26293 to 26907 regarding strain FCoV UU47) from the cats with FIP and the cats with FECoV in this study were distributed in paraphyletic groups (Figure 1). Sequence strains from 3 cats with diarrhoea but without PIF (Cats 1–3) from a multiple cat household were grouped in the same cluster. The sample-specific FCoV strain's differentiation and nucleotide polymorphism among sequences from the same cat were low (≥98%), whereas the overall sequence identification for the M gene was ≥91% among all FIPV sequences (Table 1). Mutations consisted of minor SNP changes that appeared to be randomly scattered among the sequences; few mutations resulted in amino acid changes. No geographic pattern was observed. Of the cats without FIP that harboured FECoV, the amino acid sequence identities for the M gene were 100% among cats (Cats 1–3) from the same cattery, and the overall sequence identity for the M gene was ≥91%.

Nonetheless, a striking exception was Cat 6, in which two different lineages of FCoV, one enteric and one systemic, were found that segregated apart in the M gene tree (Figure 1), with a nucleotide identity of 94% among the enteric sequence and the systemic ($n = 5$) sequences.

Five amino acid sites in the M protein suggested as potential FIPV signatures [5] were evaluated based on the reference sequence for FCoV (GenBank JN183882). Within the lineages obtained in the present study, no amino acid polymorphism was observed at position 108 or 198 (Figure 2). The amino acids at positions 120, 138, and 162 occurred with no specific pattern in the FIPV and FECoV sequences: Val120 in 100% (5/5) of FECoV and in 91.4% (32/35) of FIPV; Ile120 in 8.6% (3/35) of FIPV; Ile138 in 34.3% (12/35) of FIPV; Val138 in 80% (4/5) of FECoV and 65.7% (23/35) of FIPV; Leu138 in 20% (1/5) of FECoV; Ala162 80% (4/5) of FECoV and in 91.4% (32/35) of FIPV; Val162 in 20% (1/5) of FECoV and 8.6% (3/35) of FIPV.

TABLE 1: Feline coronavirus membrane (M) gene sequence identities (positions from 26293 to 26907 regarding strain FCoV UU47) from different samples of a same cat with FIP.

Cat	% sequence identity[a]	SD	Number of sequences	GenBank accession number
Cat 5	99.9	0.001	$n = 6$	JQ627055-60
Cat 6	98.0	0.028	$n = 6$	JQ627061-66
Cat 7	99.6	0.000	$n = 2$	JQ627067-68
Cat 8	100.0	0.000	$n = 7$	JQ627069-75
Cat 11	99.9	0.001	$n = 7$	JQ627078-84
Cat 12	99.9	0.001	$n = 3$	JQ627085-87

[a]The percentage of the sequence identity was determined by comparison with the consensus sequences of the FCoV obtained from different samples of the same cat. SD: standard deviation.

3.3. Histopathologic Analysis. A histopathological analysis was performed for 8 of the 10 necropsied cats. HE-stained sections typically showed localised inflammation with macrophages, neutrophils, lymphocytes, and plasma

TABLE 2: Histopathological analysis and results of FCoV mRNA RT-PCR in diseased cats with FIP.

Cat (n = 8)	Histopathological findings	Positive samples for mRNA FCoV
Cat 6	Pyogranulomas in lung, kidneys, cerebrum, and cerebellum Mild-to-moderate, subacute, multifocal fibrinous pleuritis Vasculitis in heart, lung, omentum, kidneys, cerebrum, and cerebellum	Cerebrum, cerebellum, lung, thymus, spleen, stomach, mesenteric lymph node, kidneys, aqueous humour, and faeces
Cat 7	Pyogranulomas in liver, kidneys, cerebrum, and cerebellum Vasculitis in cerebrum	Cerebellum, large intestine, and large intestine content
Cat 8	Severe, subacute, diffuse fibrinous pleuritis and peritonitis	Lung, thoracic lymph node, thymus, liver, spleen, stomach, mesenteric lymph node, peripancreatic lymph node, kidneys, large and small intestines, small intestine content, urinary bladder, and abdominal effusion
Cat 9	Diffuse, severe, nonsuppurative meningoencephalitis	Aqueous humour right eye, large intestine, and large intestine content
Cat 10	Moderate, subacute, diffuse fibrinous pleuritis	Mesenteric lymph node, large and small intestines contents, and abdominal effusion
Cat 11	Subacute, multifocal fibrinous peritonitis Moderate, diffuse interstitial pneumonia Pyogranulomas in kidneys (with bacteria) and liver	Cerebrum, aqueous humour left eye, mesenteric lymph node, and large intestine
Cat 12	Subacute, focally extensive fibrinous pleuritis Pyogranulomas in kidneys	Cerebrum, cerebellum, aqueous humour left eye, and thoracic effusion
Cat 13	Moderate, multifocal granulomatous pleuritis Severe, granulomatous, interstitial nephritis, associated with coalescing areas of necrosis	Cerebrum, aqueous humour left eye, lung, thoracic effusion, mesenteric lymph node, large and small intestines contents, kidneys, and abdominal effusion

cells. Vascular lesions were found surrounded by a proliferation of inflammatory cells. Focal accumulations of inflammatory cells and necrotic-proliferative lesions were observed in granulomatous lesions. Table 2 shows the main histopathological features and the FCoV replication sites for each cat.

4. Discussion and Conclusions

In this investigation, both double and single FCoV pathotype infections have been found in cats with feline infectious peritonitis, which supports both hypotheses of a viral

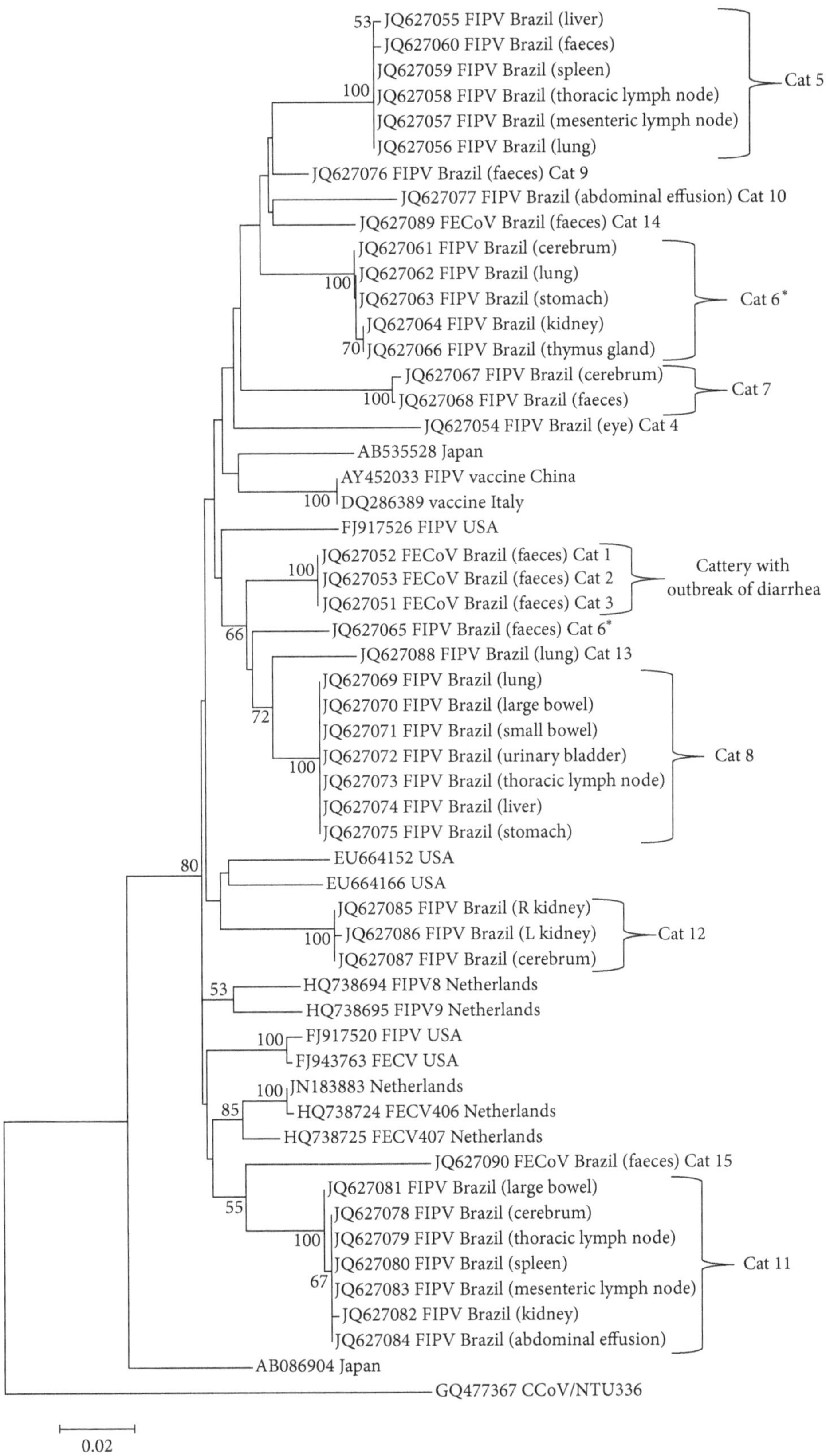

FIGURE 1: Neighbour-joining MCL phylogenetic tree of the M gene partial sequences of FCoV (positions from 26293 to 26907 regarding strain FCoV UU47). The tree was constructed using a canine coronavirus sequence as an outgroup (GQ477367). Numbers on the nodes indicate the bootstrap support from 1,000 replications. Only bootstrap values >50 are shown. The scale bar represents the number of substitutions per nucleotide. The numbers from 1 to 15 identify each cat.

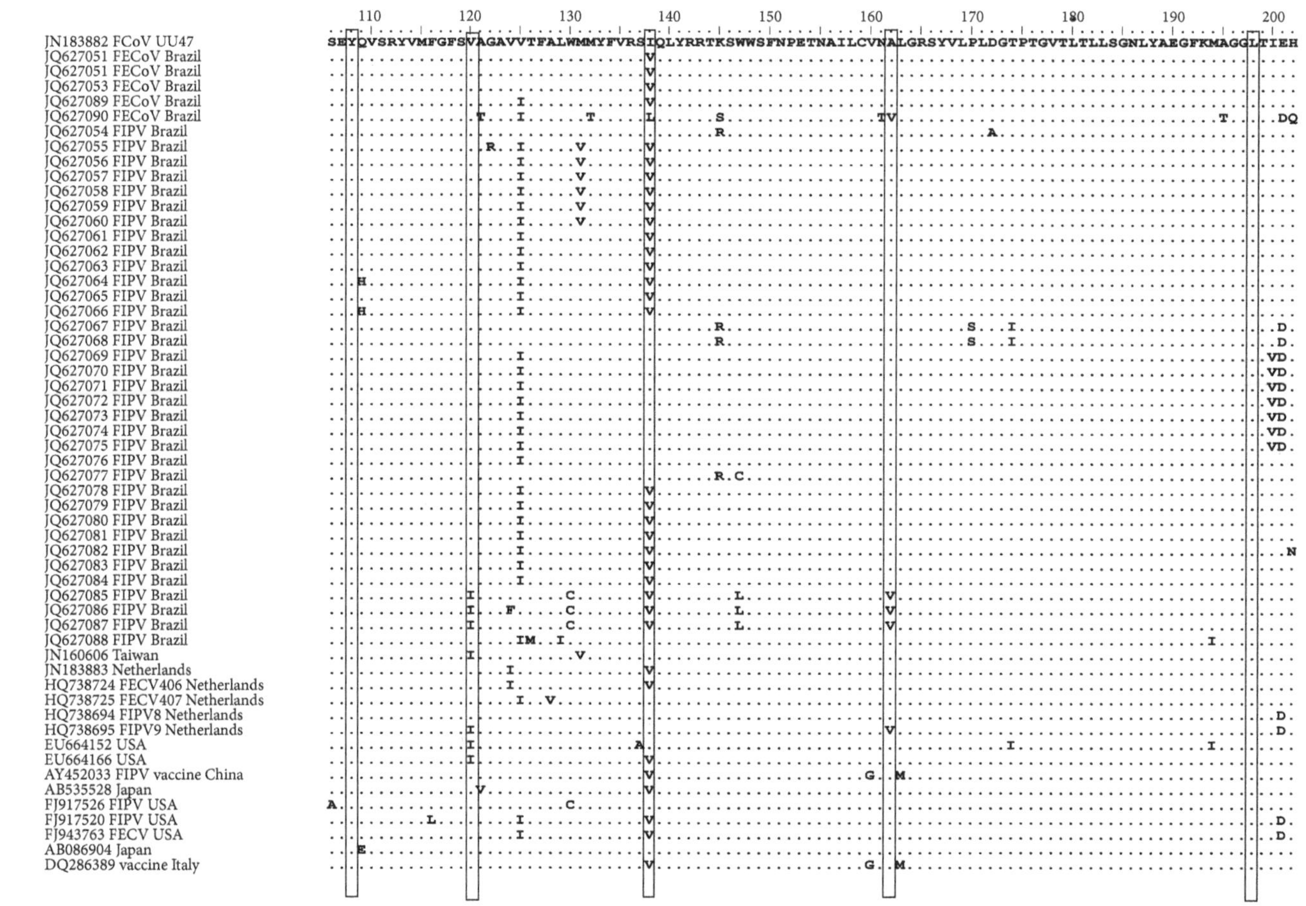

FIGURE 2: Alignment of the amino acid sequences of partial M proteins of the FCoVs compared with the feline coronavirus reference sequence (GenBank accession number JN183882) and other FCoV sequences from GenBank. The 5 aa residues at positions 108, 120, 138, 162, and 198 suggested as potential diagnostic sites [5] are boxed.

pathogenesis of the disease based on the M gene phylogeny from FCoV strains detected in naturally infected cats.

A phylogenetic analysis showed that nucleotide sequences of the FIPV and FECoV M genes do not segregate in a biotypical pattern, a distribution consistent with the in vivo mutation transition hypothesis, which postulates that a de novo virus mutation occurs in vivo, giving rise to highly virulent strains without the need for exogenous highly virulent strains. A similar pattern was observed in a previous study that also examined the M gene [8] which determined that FIPVs originate from FECVs by the accumulation and selection of point mutations [1, 2, 7]. The internal mutation hypothesis has been widely accepted and is mainly supported by the close similarities between FECoV and FIPV and the low incidence of FIP outbreaks, despite the high proportion of FCoV-seropositive cats [6, 15–17].

Although no disease-specific clusters of FCoVs were found, samples from Cat 6 were particularly informative, as two different strains of FCoV, one enteric and one systemic, can be clearly observed in Figure 1, which, in contrast to the other sampled individuals, is in agreement with the two different pathotypes hypothesis. The source for different FCoVs lineages in a cat may be a superinfection [5], but in an experimental study in which cats were infected with two variants of FIPV, a variant prevailed in each cat [7]. Cat 6 might thus have acquired at least two lineages, one with tropism for the intestinal epithelium and the other with a macrophage tropism and a systemic spread that led to the development of the disease.

The full length genomic sequence of the viruses found in two different tissues of a cat with classical FIP, one enteric (jejunum) and one nonenteric (liver), revealed a 100% nucleotide identity [10], a finding that questions the well accepted "internal mutation theory" of FIPV pathogenicity. Nonetheless, it must be taken into account that consensus sequencing, without prior cloning, can mask minority virus populations, and further viral lineages could be present at lower levels within an animal. The M gene mRNA that was detected in the faeces from Cat 6 is a further indication that this cat had two active infections, one systemic and the other enteric.

The current belief is that cats with FIPV do not transmit this pathotype to other cats [2], but it is theoretically possible for cats with an infection in the intestinal wall or kidneys to shed FIPV in the faeces or urine, respectively. The identity among the sequences obtained from the stool or intestines with the sequences of other tissues in cats with FIP in this study was ≥99.9%, indicating that the FIPV pathotype can indeed be spread via faeces and that a cat with FIP can excrete FCoV strains with no distinction between FECoV and FIPV. Accordingly, mutations in the 3c gene identical to the FIPVs from tissues were present in the faeces of some cats, thus making horizontal transmission theoretically possible in certain circumstances [7, 18] and supporting the two-pathotype hypothesis.

A sample of the urinary bladder from a cat (Cat 8) was positive for M gene mRNA; this finding shows that the urinary shedding of FCoV is also plausible. In cats, the infectivity of urine for FCoV has previously been reported [19]. Likewise, human patients with severe acute respiratory syndrome (SARS) caused by the HCoV-SARS coronavirus have been reported to shed the virus via urine and faeces [20, 21]. Furthermore, avian coronavirus also displays faecal excretion and replication in the kidneys of domestic fowl [22]. These reports not only show that FCoV might be shed via the urinary tract but also that this is a conserved feature for coronaviruses.

The phylogenetic analysis has shown that the nucleotide sequences of FCoV generally clustered according to the cattery, irrespective of their pathotypes [9]. In some circumstances, multiple FCoVs lineages can be observed in the same cattery, due to the elevated admission of new individuals in cases of open catteries or shelters [8]. A unique genetic fingerprint was observed in sequences obtained from cats (Cats 1–3) of the same cattery that underwent an outbreak of diarrhoea, indicating that coronavirus infection most likely originated from a single founder virus within this closed group of cats. Catteries and closed multicat environments usually have one major enzootic strain of coronavirus that persists over long periods of time, and these major enzootic strains are dominant even with exposure to other strains [1, 2, 6, 7, 23].

A phylogeographic pattern was not observed among the FCoVs studied herein compared with sequences from other countries, but a pronounced mutational drift (7–10%) was found in strains from the same geographic region, quite similar to the 6–16% reported for cats from distant areas of the western USA [7]. As this is the first report on FCoV diversity in Brazilian cats, further comparisons with other geographic areas within the country are an issue for future research. Recombination and a high mutation rate are common phenomena among coronaviruses, which provide a mechanism for the rapid emergence of new viral strains with dramatically altered tropisms and pathogenicity, which can have a significant impact on the host disease [2, 5–7, 9].

FCoV strains from FIP-positive cats, as determined by a classical pathological or immunohistochemistry diagnosis, have been reported as displaying YIVAL/YIIAL in the M protein (positions 108, 120, 138, 162, and 198) [5], but such markers were absent in all FECoV and FIPV putative M sequences recovered in the present investigation, as previously described [8, 18], which strongly argues against the currently accepted criteria for FIPV/FECoV differentiation.

As both hypotheses have been found as plausible according to these results, this could mean that FIPV can both emerge endogenously and be transmitted to different cats as a "ready" virulent pathotype, which has major implications for the understanding of the dynamics of viral transmission.

Conflict of Interests

The authors declare that they have no conflict of interests.

Acknowledgments

Funding for this study was provided by Fundação de Amparo à Pesquisa do Estado de São Paulo, Brazil (Grants nos. 09/17535-9 and 10/07492-8) and Conselho Nacional de Desenvolvimento Científico e Tecnológico (Grant nos. 300513/2010-0). The authors are also grateful to the veterinarians and cat owners who provided FIP cases and cat faecal samples for this study.

References

[1] A. M. Poland, H. Vennema, J. E. Foley, and N. C. Pedersen, "Two related strains of feline infectious peritonitis virus isolated from immunocompromised cats infected with a feline enteric coronavirus," *Journal of Clinical Microbiology*, vol. 34, no. 12, pp. 3180–3184, 1996.

[2] H. Vennema, A. Poland, J. Foley, and N. C. Pedersen, "Feline infectious peritonitis viruses arise by mutation from endemic feline enteric coronaviruses," *Virology*, vol. 243, no. 1, pp. 150–157, 1998.

[3] A. Kipar, H. May, S. Menger, M. Weber, W. Leukert, and M. Reinacher, "Morphologic features and development of granulomatous vasculitis in feline infectious peritonitis," *Veterinary Pathology*, vol. 42, no. 3, pp. 321–330, 2005.

[4] H. L. Dewerchin, E. Cornelissen, and H. J. Nauwynck, "Replication of feline coronaviruses in peripheral blood monocytes," *Archives of Virology*, vol. 150, no. 12, pp. 2483–2500, 2005.

[5] M. A. Brown, J. L. Troyer, J. Pecon-Slattery, M. E. Roelke, and S. J. O'Brien, "Genetics and pathogenesis of feline infectious peritonitis virus," *Emerging Infectious Diseases*, vol. 15, no. 9, pp. 1445–1452, 2009.

[6] A. A. P. M. Herrewegh, M. Mähler, H. J. Hedrich et al., "Persistence and evolution of feline coronavirus in a closed cat-breeding colony," *Virology*, vol. 234, no. 2, pp. 349–363, 1997.

[7] N. C. Pedersen, H. Liu, K. A. Dodd, and P. A. Pesavento, "Significance of coronavirus mutants in feces and diseased tissues of cats suffering from feline infectious peritonitis," *Viruses*, vol. 1, pp. 166–184, 2009.

[8] H. W. Chang, H. F. Egberink, and P. J. M. Rottier, "Sequence analysis of feline coronaviruses and the circulating virulent/avirulent theory," *Emerging Infectious Diseases*, vol. 17, no. 4, pp. 744–746, 2011.

[9] H. W. Chang, R. J. de Groot, H. F. Egberink, and P. J. M. Rottier, "Feline infectious peritonitis: insights into feline coronavirus pathobiogenesis and epidemiology based on genetic analysis of the viral 3c gene," *Journal of General Virology*, vol. 91, no. 2, pp. 415–420, 2010.

[10] C. Dye and S. G. Siddell, "Genomic RNA sequence of feline coronavirus strain FCoV C1Je," *Journal of Feline Medicine and Surgery*, vol. 9, no. 3, pp. 202–213, 2007.

[11] A. Kipar, M. L. Meli, K. E. Baptiste, L. J. Bowker, and H. Lutz, "Sites of feline coronavirus persistence in healthy cats," *Journal of General Virology*, vol. 91, no. 7, pp. 1698–1707, 2010.

[12] F. A. Simons, H. Vennema, J. E. Rofina et al., "A mRNA PCR for the diagnosis of feline infectious peritonitis," *Journal of Virological Methods*, vol. 124, no. 1-2, pp. 111–116, 2005.

[13] T. A. Hall, "Bioedit: a user-friendly biological sequence alignment editor and analysis program for Windows 95/98/NT," *Nucleic Acids Symposium Series*, vol. 41, pp. 95–98, 1999.

[14] K. Tamura, D. Peterson, N. Peterson, G. Stecher, M. Nei, and S. Kumar, "MEGA5: molecular evolutionary genetics analysis using maximum likelihood, evolutionary distance, and maximum parsimony methods," *Molecular Biology and Evolution*, vol. 28, pp. 2731–2739, 2011.

[15] A. H. Sparkes, T. J. Gruffydd-Jones, and D. A. Harbour, "Feline coronavirus antibodies in UK cats," *Veterinary Record*, vol. 131, no. 10, pp. 223–224, 1992.

[16] A. Pratelli, "Comparison of serologic techniques for the detection of antibodies against feline coronaviruses," *Journal of Veterinary Diagnostic Investigation*, vol. 20, no. 1, pp. 45–50, 2008.

[17] B. S. Holst, L. Englund, S. Palacios, L. Renström, and L. T. Berndtsson, "Prevalence of antibodies against feline coronavirus and *Chlamydophila felis* in Swedish cats," *Journal of Feline Medicine and Surgery*, vol. 8, no. 3, pp. 207–211, 2006.

[18] N. C. Pedersen, H. Liu, J. Scarlett et al., "Feline infectious peritonitis: role of the feline coronavirus 3c gene in intestinal tropism and pathogenicity based upon isolates from resident and adopted shelter cats," *Virus Research*, vol. 165, pp. 17–28, 2012.

[19] W. D. Hardy Jr. and A. I. Hurvitz, "Feline infectious peritonitis: experimental studies," *Journal of the American Veterinary Medical Association*, vol. 158, no. 6, supplement 2, article 994, 1971.

[20] K. H. Chan, L. L. L. M. Poon, V. C. C. Cheng et al., "Detection of SARS coronavirus in patients with suspected SARS," *Emerging Infectious Diseases*, vol. 10, no. 2, pp. 294–299, 2004.

[21] W. C. Yam, K. H. Chan, L. L. M. Poon et al., "Evaluation of reverse transcription-PCR assays for rapid diagnosis of severe acute respiratory syndrome associated with a novel coronavirus," *Journal of Clinical Microbiology*, vol. 41, no. 10, pp. 4521–4524, 2003.

[22] D. Cavanagh, "Coronavirus avian infectious bronchitis virus," *Veterinary Research*, vol. 38, no. 2, pp. 281–297, 2007.

[23] D. D. Addie, I. A. T. Schaap, L. Nicolson, and O. Jarrett, "Persistence and transmission of natural type I feline coronavirus infection," *Journal of General Virology*, vol. 84, no. 10, pp. 2735–2744, 2003.

26

Actinobaculum suis Detection Using Polymerase Chain Reaction

Cristina Román Amigo,[1] Debora Dirani Sena de Gobbi,[1] Vasco Túlio de Moura Gomes,[1] Danilo do Prado Perina,[2] Pedro Henrique Nogueira de Lima Filsner,[1] Barbara Letícia Pereira Costa,[1] Maria Garcia Spindola,[1] Thais Sebastiana Porfida Ferreira,[1] Paulo Eduardo Brandão,[1] and Andrea Micke Moreno[1]

[1] *Departamento de Medicina Veterinária Preventiva e Saúde Animal, Faculdade de Medicina Veterinária e Zootecnia (FMVZ), Universidade de São Paulo (USP), Avenida Professor Dr. Orlando Marques de Paiva 87 Cidade Universitária, 05508 270 São Paulo, SP, Brazil*

[2] *Departamento de Zootecnia, Escola Superior de Agricultura "Luiz de Queiroz" (ESALQ), Universidade de São Paulo (USP), Avenida Pádua Dias 11, Agronomia, 13418-900 Piracicaba, SP, Brazil*

Correspondence should be addressed to Andrea Micke Moreno, morenoam@usp.br

Academic Editors: B. Harrach and M. F. Landoni

Actinobaculum suis is an important agent related to urinary infection in swine females. Due to its fastidious growth characteristics, the isolation of this anaerobic bacterium is difficult, thus impairing the estimation of its prevalence. The purpose of this study was to develop and test a polymerase chain reaction (PCR) for the detection and identification of *A. suis* and then compare these results with traditional isolation methods. Bacterial isolation and PCR were performed on one hundred and ninety-two urine samples from sows and forty-five preputial swabs from boars. The results indicate that this PCR was specific for *A. suis*, presenting a detection limit between 1.0×10^1 CFU/mL and 1.0×10^2 CFU/mL. *A. suis* frequencies, as measured by PCR, were 8.9% (17/192) in sow urine samples and 82.2% (37/45) in preputial swabs. Assessed using conventional culturing techniques, none of the urine samples were positive for *A. suis*; however, *A. suis* was detected in 31.1% (14/45) of the swabs. This PCR technique was shown to be an efficient method for the detection of *A. suis* in urine and preputial swabs.

1. Introduction

Actinobaculum suis is a Gram-positive anaerobic rod bacterium involved in serious forms of urinary infection in gilt swine that result in hematuria, cystitis, and pyelonephritis, which can cause animal death. Sow infection occurs through contact with a contaminated environment or through natural mating with carrier boars. A high number of swine males are colonized by *A. suis* in their preputial diverticula, and this colonization begins in the first weeks of life [1].

Due to its slow fastidious growth, *A. suis* has been difficult to isolate, a fact which may have impaired estimates of its prevalence. Conventional culturing techniques for the identification of anaerobic bacteria can be time-consuming, are not always economically feasible and are beyond the capabilities of some smaller diagnostic laboratories [2]. As an alternative to direct bacterial isolation, indirect immunofluorescence (IF) has been used for *A. suis* detection [3–7]. However, the disadvantages of the IF technique—such as the need for animals for antibody production, the paucity of antibody production laboratories for this agent, and the requirement of specialized equipment and personnel—make polymerase chain reaction (PCR) an affordable and promising alternative tool for the detection of *A. suis*. Although PCR has not been used as a diagnostic method for this bacterium in pigs, this mechanism is already being applied to detect other species of the genus *Actinobaculum* sp. Bank et al. [8] described a PCR technique for the detection of *Actinobaculum schaalii* in human urine and found PCR to be a rapid and reliable method of detection, which contributed to more effective treatment and faster recovery of patients.

The present study aims to develop a PCR strategy for the detection and identification of *A. suis* in pure cultures, urine samples, and preputial swabs; evaluate the PCR specificity and limits of detection; and compare the PCR results with those obtained using direct bacterial isolation techniques.

2. Material and Methods

2.1. Sample Collection. One hundred and ninety-two urine samples from sows and forty-five swabs of preputial diverticula from boars were collected from three swine herds in São Paulo State, Southeastern Brazil. Samples were kept at 4°C until processing.

2.2. Bacteriological Examination. Urine samples (10 mL) were centrifuged at 4,000 ×g for 10 minutes, and the obtained pellet or preputial swabs were spread in 5% sheep blood agar supplemented with colistin sulphate (10 mg/L), nalidixic acid (15 mg/L) and metronidazole (50 mg/L). All antimicrobial powders were obtained from Sigma Chemical (St. Louis, MO, USA.). The plates were incubated in anaerobic conditions at 37°C for 72 hours. The colonies presenting a characteristic dry, greyish-white, flattened, opaque surface, without hemolysis, were submitted for biochemical tests and the PCR described below. Morphology, catalase and urease production, hippurate hydrolysis, nitrate reduction, and the fermentation of glucose, starch, lactose, maltose, and trehalose were all tested.

2.3. DNA Extraction. Purified DNA was recovered according to the Boom et al. [9] protocol for DNA extraction, following previous enzymatic treatment for 60 min at 37°C with 10 μg of lysozyme (USBiological, Swampscott, MA/USA) and 400 μg of proteinase K (LGC Biotecnologia, Cotia, SP/Brazil), and was then stored at −20°C.

2.4. Primer Design. A pair of specific primers for *A. suis* detection was designed using the 16S ribosomal RNA-coding sequence described by Ludwig et al. [10] (GenBank accession number S83623.1), using Primer BLAST (http://www.ncbi.nlm.nih.gov/tools/primer-blast/index.cgi?LINK_LOC=BlastHome).

Putative primers suggested by Primer BLAST and those with lower identity with non-*A. suis* sequences were selected, resulting in the pair Acs-1 and Acs-2 (Table 1) (Tms 59.45 and 60.18°C, resp.; positions 86 to 217 of S83623.1).

2.5. Polymerase Chain Reaction. Multiple PCR conditions were evaluated, and optimum conditions used for all subsequent tests were: 50 μL reaction containing 1.5 mM of $MgCl_2$, 5.0 μL of PCR Buffer, 200 mM dNTP, 20 pmol of each *primer* (Table 1), 1.0 U of *Taq* DNA polymerase (Fermentas Inc., Glen Burnie, Maryland/USA), 5 μL of DNA template, and ultrapure water. PCR was carried out for 35 cycles consisting of denaturation for 1 min at 94°C, annealing for 1 min at 50°C, and extension for 1 min at 72°C.

The amplified products were detected by means of electrophoresis at 80 V in 1.5% agarose gel stained with Blue Green (LGC Biotecnologia, Cotia, São Paulo/Brazil) for 40 min and were photographed under UV transillumination with the ImageMaster Photo Documentation System (GE Healthcare do Brazil Ltda., São Paulo/Brazil). A 100 bp DNA ladder (New England BioLabs Inc., Ipswich, MA/USA) was used for band size determination.

Table 1: Primer design for *A. suis* PCR detection.

Primer	Sequence (5′-3′)	Amplicon size (bp)
Acs1	CGTGGGTAACCTGCCCTCAACTG	133
Acs2	CAAACTGATAGGCCGCGAGCCC	

2.6. Detection Limit. The detection limit of the PCR assay was determined by using a 10-fold serial dilution of known concentrations (1×10^1 to 1×10^{10} CFU/mL) of *A. suis* strain LSSU9/11 in phosphate buffered saline (PBS, LGC Biotecnologia, Cotia, São Paulo/Brazil).

2.7. Analytical Specificity. To determine the analytical specificity of the assay, 14 clinical strains of *A. suis* and the LSSU9/11 strain were tested. Phylogenetically related and clinically relevant bacterial strains, including 22 species described in Table 2, were also tested.

2.8. DNA Sequencing. PCR products obtained from three *A. suis* strains (the LSSU9/11 strain and two preputial strains) were gel-purified using the AxyPrep Gel Extraction Kit (Axygen Biosciences, Union City, CA/USA) and were then sequenced with the Acs-1 and Acs-2 (Table 1) primers using BigDye 3.1 (Applied Biosystems, Foster City, CA, USA) and ABI 3500 XL genetic analyzer (Applied Biosystems, Foster City, CA, USA), according to the manufacturer's instructions. Sequences were then submitted to blastn analysis.

2.9. Statistical Analysis. The agreement between the PCR and isolation results was estimated using the Kappa test [11].

3. Results

PCR using primers specifically designed for *A. suis* showed a detection limit between 1×10^1 CFU/mL and 1×10^2 CFU/mL and generated a 133 bp band. None of the twenty-three strains from different species tested were positive according to PCR, whereas all fourteen *A. suis* strains isolated from urine by culture technique were positive. Sequencing of amplicons obtained from three *A. suis* strains showed a 98% similarity with the sequence of *A. suis* 16S (NR 044760.1) deposited in GenBank and only a 90% similarity when compared with three *Actinobaculum massiliense* isolates.

Among the 237 samples processed, PCR detected 22.8% (54/237) of positives for *A. suis*, while traditional culturing indicated only 5.9% (14/237) of positives (Table 3). From the urine samples, PCR detected *A. suis* in 8.9% (17/192) of the samples, and the isolation procedure did not identify any positive samples. From the preputial swabs, *A. suis* was detected by PCR in 82.2% (37/45) of the samples, and isolated in 31.1% (14/45). The analysis of agreement between

TABLE 2: Bacteria species used to test analytical specificity of PCR for *Actinobaculum suis*.

Species	Source/identification
Actinobaculum suis	Clinical isolates (14)
Actinobacillus pleuropneumoniae	ATCC 27089
Arcanobacterium pyogenes	ATCC 19411
Arcobacter butzleri	ATCC 49616
Arcobacter cryaerophilus	ATCC 43158
Bordetella bronchiceptica	ATCC 4617
Brachyspira hyodysenteriae	ATCC 27164
Brachyspira pilosicoli	ATCC 51139
Campylobacter coli	ATCC 43478
Campylobacter jejuni	ATCC 33292
Clostridium perfringens	ATCC 12922
Erysipelothrix rhusiopathiae	ATCC 19414
Escherichia coli	ATCC 11105
Haemophilus parasuis	Clinical isolate
Klebsiella pneumoniae	ATCC 10031
Listeria monocytogenes	ATCC 7644
Mycoplasma hyopneumoniae	ATCC 25095
Mycoplasma hyorhinis	ATCC 17981
Pasteurella multocida	ATCC 43137
Salmonella typhimurium	ATCC 14028
Staphylococcus aureus	ATCC 25923
Staphylococcus hycus	Clinical isolates
Streptococcus suis	Clinical isolates

TABLE 3: Results of PCR and isolation of *A. suis* from urine and preputial swabs.

Sample	PCR	Isolation	
		Positive	Negative
Urine	Positive	0	17 (8.9%)
	Negative	0	175 (91.1%)
Preputial swab	Positive	14 (31.1%)	23 (51.1%)
	Negative	0	8 (17.8%)

techniques encompassing all samples showed a Kappa value of 0.358, which is considered a weak level of agreement.

4. Discussion

Considering the difficulties involved in isolating bacteria due to the growth features of *A. suis* in veterinary diagnostic laboratories—the need for antimicrobial supplemented media, time-consuming incubation (72 hours), and laborious biochemical tests—the importance and prevalence of this agent in swine herds in Brazil and worldwide are often underestimated, because of the low-sensitivity detection methods currently in use.

To date, there have been no reports on the use of molecular tests for the detection of *A. suis* in swine. Bank et al. [8] described a PCR protocol for the detection of *Actinobaculum shaalii* in human urine samples, using specific primers for the gyrase B (*gyr*B) gene. For the present this study, the primers were designed using the 16S ribosomal RNA sequence deposited in GenBank and described by Ludwig et al. [10], which is a highly conserved gene in bacterial genera, widely used in targeted detection and typing.

The detection limit of the PCR assay described herein was between 10 and 100 CFU/mL, which is compatible with several publications concerning molecular diagnostic tools but inferior to that described by Bank et al. [8], who reported 1.5×10^3 to 1.5×10^4 CFU/mL of *Actinobaculum shaalii* in urine samples using real-time PCR. The evaluation of the analytical specificity using different swine pathogens, including *Arcanobacterium pyogenes*, the phylogenetically closest bacterium to the *Actinobaculum* genus [12], showed no reaction. Sequences from amplicons obtained with these new primers matched *A. suis* sequences. Furthermore, when primers were tested in clinical samples, nonspecific bands were not observed.

Because the aim of the present study was not to evaluate the prevalence of *A. suis* in urine or preputial swabs, but rather to compare the two methodologies tested, a statistically significant sampling was not carried out. Nonetheless, the comparison of the results obtained herein with other *A. suis* frequency reports is key to determining the potential use of PCR in future research involving this bacterium.

Considering the presence of *A. suis* in the urine samples analyzed, it was found that the isolation method did not detect any samples positive for *A. suis* among the 192 samples processed, while PCR detected 8.9%. Reis et al. [13], and Menin et al. [14] isolated the agent from 2.0% (1/60) and 4.0% (37/922) of the cases examined in Brazil. Vaz et al. [6] and Porto et al. [4] reported *A. suis* prevalence rates of 16.8% (17/101) and 31.4% (11/35), respectively, using IF in Brazilian herds. The frequency found in the present study lies within the ranges previously described.

From the preputial swab samples, isolation demonstrated 31.1% (14/45) positivity for *A. suis*, while PCR detected 82.2% positivity (37/45). These values are in accordance with prevalence studies previously conducted in Brazil, which reported rates of 53.8% (21/39) by means of isolation and 78.0% (75/96) by means of IF [5, 15].

Other groups have previously reported the occurrence of *A. suis* in boar preputial swabs around the world. These include Pijoan [16], with a 60.5% (23/38) positivity rate in the United States samples, and Jones and Dagnall [17], who indicated 89.0% (200/224) positivity for *A. suis* in the United Kingdom samples, both using isolation procedures. Sobestiansky et al. [5] reported 67.0% (52/78) positive swabs in Portugal, and 76.0% (16/21) positive swabs in Argentina by means of IF.

In this study, a comparison between the PCR technique developed here and the isolation and IF techniques was not possible. However, the results indicate a higher efficacy for the PCR method compared to isolation, as the number of positives detected by PCR in preputial swabs and urine were comparable to the rates observed using IF. Presently, use of molecular tools is widespread in research and veterinary diagnostic laboratories and is considered accessible and affordable.

The Kappa value of 0.358 indicates a very weak concordance between PCR and isolation methods, indicating that PCR is a very efficient tool for epidemiological and diagnostic studies of *A. suis* infections in swine herds when compared with the traditional isolation method. This is partly due to the ability of PCR to detect specific genome fragments from viable as well as dead bacteria. This result is even more important when considering this agent's previously described growth traits and the absence of nonspecific PCR amplicons for all samples tested.

In conclusion, the PCR developed and tested in this study is a fast and reliable tool for *A. suis* detection, even when the agent is present in small quantities together with other bacteria in its original environment, such as the urinary tract or preputial diverticula.

Ethical Approval

All procedures using animals were approved by the "Ethic Committee in the use of animals" of the School of Veterinary Medicine and Animal Science of University of São Paulo (Protocol no. 2412/2011).

Conflict of Interests

None of the authors of this paper has a financial or personal relationship with other people or organizations that could inappropriately influence or bias the content of the paper.

Acknowledgment

This study was supported by CAPES—Coordenação de Aperfeiçoamento de Pessoal de Nível Superior.

References

[1] D. J. Taylor, "Miscellaneous bacterial infections (*Actinobaculum suis*)," in *Diseases of Swine*, B. E. Straw, J. J. Zimmerman, S. D'Allaire, and D. J. Taylor, Eds., pp. 837–839, Iowa State University Press, Ames, Iowa, USA, 9th edition, 2006.

[2] R. L. Walker, R. T. Greene, and T. M. Gerig, "Evaluation of four commercial anaerobic systems for identification of *Eubacterium suis*," *Journal of Veterinary Diagnostic Investigation*, vol. 2, no. 4, pp. 318–322, 1990.

[3] N. Langfeldt, M. Wendt, and G. Amtsberg, "Vergleichende Untersuchungen zum Nachweis von *Corynebacterium suis*—Infektion beim Schwein mit Hilfe der indirekten Imunofluoreszenz und der Kultur," *Berliner und Münchener Tierärztliche Wochenschrift*, vol. 103, pp. 273–276, 1990.

[4] R. N. G. Porto, J. Sobestiansky, M. P. C. Matos, and M. L. Gambarini, "Aspectos físico, químicos e microbiológicos da urina de matrizes suínas descartadas," *Ciência Rural*, vol. 33, no. 2, pp. 319–324, 2003.

[5] J. Sobestiansky, M. Wendt, R. Perestrelo, and A. Ambrogi, "Studies on the prevalence of *Eubacterium suis* in boars on farms in Brazil, Portugal and Argentina by indirect immunofluorescence technique," *Deutsche Tierarztliche Wochenschrift*, vol. 100, no. 12, pp. 463–464, 1993.

[6] E. K. Vaz, J. Sobestiansky, S. M. Brum, E. C. Zago, and M. E. V. Tonnemann, "Ocorrência de *Actinomyces suis* em fêmeas em produção provenientes de granjas com transtornos reprodutivos localizadas no planalto catarinense—Santa Catarina," *Ciência Rural*, vol. 27, no. 3, pp. 447–449, 1997.

[7] M. Wendt and C. Vesper, "Occurrence of *Eubacterium suis* in breeding herds," in *Proceedings of 12th International Pig Veterinary Society Congress*, p. 349, Deen Haag, The Netherlands, 1992.

[8] S. Bank, A. Jensen, T. M. Hansen, K. M. Søby, and J. Prag, "*Actinobaculum schaalii*, a common uropathogen in elderly patients, Denmark," *Emerging Infectious Diseases*, vol. 16, no. 1, pp. 76–80, 2010.

[9] R. Boom, C. J. A. Sol, M. M. M. Salimans, C. L. Jansen, P. M. E. Wertheim-van Dillen, and J. van der Noordaa, "Rapid and simple method for purification of nucleic acids," *Journal of Clinical Microbiology*, vol. 28, no. 3, pp. 495–503, 1990.

[10] W. Ludwig, G. Kirchhof, M. Weizenegger, and N. Weiss, "Phylogenetic evidence for the transfer of *Eubacterium suis* to the genus *Actinomyces* as *Actinomyces suis* comb. nov.," *International Journal of Systematic Bacteriology*, vol. 42, no. 1, pp. 161–165, 1992.

[11] R. D. Smith, *Veterinary Clinical Epidemiology*, CRC Press, London, UK, 1995.

[12] P. A. Lawson, E. Falsen, E. Åkervall, P. Vandamme, and M. D. Collins, "Characterization of some *Actinomyces*-like isolates from human clinical specimens: reclassification of *Actinomyces suis* (Soltys and Spratling) as *Actinobaculum suis* comb. nov. and description of *Actinobaculum schaalii* sp. nov.," *International Journal of Systematic Bacteriology*, vol. 47, no. 3, pp. 899–903, 1997.

[13] R. Reis, M. Nakajima, E. F. Nascimento, I. B. F. Ferraz, and R. C. Leite, "Infecções urinárias em porcas," *Arquivo Brasileiro de Medicina Veterinária e Zootecnia*, vol. 44, no. 5, pp. 363–376, 1992.

[14] A. Menin, C. Reck, J. C. Capelli, S. M. Ferraz, and E. K. Vaz, "Diagnóstico de infecção urinária em fêmeas suínas produtivas em granjas comerciais no sul do Brasil," *Ciência Animal Brasileira*, vol. 9, no. 1, pp. 199–206, 2008.

[15] S. J. Oliveira, D. E. S. N. Barcellos, and S. M. Borowky, "Urinary tract infections in two pig breeding herds, with emphasis on the presence of *Corynebacterium suis*," in *Proceedings of 10th International Pig Veterinary Society Congress*, p. 304, Rio de Janeiro, Brazil, 1988.

[16] C. Pijoan, A. Lastra, and A. Leman, "Isolation of *Corynebacterium suis* from the prepuce of boars," *Journal of the American Veterinary Medical Association*, vol. 183, no. 4, pp. 428–429, 1983.

[17] J. E. T. Jones and G. J. R. Dagnall, "The carriage of *Corynebacterium suis* in male pigs," *The Journal of Hygiene*, vol. 93, no. 2, pp. 381–388, 1984.

Effects of Electrical Stimulation on Meat Quality of Lamb and Goat Meat

Omer Cetin,[1] Enver Baris Bingol,[1] Hilal Colak,[1] and Hamparsun Hampikyan[2]

[1] *Department of Food Hygiene and Technology, Faculty of Veterinary Medicine, Istanbul University, Avcilar, 34320 Istanbul, Turkey*
[2] *The School of Vocational Studies, Beykent University, Buyukcekmece, 34500 Istanbul, Turkey*

Correspondence should be addressed to Enver Baris Bingol, bingolb@istanbul.edu.tr

Academic Editors: P. O. Hasselgren and G. Leitner

Effect of various voltage of electrical stimulation (ES) on meat quality of lamb and goat was investigated by using a total of 36 animals at 3–5 years old. Constant 50 Hz frequency and 50, 100, and 250 V, 90 sec of ES were administered to 1/2 carcasses and were examined according their textural, physicochemical, and sensorial characteristics. ES decreased the pH values of lamb and goat meat, and accelerated the rigor mortis ($P < 0.05$). Additionally, ES enhanced the water activity, water-holding capacity, and drip loss of both animals. Shear force varied between lamb and goat meat, and tenderness was improved depending on voltage range used ($P < 0.001$). ES caused difference in instrumental colour (CIE L^*, a^*, b^*) values of lamb and goat meat compared with the control groups ($P < 0.05$) during aging period at 4°C. Sensorial characteristics were also improved with various levels of ES treatments. In conclusion, ES had positive effects on meat quality of lamb and goat, in contrast to undesirable consumer preferences.

1. Introduction

Organoleptical properties such as colour, texture, and flavour are important criterions determining the meat quality. These properties are related to age, gender, race, nutrition, nursing, anatomical, and technological characteristics [1, 2].

Electrical stimulation (ES) is an innovation being used in the meat industry to increase meat tenderness and colour of beef, lamb, and goat carcasses [3–5]. ES is a procedure that depends on electric current passing through hot carcass immediately after slaughtering [6]. Passing of voltage lower than 100 volts is known as low-voltage electrical stimulation (LVES) and treatments with higher than 100 volts as high-voltage electrical stimulation (HVES). Although increase in efficacy is reported with increase in voltage, it is risky for workers to stimulate with high voltage. Nowadays, high-voltage electrical stimulation studies are limited [2, 7]. The electric current flowing through the muscle tissue causes pH decline by increasing postmortem glycolysis. It also partially decreases the microbial total count of the carcasses by preventing cold shortening and improving some quality parameters such as colour, tenderness, and flavour [2, 3, 8].

Sheep and goat meat are important sources of protein in our country as in the world [9–11]. Approximately 159,000 tons of the total red meat production of slaughtered animals (780,718 tons) in 2010 was obtained from small ruminants. According to this, about 20% of the total production in 2010 was produced from sheep and goat meat [12].

Goat meat is tough as it contains less fat, so it is not generally preferred by consumers. Sheep meat is more tender than goat's meat; however, with the age of the sheep, a typical mutton flavour decreases its preferences by consumers [9, 11]. There are various applications to avoid the limiting properties of goat's and sheep's meat; in our days, low- and high-voltage ES applications become an ideal application area to minimize these negative effects of both meats [3, 5, 13].

This study was conducted to investigate the effects of various voltage of electrical stimulation on meat quality of lamb and goat meat.

2. Materials and Methods

2.1. Materials. A total of 18 Kivircik breed lambs and 18 Malta goats between 3 and 5 years old, which are at the same age period, same breed, and are subjected to the same feeding process, were processed by the approval of the Ethic Committee of the Istanbul University, Turkey (approval number: 58/26.05.2011).

2.2. Preslaughter and Slaughtering Process. Animals were transported to the slaughterhouse from farm one day before the slaughter and were held in different shelters. During this period, they were provided with *ad libitum* water and kept without feed for 24 h before slaughter. After the rest period, animals were put through health detection and sent for slaughter without any stress.

The animals were stunned applying 220–250 V, 1.0–1.3 A, and 1–3 seconds of electroshock and then slaughtered by Halal method. Following exsanguinations, dressing, and evisceration processes, the carcasses were halved by splitting along the vertebral column approximately in 30–45 min postslaughter period, and one side of the carcasses was kept for ES treatment.

Both animal groups (lamb and goat) were divided into three subgroups according to ES. Half-carcasses were stimulated with 17 impulses (1.8 s duration each, with a 1.8 s interval between pulses) constant voltage (AC) at 2.5 amps, and 50 Hz. Half-carcasses in the first group were stimulated with low voltage (LVES; 50 V, 50 Hz for 90 s), the second ones were stimulated with medium voltage (MVES; 100 V, 50 Hz for 90 s), and the third ones were stimulated with high voltage (HVES; 250 V, 50 Hz for 90 s). ES was applied to the right sides of each carcass, and the corresponding left carcasses were used as controls (no electrical stimulation, NES). After electrical stimulation, all the half-carcasses were maintained at 0–4°C air flow 1–1.5 ms^{-2}.

2.3. Sampling and Measurements. During the first 24 hours, carcasses were held at the cold chain (4°C) and at the end of the first day; samples were taken from the back (*M. longissimus dorsi*, LD) muscles of splitted carcasses and were examined according their textural (Warner-Bratzler shear force), physicochemical (instrumental colour, pH, water holding capacity (WHC), water activity (a_w), and drip loss (DL)), and sensorial characteristics (colour, odour, appearance, and tenderness).

2.4. Determination of pH. At 1, 3, 6, and 24 h of postmortem, pH of meat samples was measured using a portable pH meter (WTW pH 340i with a probe SenTix, Weilheim, Germany). The mean of three measures in each sample was evaluated as pH value [14].

2.5. Determination of Water Activity (a_w). Water activity measurement was carried out using a water activity device (Hygrometer-Lufft, Fellbach, Germany). A 20 g of meat sample was placed in the cup of the instrument, and at the end of 3 h, values were recorded. The meter was calibrated using the manufacturer's standards. All water activity measurements were performed at room temperature (25 ± 2°C) [14].

2.6. Determination of Drip Loss (DL). Following the slaughter, the carcasses were weighed as a whole on the 0, 1, 3, and 7 days, while they were kept in the fridge at 4°C. Thereby, the drip loss was evaluated by subtracting the values from the previous day's values using a digital scale [15].

2.7. Determination of Water-Holding Capacity (WHC). To measure the water-holding capacity, 300 mg meat samples were collected from control and treated sides of the carcasses on the 1, 3, and 7 days of the postmortem phase and placed on Whatman no. 1 filter paper. The samples were kept between glass slips and under a fixed weight of 1 kg for 20 minutes. At the end of the waiting period, the filter paper was taken. The impressions released by the water were measured using millimetric paper and calculated by appropriate formulas [16],

$$\text{Water holding capacity} = \frac{\text{Range of dispersion } (\text{cm}^2)}{\text{total area } (\text{cm}^2)}. \quad (1)$$

2.8. Instrumental Colour Measurement. The surface colour of meat samples at five different locations on each muscle and averages were determined at each sampling day in terms of L^* (lightness), a^* (redness), and b^* (yellowness) values using colour difference meter [17]. Samples were placed in a special cup, which fitted well with the sample port of the colorimeter, to protect it from the interference of outside light. The colour of each sample was measured using a Colorflex HunterLab Spectrophotometer (Hunter Associates Laboratory Inc., Reston, VA, USA). Colour was evaluated using a diffuse illumination (D65 2° observer) with 8 mm viewing aperture and a 25 mm port size with the specular component excluded.

2.9. Instrumental Texture Measurement. Warner-Bratzler shear force values were determined from *M. longissimus dorsi* on the 1, 3, and 7 days of stored meat under refrigerated conditions by using Instron Texture Analyzer model 3343 device (USA) equipped with a Warner-Bratzler shear force system [18]. Shear force was perpendicular to the length of the 2 cm thick chops stakes which were parallel to the muscle fibre orientations, and force required to shear was recorded in kilograms. For each sample, eight to ten replicates were made, and a mean value was calculated for using in statistical analysis.

2.10. Sensory Evaluation. Eight semitrained panelists, staff of Istanbul University, Food Hygiene and Technology Department, who had previously participated in training sessions to become familiar with the sensory characteristics of meat [19, 20] were requested to score the sensory attributes (red-colour, animal odour intensity, tenderness, and general appearance acceptability) on the basis of nine-point hedonic rating scales. The scales included 1 = extremely unacceptable, 2 = very much unacceptable, 3 = moderately unacceptable, 4 = slightly unacceptable, 5 = between acceptable and unacceptable, 6 = slightly acceptable, 7 = moderately acceptable, 8 = very much acceptable, and 9 = extremely acceptable [21]. The panelists were trained in two separate sessions approximately 2 hours for the evaluation of selected attributes. Training sessions were conducted to acquaint panelists with the products and attributes to be evaluated and were followed by an open-discussion session to familiarise panelists with the attributes and the scale to be used.

Samples chosen for sensory analyses were served to the panel members, who were seated in individual booths in a temperature-controlled and light-controlled room (fluorescent lighting of 2000 lx; Philips 40 W Cool White), receiving a set of 8 samples served in a complete randomised order. Each sample was labelled, at random, with a two-digit code number [22]. Sensory panel was carried out triplicate in two sessions.

2.11. Statistical Analyses. The general linear model procedure (PROC GLM) of SPSS 13.0 program was used in the statistical analyzes of electrically stimulated lamb and goat meat [23]. Least squares procedures were used to analyze data for pH, water activity, WHC, drip loss, surface colour (CIE L^*, a^*, b^* values), shear force, and sensory characteristics. The model used in the analyses of these characteristics included the fixed effects of ES and aging period. Significance of differences was defined as $P < 0.05$, and paired Student t-tests were used for comparison of the means in both animals.

3. Results and Discussion

The pH values obtained from carcass halves through the measurements at the 1, 3, 6, and 24 h are given in Table 1. In all groups treated with various levels of voltage, a considerable pH decrease relating the control group was observed in lamb and goat carcasses, and difference among the results of the groups was found statistically significant ($P < 0.05$).

According to these results, it was found that the pH values obtained from electrically stimulated lamb carcasses were lower than the goat ones, but not significantly different during the whole aging period (Table 6).

Similarly, it is reported in many studies that electrical stimulation accelerates the ATP and glycogen break down and causes a rapid pH decrease [3, 4, 9]. Kahraman and Ergun [4] stated that the pH values in *longissimus dorsi* muscle of lamb carcasses showed a significant correlation ($P < 0.05$) between ES and NES groups, but no significant differences were recorded between LVES (50 V, 100 Hz for 120 s) and MVES (100 V, 100 Hz for 120 s) treated lambs ($P > 0.05$). Ferguson et al. [8] determined that ES (300 V, 20 min) caused a significant difference in pH decline of electrically stimulated Merinos breed sheep. Similar results in pH have been reported by Polidori et al. [5] and Morton et al. [24] in lamb carcasses. Cetin and Topcu [9] reported also that the pH values of electrically stimulated goat carcasses were lower than the ones from the nonstimulated ones. Additionally, Biswas et al. [3] emphasized that significant improvement was observed on goat carcasses which were electrically stimulated with different voltages (35, 110, 330, 550, and 1100) and 50 Hz frequency. These results suggested that the ES treatment caused an acceleration of glycolysis and subsequent early rigor mortis development.

Water activity was enhanced with the range of voltage used and was higher than the control groups of both animal species (Table 2). The a_w value was decreased during the aging period depending on the ES used and was significantly different ($P < 0.05$) in lamb and goat meat (Table 6). Cetin and Topcu [9] also remarked that water activity values of electrically stimulated goat meat were higher than the control ones; however, any significant difference ($P > 0.05$) was observed between the control and the ES-treated lamb carcasses in a study conducted by Kahraman [25].

Water-holding capacity increased with the range of voltage used for ES (Table 3). The WHC values decreased with the aging period and differed in lamb and goat meat (Table 6). The effect of ES on water-holding capacity and protein denaturation is dependent on the muscle considered [16]. The number of components that bind water change postmortem with the loss of ATP drops in pH, proteolysis, and protein denaturation [15]. Kahraman and Ergun [4] determined that WHC was significantly greater for stimulated lamb carcasses ($P < 0.05$) and revealed that MVES (100 V, 100 Hz for 120 s) was more effective than LVES (50 V, 100 Hz for 120 s) only at 1 day of postslaughter period ($P < 0.05$). The authors indicated also that these results supported the theory that ES significantly increased drip loss. Cetin and Topcu [9] stated that WHC values of ES-treated goat decreased in aging period but were not significantly different to control ones. Similarly, Strydom et al. [26] determined that ES-treated (400 V) Cholaris breed lamb showed lower WHC than control group although no significant difference was observed. Contrary to these, Biswas et al. [3] reported that electrically stimulated Bengal goats showed significant differences ($P < 0.05$) with respect to water-holding capacity.

It has been observed that drip loss was enhanced with the range of voltage used and was higher than the control groups (Table 4). DL increased during the aging period depending on ES used and was significantly different ($P < 0.05$) in lamb and goat meat (Table 6). Cetin and Topcu [9] indicated that drip loss amount obtained from the ES-treated goat carcasses was greater and significantly different ($P < 0.01$) than control group. However, Bond et al. [27] stated that ES did not change the drip loss of 200 V applied sheep. Drip loss is formed over time as the meat is tenderised. When proteins degrade at postmortem, they release the binding water in muscles. ES ensures early rigor, protects the enzymes that tenderise meat, and promotes the protein degradation by resulting in increase in the drip loss [15, 16].

An evident improvement of shear force compared with control groups was observed in ES-treated lamb and goat meat, and difference between the results relating the animal groups was found important ($P < 0.001$) during aging period (Table 5). Shear force of meat varied between lamb and goat, and lamb meat was defined more tender than goat one (Table 6). The improved tenderness associated with ES has been attributed to the prevention of cold shortening, increased proteolysis, and physical disruption of muscle fibers [10].

Table 1: Mean and standard errors of pH values in lamb and goat meat during aging at 4°C.

Group	n	Lamb				Goat			
		1 h	3 h	6 h	24 h	1 h	3 h	6 h	24 h
Control (NES)	18	6.54 ± 0.032^{a}	6.47 ± 0.013^{a}	6.44 ± 0.052^{a}	6.19 ± 0.022^{a}	6.68 ± 0.49^{a}	6.59 ± 0.55^{a}	6.58 ± 0.51^{a}	6.32 ± 0.40^{a}
50 volt (LVES)	6	6.46 ± 0.023^{b}	6.36 ± 0.042^{b}	6.25 ± 0.033^{b}	6.08 ± 0.032^{b}	6.58 ± 0.21^{b}	6.48 ± 0.17^{b}	6.39 ± 0.39^{b}	5.79 ± 0.61^{b}
100 volt (MVES)	6	6.38 ± 0.023^{b}	6.20 ± 0.042^{c}	6.08 ± 0.033^{c}	5.98 ± 0.032^{b}	6.54 ± 0.21^{b}	6.41 ± 0.17^{b}	6.29 ± 0.39^{b}	5.72 ± 0.61^{b}
250 volt (HVES)	6	6.22 ± 0.023^{c}	5.94 ± 0.042^{d}	5.79 ± 0.033^{d}	5.60 ± 0.032^{b}	6.49 ± 0.21^{c}	6.23 ± 0.17^{c}	5.98 ± 0.39^{c}	5.68 ± 0.61^{b}
P	36	*	***	***	***	**	**	***	***

^{a,b}Values in column with different superscripts differ significantly ($P < 0.05$), (*): $P < 0.05$, (**): $P < 0.01$, (***): $P < 0.001$, (NS): not significant ($P > 0.05$).

Table 2: Mean and standard errors of water activity (a_w) values in lamb and goat meat during aging at 4°C.

Group	n	Lamb			Goat		
		Day 1	Day 3	Day 7	Day 1	Day 3	Day 7
Control (NES)	18	9.60 ± 0.052^{c}	9.58 ± 0.044^{b}	9.55 ± 0.014^{b}	9.63 ± 0.027^{b}	9.60 ± 0.024^{b}	9.58 ± 0.044
50 volt (LVES)	6	9.72 ± 0.035^{b}	9.69 ± 0.061^{ab}	9.64 ± 0.022^{a}	9.75 ± 0.055^{ab}	9.71 ± 0.035^{ab}	9.69 ± 0.056
100 volt (MVES)	6	9.75 ± 0.035^{b}	9.73 ± 0.061^{a}	9.67 ± 0.022^{a}	9.79 ± 0.055^{a}	9.75 ± 0.035^{a}	9.71 ± 0.056
250 volt (HVES)	6	9.79 ± 0.035^{a}	9.71 ± 0.061^{a}	9.64 ± 0.022^{a}	9.81 ± 0.055^{a}	9.77 ± 0.035^{a}	9.72 ± 0.056
P	36	**	*	*	*	*	NS

^{a,b}Values in column with different superscripts differ significantly ($P < 0.05$), (*): $P < 0.05$, (**): $P < 0.01$, (***): $P < 0.001$, (NS): not significant ($P > 0.05$).

Table 3: Mean and standard errors of water-holding capacity (WHC) values in lamb and goat meat during aging at 4°C (%).

Group	n	Lamb			Goat		
		Day 1	Day 3	Day 7	Day 1	Day 3	Day 7
Control (NES)	18	3.50 ± 0.057^{c}	3.36 ± 0.214	2.81 ± 0.055^{d}	3.62 ± 0.137	3.41 ± 0.250	2.90 ± 0.112^{a}
50 volt (LVES)	6	3.57 ± 0.031^{b}	3.25 ± 0.315	2.94 ± 0.082^{c}	3.77 ± 0.243	3.48 ± 0.321	3.10 ± 0.210^{b}
100 volt (MVES)	6	3.74 ± 0.031^{a}	3.34 ± 0.315	3.08 ± 0.082^{b}	3.89 ± 0.243	3.58 ± 0.321	3.16 ± 0.210^{b}
250 volt (HVES)	6	3.88 ± 0.031^{d}	3.51 ± 0.315	3.21 ± 0.082^{a}	3.98 ± 0.243	3.67 ± 0.321	3.32 ± 0.210^{c}
P	36	*	NS	**	NS	NS	*

^{a,b}Values in column with different superscripts differ significantly ($P < 0.05$), (*): $P < 0.05$, (**): $P < 0.01$, (***): $P < 0.001$, (NS): not significant ($P > 0.05$).

Table 4: Mean and standard errors of drip loss (DL) values in lamb and goat meat during aging at 4°C (%).

Group	n	Lamb			Goat		
		Day 1	Day 3	Day 7	Day 1	Day 3	Day 7
Control (NES)	18	4.02 ± 0.054^{c}	4.53 ± 0.041^{b}	5.94 ± 0.108^{c}	3.81 ± 0.104^{c}	4.25 ± 0.413^{b}	5.62 ± 0.180^{c}
50 volt (LVES)	6	5.55 ± 0.033^{b}	6.22 ± 0.024^{ab}	6.72 ± 0.081^{bc}	5.02 ± 0.227^{b}	5.81 ± 0.234^{ab}	6.50 ± 0.381^{bc}
100 volt (MVES)	6	5.78 ± 0.033^{b}	6.44 ± 0.024^{a}	7.98 ± 0.081^{b}	5.33 ± 0.227^{b}	6.14 ± 0.234^{a}	7.84 ± 0.381^{b}
250 volt (HVES)	6	5.97 ± 0.033^{a}	6.69 ± 0.024^{a}	8.45 ± 0.081^{a}	5.76 ± 0.227^{a}	6.23 ± 0.234^{a}	8.31 ± 0.381^{a}
P	36	***	**	***	***	**	***

^{a,b}Values in column with different superscripts differ significantly ($P < 0.05$), (*): $P < 0.05$, (**): $P < 0.01$, (***): $P < 0.001$, (NS): not significant ($P > 0.05$).

Table 5: Mean and standard errors of shear force values in lamb and goat meat during aging at 4°C (kg/cm^2).

Group	n	Lamb			Goat		
		Day 1	Day 3	Day 7	Day 1	Day 3	Day 7
Control (NES)	18	14.62 ± 0.094^{a}	11.65 ± 0.112^{a}	10.64 ± 0.085^{a}	15.23 ± 0.29^{a}	12.46 ± 0.25^{a}	11.56 ± 0.31^{a}
50 volt (LVES)	6	13.71 ± 0.121^{b}	10.57 ± 0.071^{b}	9.44 ± 0.046^{b}	14.43 ± 0.21^{b}	11.39 ± 0.17^{b}	10.73 ± 0.56^{b}
100 volt (MVES)	6	11.88 ± 0.121^{c}	9.49 ± 0.071^{c}	8.76 ± 0.046^{c}	12.18 ± 0.21^{c}	10.54 ± 0.17^{b}	9.64 ± 0.56^{c}
250 volt (HVES)	6	10.56 ± 0.121^{d}	8.73 ± 0.071^{d}	8.11 ± 0.046^{c}	11.06 ± 0.21^{c}	9.12 ± 0.17^{c}	8.58 ± 0.56^{d}
P	36	***	***	***	***	***	***

^{a,b}Values in column with different superscripts differ significantly ($P < 0.05$), (*): $P < 0.05$, (**): $P < 0.01$, (***): $P < 0.001$, (NS): not significant ($P > 0.05$).

TABLE 6: Functional parameters variation in lamb and goat meat during aging at 4°C.

Parameters	Storage time	Meat type	Mean	Std. error	P value
pH	1 h	Lamb	6.400	0.068	0.061
		Goat	6.573	0.040	
	3 h	Lamb	6.243^b	0.115	0.006
		Goat	6.428^a	0.076	
	6 h	Lamb	6.140^b	0.138	0.005
		Goat	6.310^a	0.125	
	24 h	Lamb	5.963	0.128	0.307
		Goat	5.878	0.149	
Shear force	Day 1	Lamb	12.693^b	0.911	0.003
		Goat	13.225^a	0.968	
	Day 3	Lamb	10.110^b	0.637	0.016
		Goat	10.878^a	0.705	
	Day 7	Lamb	9.238^b	0.541	
		Goat	10.128^a	0.649	0.023
WHC	Day 1	Lamb	3.673^b	0.086	0.031
		Goat	3.815^a	0.078	
	Day 3	Lamb	3.365	0.054	0.311
		Goat	3.535	0.057	
	Day 7	Lamb	3.010^b	0.087	0.021
		Goat	3.120^a	0.087	
a_w	Day 1	Lamb	9.715^b	0.041	0.005
		Goat	9.745^a	0.040	
	Day 3	Lamb	9.678^b	0.034	0.032
		Goat	9.708^a	0.038	
	Day 7	Lamb	9.625^b	0.026	0.046
		Goat	9.675^a	0.032	
Drip loss	Day 1	Lamb	5.330^a	0.445	0.016
		Goat	4.980^b	0.418	
	Day 3	Lamb	5.970^a	0.490	0.002
		Goat	5.608^b	0.461	
	Day 7	Lamb	7.273^a	0.575	0.000
		Goat	7.068^b	0.616	
Lightness (L^*)	Day 1	Lamb	51.778^a	1.420	0.033
		Goat	35.565^b	0.817	
	Day 3	Lamb	49.570^a	1.191	0.026
		Goat	36.653^b	1.053	
	Day 7	Lamb	47.498^a	0.903	0.026
		Goat	37.943^b	1.402	
Redness (a^*)	Day 1	Lamb	14.143^a	0.394	0.025
		Goat	14.073^b	0.726	
	Day 3	Lamb	12.938^b	0.457	0.029
		Goat	13.085^a	0.635	
	Day 7	Lamb	11.720^b	0.373	0.025
		Goat	12.088^a	0.750	
Yellowness (b^*)	Day 1	Lamb	13.025^b	0.398	0.014
		Goat	15.295^a	0.533	
	Day 3	Lamb	14.133	0.428	0.082
		Goat	16.245	0.426	
	Day 7	Lamb	15.353	0.488	0.137
		Goat	17.253	0.526	

^{a,b}Values in column with different superscripts differ significantly ($P < 0.05$).

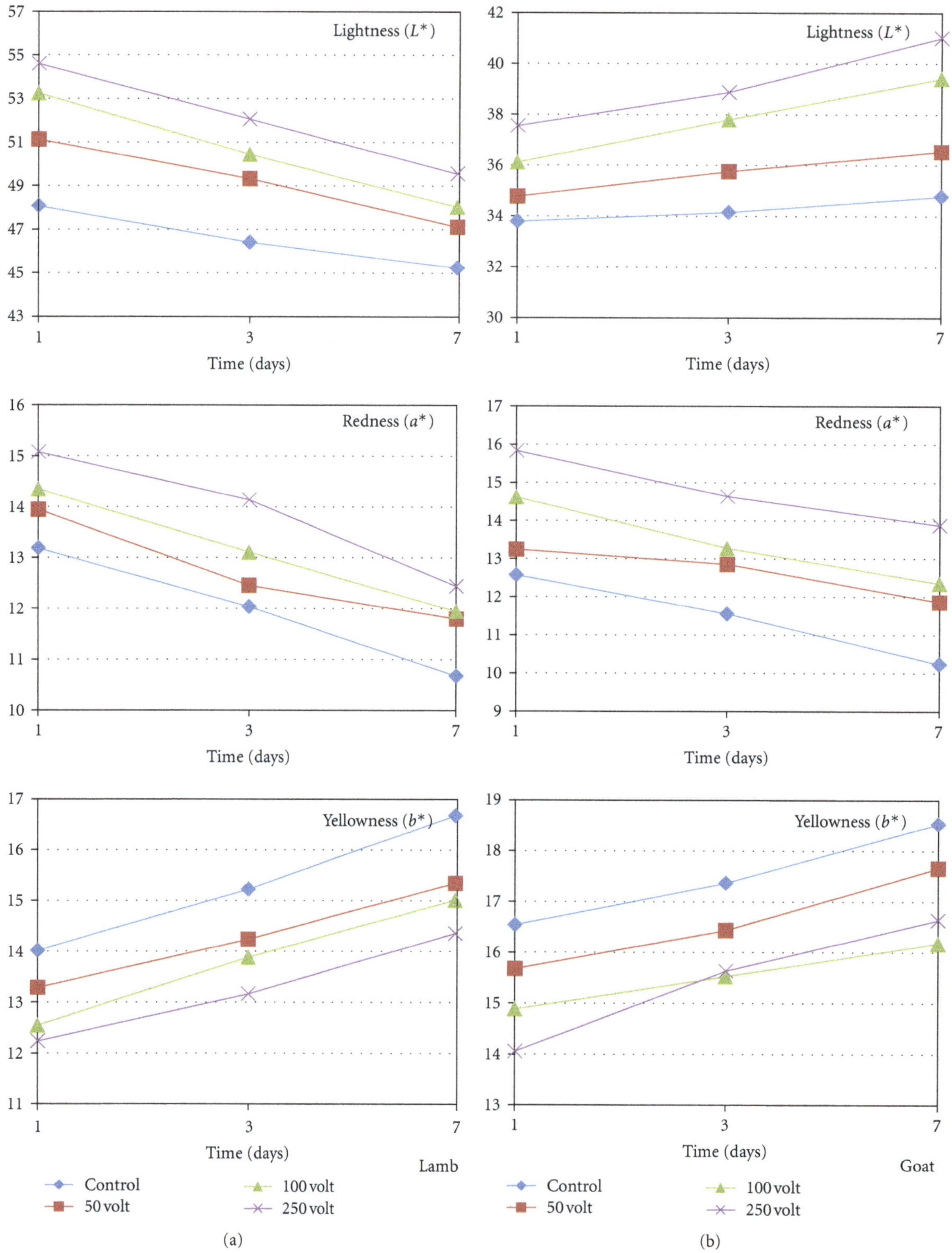

FIGURE 1: Instrumental colour (CIE L^*, a^*, b^*) of lamb and goat meat aging at 4°C.

In similar studies performed on textural properties of small ruminant carcasses, the improving effect of electrical stimulation on tenderness was clearly determined [4, 5, 9, 11, 24, 28, 29]. Kahraman and Ergun [4] stated that ES applied carcasses were more tender than NES at 1 and 7 days of postslaughter period ($P < 0.001$) and added that significant differences were found between LVES and MVES ($P < 0.05$) applied lamb. These findings were in agreement with Morton

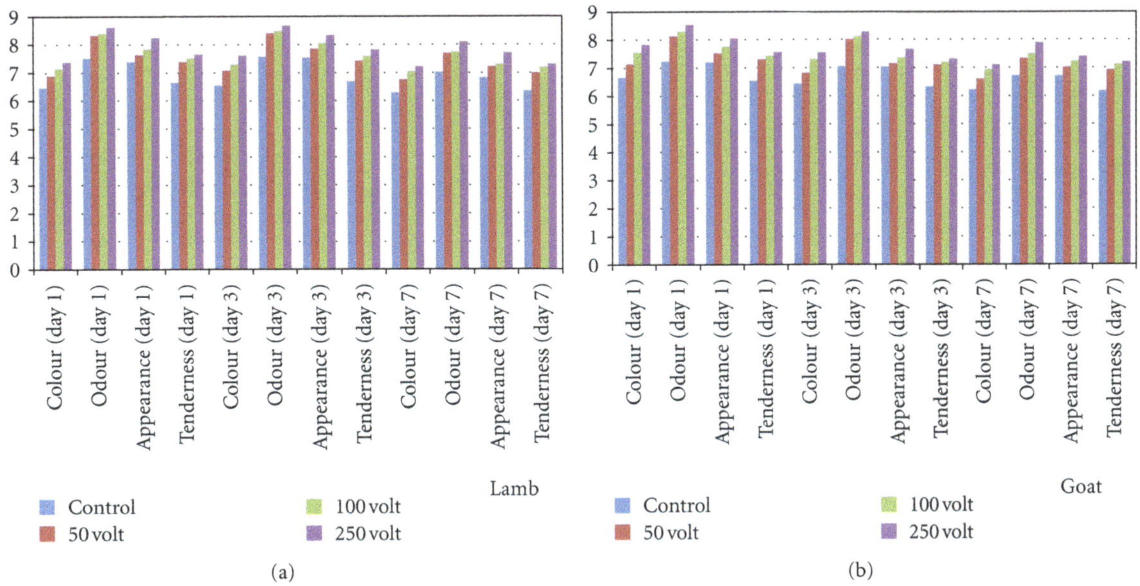

FIGURE 2: Sensory evaluation of lamb and goat meat during aging at 4°C.

et al. [24] in lamb carcasses. Yanar and Yetim [11] reported that 350 volt of electrical stimulation on 14 half-carcasses of 3–5 years old sheep improved the texture of *longissimus dorsi* muscle ($P < 0.01$) and made no considerable effect on the *semimembranosus* muscle. Similarly, Solomon and Lynch [30] emphasized that stimulated *longissimus dorsi* muscle of lamb carcasses had a significantly lower shear force value than nonstimulated one. Cetin and Topcu [9] indicated that shear force values obtained from the electrically stimulated goat carcasses were lower than nonstimulated ones. Polidori et al. [5] reported that ES remarkably affected shear force values of lamb carcasses and improved tenderness. Geesink et al. [29] notified that 1130 V of electrical stimulation positively affected shear force values of lamb meat. King et al. [10] observed that low-voltage ES was not effective on tenderness improvement in Cabrito carcasses but underlined that high-voltage ES was effective on tenderness at 1–3 days of postmortem. Additionally, Devine et al. [28] stated that electrically stimulated lambs were always more tender than nonstimulated lambs.

Various voltage treatments caused difference in instrumental colour values of lamb and goat meat compared with the control groups (Figure 1). The difference between the results of the animal groups has been significant during aging period at 4°C for L^*, a^*, and b^* values, but not significant for b^* values when compared with one another (Table 6). Lightness (L^*) and redness (a^*) increased with ES treatment, while a remarkable decrease was observed in yellowness (b^*) of lamb and goat meat compared with controls. Similarly, in an observation of Kerth et al. [6] based on 5 different muscles, ES-treated lamb muscles were brighter with a better red colour than nontreated ones. In another study, 550 V of high-voltage electrical stimulation was applied to Cabrito carcasses, and ES increased a^* and b^* values of carcasses [10]. Kahraman and Ergun [4] explained that the initial colour parameters were not affected by ES ($P > 0.05$), but at the 7th day of aging period, significant differences were found in the redness (a^*) values among the groups ($P < 0.01$). Cetin and Topcu [9] stated also that colour improvement was observed with ES treatment in goat carcasses, while significant differences were obtained ($P < 0.01$) only in L^* value at the 7th day of aging. Opposite to the findings, Gadiyaram et al. [31] determined that ES had no significant effect on colour of castrated goat meat. This may be explained that ES reduces the colour stability, as defined by the rate of metmyoglobin accumulation in the surface layer of meat [32].

Sensorial characteristics were improved with various levels of ES treatments. Significant difference was observed between ES and control groups ($P < 0.05$) during aging at 4°C, and red colour, odour intensity, and tenderness of both meats were particularly enhanced depending on voltage range used (Figure 2). Cetin and Topcu [9] found that sensorial characteristics were improved in the ES groups and were significantly different ($P < 0.01$) in raw samples. Yanar and Yetim [11] investigated that ES remarkably improved ($P < 0.01$) the tenderness of *longissimus dorsi* muscle in sheep meat. Contrary to these, Kerth et al. [6] evaluated that ES had no effect on sensorial characteristics of five different muscles of Hampshire × Rambouillet crossbred lambs ($P > 0.05$) but pointed out that the percentage of loin chops rated slightly tender or better was improved 30 to 34% by electrical stimulation ($P < 0.05$).

4. Conclusion

Meat quality can be influenced by preslaughter and postslaughter factors. Electrical stimulation is one of the postslaughter methods to be used for increasing the meat quality.

An obvious pH decrease and improvement in tenderness, colour, and sensorial characteristics can occur in lamb and goat meat by applying various voltage of electrical stimulation.

It is concluded that the electrical stimulation is a useful tool in the solution of cold-shortening problem of meat and in obtaining more tender and high-quality meat.

References

[1] B. Eroglu and O. Cetin, "The effect of low voltage electrical stimulation on M. longissimus dorsi thoracis," *Journal of Faculty of Veterinary Medicine, Istanbul University*, vol. 37, no. 1, pp. 53–62, 2011.

[2] B. Nazli, O. Cetin, E. B. Bingol, T. Kahraman, and O. Ergun, "Effects of high voltage electrical stimulation on meat quality of beef carcasses," *Journal of Animal and Veterinary Advances*, vol. 9, no. 3, pp. 556–560, 2010.

[3] S. Biswas, A. K. Das, R. Banerjee, and N. Sharma, "Effect of electrical stimulation on quality of tenderstretched chevon sides," *Meat Science*, vol. 75, no. 2, pp. 332–336, 2007.

[4] T. Kahraman and Ö. Ergun, "Effects of Electrical Stunning and Electrical Stimulation on Kivircik Carcass Quality," *Kafkas Universitesi Veteriner Fakultesi Dergisi*, vol. 15, no. 3, pp. 461–464, 2009.

[5] P. Polidori, S. Lee, R. G. Kauffman, and B. B. Marsh, "Low voltage electrical stimulation of lamb carcasses: effects on meat quality," *Meat Science*, vol. 53, no. 3, pp. 179–182, 1999.

[6] C. R. Kerth, T. L. Cain, S. P. Jackson, C. B. Ramsey, and M. F. Miller, "Electrical stimulation effects on tenderness of five muscles from Hampshire × Rambouillet crossbred lambs with the callipyge phenotype," *Journal of Animal Science*, vol. 77, no. 11, pp. 2951–2955, 1999.

[7] I. H. Hwang, C. E. Devine, and D. L. Hopkins, "The biochemical and physical effects of electrical stimulation on beef and sheep meat tenderness," *Meat Science*, vol. 65, no. 2, pp. 677–691, 2003.

[8] D. M. Ferguson, B. L. Daly, G. E. Gardner, and R. K. Tume, "Effect of glycogen concentration and form on the response to electrical stimulation and rate of post-mortem glycolysis in ovine muscle," *Meat Science*, vol. 78, no. 3, pp. 202–210, 2008.

[9] O. Cetin and T. Topcu, "Effects of electrical stimulation on meat quality in goat carcasses," *Journal of Food, Agriculture and Environment*, vol. 7, no. 3-4, pp. 101–105, 2009.

[10] D. A. King, K. L. Voges, D. S. Hale, D. F. Waldron, C. A. Taylor, and J. W. Savell, "High voltage electrical stimulation enhances muscle tenderness, increases aging response, and improves muscle color from cabrito carcasses," *Meat Science*, vol. 68, no. 4, pp. 529–535, 2004.

[11] M. Yanar and H. Yetim, "The effects of electrical stimulation on the sensory and textural quality properties of mutton carcasses," *Turkish Journal of Veterinary and Animal Sciences*, vol. 27, no. 2, pp. 433–438, 2003.

[12] Turkish Statistical Institute, "Red meat production statistics—number of slaughtered sheep, goat and bovine animals by types and races and quantity of meat production," 2011, http://www.tuik.gov.tr/.

[13] M. Yanar, H. Yetim, and H. W. Ockerman, "Effects of blade tenderization on some quality characteristics of the muscles of mature ewes," *European Food Research and Technology*, vol. 209, no. 3-4, pp. 197–200, 1999.

[14] W. Horwitz, R. Albert, M. J. Deutsch, and J. N. Thompson, "Precision parameters of methods of analysis required for nutrition labeling. Part I. Major nutrients," *Journal of the Association of Official Analytical Chemists*, vol. 73, no. 5, pp. 661–680, 1990.

[15] Y. Yıldırım, "Et Endüstrisi," *Kozan Ofset Matbaacılık Sanayi ve Ticaret Ltd.Şti Ankara, Turkey*, pp. 239–245, 1996.

[16] M. J. A. Den Hertog-Meischke, F. J. M. Smulders, J. G. Van Logtestijn, and F. Van Knapen, "The effect of electrical stimulation on the water-holding capacity and protein denaturation of two bovine muscles," *Journal of Animal Science*, vol. 75, no. 1, pp. 118–124, 1997.

[17] AMSA, *Guidlines for Meat Color Evaluation*, National Live Stock and Meat Board, Chicago, Ill, USA, 1991.

[18] B. Ekiz, A. Yilmaz, M. Ozcan et al., "Carcass measurements and meat quality of Turkish Merino, Ramlic, Kivircik, Chios and Imroz lambs raised under an intensive production system," *Meat Science*, vol. 82, no. 1, pp. 64–70, 2009.

[19] International Organization for Standardization (ISO) 6658-1985, *Sensory Analysis—Methodology—General Guidance*, International Organization for Standardization, Paris, France, 1985.

[20] International Organization for Standardization (ISO) 8586-1, *Sensory Analysis—General Guidance for the Selection, Training and Monitoring of Assessors. Part 1: Selected Assessors*, International Organization for Standardization, Genève, Switzerland, 1993.

[21] S. Ranganna, *Handbook of Analysis and Quality Control for Fruit and Vegetable Products*, TATA, McGraw-Hill, New Delhi, India, 2nd edition, 1994.

[22] International Organization for Standardization (ISO) 8589, *Sensory Analysis—General Guidance for Design of Test Rooms*, International Organization for Standardization, Paris, France, 1998.

[23] SPSS, *SPSS for Windows, Release no. 16.0*, LEAD Technologies Inc, 2008.

[24] J. D. Morton, R. Bickerstaffe, M. P. Kent, E. Dransfield, and G. M. Keeley, "Calpain-calpastatin and toughness in M. longissimus from electrically stimulated lamb and beef carcasses," *Meat Science*, vol. 52, no. 1, pp. 71–79, 1999.

[25] T. Kahraman, *Effects of low voltage electrical stimulation on meat quality of small ruminants*, Ph.D. thesis, Istanbul University Health Science Institute, Istanbul, Turkey, 2007.

[26] P. E. Strydom, L. Frylinck, and M. F. Smith, "Should electrical stimulation be applied when cold shortening is not a risk?" *Meat Science*, vol. 70, no. 4, pp. 733–742, 2005.

[27] J. J. Bond, L. A. Can, and R. D. Warner, "The effect of exercise stress, adrenaline injection and electrical stimulation on changes in quality attributes and proteins in *Semimembranosus* muscle of lamb," *Meat Science*, vol. 68, no. 3, pp. 469–477, 2004.

[28] C. E. Devine, T. E. Lowe, R. W. Wells et al., "Pre-slaughter stress arising from on-farm handling and its interactions with electrical stimulation on tenderness of lambs," *Meat Science*, vol. 73, no. 2, pp. 304–312, 2006.

[29] G. H. Geesink, M. H. D. Mareko, J. D. Morton, and R. Bickerstaffe, "Effects of stress and high voltage electrical stimulation on tenderness of lamb *M. longissimus*," *Meat Science*, vol. 57, no. 3, pp. 265–271, 2001.

[30] M. B. Solomon and G. P. Lynch, "Combined effects of ES, carcass posture and insulated bags on ram lamb tenderness," *Journal of Muscle Foods*, vol. 2, pp. 279–288, 1991.

[31] K. M. Gadiyaram, G. Kannan, T. D. Pringle, B. Kouakou, K. W. McMillin, and Y. W. Park, "Effects of postmortem carcass

electrical stimulation on goat meat quality characteristics," *Small Ruminant Research*, vol. 78, no. 1–3, pp. 106–114, 2008.

[32] E. Wiklund, J. M. Stevenson-Barry, S. J. Duncan, and R. P. Littlejohn, "Electrical stimulation of red deer (*Cervus elaphus*) carcasses—effects on rate of pH-decline, meat tenderness, colour stability and water-holding capacity," *Meat Science*, vol. 59, no. 2, pp. 211–220, 2001.

28

Effect of Calcium Soap of Fatty Acids Supplementation on Serum Biochemical Parameters and Ovarian Activity during Out-of-the-Breeding Season in Crossbred Ewes

Hayat H. M. El-Nour,[1] Soad M. Nasr,[2] and Walid R. Hassan[3]

[1] *Department of Biology, Animal Reproduction Research Institute, El-Ahram, Giza, Egypt*
[2] *Department of Parasitology and Animal Diseases, National Research Center, El-Behouse Street, P.O. Box 12622, Dokki, Giza, Egypt*
[3] *Ultrasonography Unit, Animal Reproduction Research Institute, El-Ahram, Giza, Egypt*

Correspondence should be addressed to Soad M. Nasr, soadnasr@yahoo.com

Academic Editors: S. Behboudi and C. C. Chang

This experiment aimed to evaluate the effect of calcium soap of fatty acid (CSFA) supplementation on serum biochemical and hormones and ovarian activity during out-of-the-breeding season in ewes. Twelve crossbred ewes, 2-3 years of age and weighting 45–55 kg, were allocated into two equal groups. The first group was control and the other was treated with 50 g/head of CSFA. All ewes were fed basal diet and treated with 60 mg of medroxy progesterone acetate intravaginal sponge for 12 day. At the third day of sponge removal, the CSFA-treated group was given 50 g/head of CSFA daily for two estrous cycles. During the estrus phase, ovarian activity was detected using ultrasonography in both groups. All ewes were then subjected to natural breeding and conception rate. Blood samples were collected from all ewes during treatment period. Results revealed significant ($P < 0.05$) increases in serum cholesterol, triglycerides, low-density lipoprotein cholesterol, glucose, and progesterone levels with decrease in calcium and phosphorous levels in treated group. In treated group, normal-size ovaries and more than one follicle on the ovaries were detected and pregnancy rate increased. In conclusion, CSFA supplementation was effective to maintain the reproductive performance when ewes were out of the breeding season.

1. Introduction

The normal breeding season of sheep is between June and July and they undergo postpartum anestrus during the spring [1, 2] which results in only one offspring per year. As a result, much of the attempts to increase the productivity of small ruminants in the semiarid regions were concentrated on either increasing twinning rate or having two parturitions per year. Nutrition plays a key role in regulating the reproductive performance in farm animals. Restriction of energy intake has a major role in increasing the length of postpartum anestrus in sheep and cattle [3]. Well-fed postpartum Awassi ewes returned to estrus earlier, indicating the possibility of lambing every six months [2]. Increased glucose availability is one of the "immediate nutrient" effects on ovulation rate [4]. Glucose entry rate explained 63% of the variation in the ovulation rate of ewes that were infused with glucose. Energy intake is one of the most important factors influencing reproductive performance of sheep. Fat is usually used as a generic term to describe compounds that have a high contents of long chain fatty acids (FAs) including triglycerides, phospholipids, nonesterified FAs, and salts of long chain FAs [5]. In ruminants, fat diet can increase the caloric density without reducing the fiber contribution and it can also increases energy consumption and utilization efficiency [6]. Greater dietary fat ingestion has direct effects on ovarian structures [7]. Calcium soaps of fatty acids supplementation increase the number and size of ovarian follicles in estrous cyclic ewes and increase the circulating progesterone concentration [8]. In ewes fed supplemental fat, there are reports of increased plasma concentrations of cholesterol, triglycerides, high-density lipoprotein cholesterol (HDL-C), low-density lipoprotein cholesterol (LDL-C), and progesterone [9, 10]. The first author recorded that increased consumption of fats by cows resulted in increases in the number of ovarian follicles, increase in the number and size of corpora lutea, stimulation of postpartum ovarian activity, and improved pregnancy rate in goats [11, 12]. Calcium salts of fatty acids (CSFAs) are readily available and easily incorporated into ruminant diets; affordability will depend largely upon duration and amount of supplementation [13]. The precise mechanism through which fat supplementation modifies ovarian physiology in ruminants remains undetermined completely. Limited information is available regarding the response of sheep to supplemental fat. Therefore, the objective of this research is to study the effect of calcium soap of fatty acids (CSFAs) supplementation on some biochemical and hormonal changes and reproductive performance (ovarian activity and of crossbred ewes during out-of-the-breeding season using ultrasonography).

2. Materials and Methods

The present study was carried out at Departments of Biology, Animal Reproduction Research Institute, El-Ahram, Giza, Egypt and Parasitology and Animal Diseases, National Research Center, Dokki, Giza, Egypt during March until August 2006.

2.1. Animals. Twelve sexually mature native crossbred (Barki × Rahmani) ewes of 2-3 years of age and weighting 45–55 kg were used. Animals were housed under conditions of natural day light and temperature. Ewes were offered maintenance ration according to the management system of the Animal Reproduction Research Institute (ARRI). Ewes were fed a basal diet containing ground yellow corn 31%, soybean meal 16%, sunflower meal 23%, wheat bran 20.7%, molasses 5%, lime stone 2%, common salt 2%, and mineral mixture 0.3%. In addition, green berseem (*Trifolium alexanderinum*) was added. Water was offered *ad libitum*. Ewes proved to be clinically healthy and free from external or internal parasites.

2.2. Experimental Procedure. Ewes were synchronized by using intravaginal sponge containing 60 mg medroxy progesterone acetate for 12 days. The third day of sponge removal, all ewes were randomly allocated into two equal groups (6 ewes/group). The first group was supplemented with 50 g of calcium soaps of palm oil fatty acids/head/day (Magnabac: calcium soaps of palm oil fatty acids (protected fat); Norel, Spain) for 34 days (two estrous cycles) according to Abd El-Rahman et al. [12]. The second group was kept as a control (received no treatment). The ovarian activity was detected by ultrasonography in both control and CSFA-treated ewes during estrus phase. Ewes were naturally inseminated by three good fertile rams (1 ram/4 ewes) after the end of the treatment by one month. Ultrasonography was performed for all ewes after one month to detect ovarian activity and was repeated again after the end of the treatment by three months to detect pregnancy rate.

2.3. Blood Samples. Ten mL of blood was collected from jugular vein from each ewe in the early morning before ration was offered at time zero (before treatment), on day 10 from the first and second estrous cycles, and after 30 days of CSFA-treatment withdrawal. Each whole blood sample was allowed to clot for 30 minutes in a plain centrifuge tube and centrifuged for serum separation at 2000 ×g for 15 minutes. Serum was transferred carefully into clean dry vials and stored at −20°C until further biochemical and hormonal analyses.

2.4. Biochemical Analyses. Enzymatic determination of serum total cholesterol [14], triglycerides [15], HDL-C [16], and glucose [17] was performed. Serum LDL-C level was calculated according to the following equation of Friedewald et al. [18]:

$$\text{Concentration of LDL-C in serum (mg/dL)} = \text{Total Cholesterol} - \text{HDL-C} - \left(\frac{\text{Triglycerides}}{5}\right). \quad (1)$$

Serum calcium [19] and inorganic phosphorus [20] were determined. All test kits were supplied by bioMérieux, France except calcium kit supplied by RANDOX, Laboratories Ltd, United Kingdom. Measurements were performed by a Spectrophotometer model T80, UV/Visible, double beam, UK.

2.5. Hormones Assay. Serum progesterone and insulin assay were performed using ELISA technique (DRG Instruments GnbH, Germany) according to Katt et al. [21] and Judzewitsch et al. [22], respectively. Total thyroxine (T4) was determined in serum using ELISA technique (DRG International Inc., USA) according to Wisdom [23].

2.6. Ultrasonography. It was performed using a real time B-mode Scanner (Vet son, Kontron, France) equipped with 5L Vet linear-array rectal out-adapted frequency transducer ranged between 3–7 MHz. The data were printed out on thermal paper (Sony thermal video printer, France). Ultrasonic gel was used to cover the short distance between the transducer scan head and the animal. This prevent air interface and hence produces good quality image and minimizes image artifacts. The diameter of follicles was measured through a built caliper system inside the machine.

2.7. Statistical Analysis. All data were subjected to statistical analysis including the calculation of the mean and standard error according to Snedecor and Cochran [24]. Data were analyzed by one-way ANOVA implying a randomized complete block design. The difference between treatments was further compared by Duncan multiple range test using 3.03 version of Cost.

TABLE 1: Serum lipid profile and glucose levels of CSFA-treated and control ewes during out-of-breeding season (mean ± SE, $N = 6$).

Parameters	Periods groups	Before treatment	Day 10 of first cycle	Day 10 of second cycle	Day 30 after with drawl
Cholesterol (mg/dL)	Control	91.20 ± 3.12^a	83.06 ± 0.84^b	85.71 ± 1.77^b	87.72 ± 1.44^b
	CSFA	94.45 ± 0.98^a	98.52 ± 3.60^a	94.55 ± 2.47^a	109.14 ± 1.38^a
	Sig.	NS	**	*	***
Triglycerides (mg/dL)	Control	81.30 ± 1.42^b	72.44 ± 4.05^b	64.64 ± 3.3^b	73.67 ± 3.44^b
	CSFA	87.58 ± 1.68^a	91.47 ± 2.92^a	85.39 ± 2.77^a	88.36 ± 2.09^a
	Sig.	*	**	***	**
HDL-Chol (mg/dL)	Control	59.47 ± 2.34^a	55.16 ± 1.02^a	57.69 ± 1.81^a	58.33 ± 1.29^b
	CSFA	57.31 ± 2.68^a	55.36 ± 2.35^a	58.54 ± 2.39^a	70.69 ± 2.14^a
	Sig.	NS	NS	NS	***
LDL-Chol (mg/dL)	Control	19.57 ± 2.04^a	14.97 ± 1.68^b	14.43 ± 1.16^a	13.33 ± 1.64^b
	CSFA	19.62 ± 1.47^a	25.31 ± 1.01^a	16.92 ± 0.77^a	20.59 ± 1.26^a
	Sig.	NS	***	NS	**
Glucose (mg/dL)	Control	47.81 ± 5.81^a	42.09 ± 3.96^b	63.20 ± 3.24^b	47.09 ± 3.98^a
	CSFA	52.35 ± 2.84^a	53.78 ± 2.28^a	99.78 ± 4.16^a	50.11 ± 2.02^a
	Sig.	NS	*	***	NS

Means with different superscripts letters in the same column are significantly different at $P < 0.05$. *: significant, **: highly significant, ***: very highly significant, NS: nonsignificant.
SE: standard error. CSFA: calcium soap of fatty acid.
HDL-C: high-density lipoprotein cholesterol. LDL-C: Low-density lipoprotein cholesterol.

3. Results

3.1. Biochemical Parameters

3.1.1. Serum Lipid Profile. In Table 1 there was significant ($P < 0.05$) increase in serum total cholesterol, triglycerides, and low-density lipoprotein cholesterol (LDL-C) levels during treatment of CSFA ewes when compared with nontreated ewes. Serum high-density lipoprotein cholesterol (HDL-C) showed significant ($P < 0.05$) increase after withdrawal of CSFA-treated ewes than control nontreated ewes.

3.1.2. Serum Glucose. On day 10 from the first and the second estrous cycles, serum glucose levels were markedly elevated ($P < 0.05$) in CSFA-treated ewes than control nontreated ewes as shown in Table 1.

3.1.3. Serum Calcium, Phosphorus, and Calcium/Phosphorus Ratios. There was no statistical difference in serum calcium levels in CSFA-treated groups and control group. While serum phosphorous level showed significant ($P < 0.05$) increase after one month of CSFA treatment while calcium/Phosphorous (Ca/P) ratio showed significant ($P < 0.05$) decrease at the same time (Table 2).

3.2. Serum Hormones. In all periods of treatment with CSFA, progesterone levels revealed significant ($P < 0.05$) increase in serum of CSFA-treated ewes compared to control ewes. No effects of CSFA on serum insulin and thyroxin levels were noticed during the periods of treatment (Table 3).

3.3. Reproductive Performance

3.3.1. Examination of the Ovaries. According to results obtained by ultrasonography, examination of the ovaries of the CSFA-treated ewes showed presence of normal size ovaries and more than one follicle on the ovaries (100%). The follicles were rounded in shape with thin echogenic wall and had echoic cavity. Examination of the control group showed presence of smooth small ovaries in four ewes (66%) which appeared hypoechoic and circumscribed area without any follicles. There were small follicles in two ewes (34%) as shown in Figures 1 and 2.

3.3.2. Pregnancy Rate. Pregnancy rates were 50% and 17% in CSFA-treated and control groups, respectively, using ultrasonography (Figures 1 and 3).

4. Discussion

In the present work, the effect of CSFA supplementation on some biochemical parameters: lipid profile, glucose, calcium, and phosphorus levels; hormones: progesterone, insulin, and T4; and reproductive performance: ovarian activity and pregnancy rate using ultrasonography were studied in ewes during out-of-the-breeding season.

In our study, there was significant increase in serum total cholesterol, triglycerides, and LDL-C concentrations in CSFA-treated ewes than control ones. Serum HDL-C showed significant increase after withdrawal. An increase in dietary lipids leads to elevation of plasma total cholesterol and the supply of lipoproteins which play significant role in

TABLE 2: Serum calcium, phosphorus, and calcium/phosphorus ratio concentrations of CSFA-treated and control ewes during out-of-breeding season (mean ± SE, $N = 6$).

Parameters	Periods groups	Before treatment	Day 10 of first cycle	Day 10 of second cycle	Day 30 after with drawl
Calcium (mg/dL)	Control	9.78 ± 0.30^a	10.03 ± 0.20^a	9.35 ± 0.24^a	8.50 ± 0.22^a
	CSFA	10.23 ± 0.18^a	9.79 ± 0.37^a	9.95 ± 0.40^a	8.67 ± 0.25^a
	Sig.	NS	NS	NS	NS
Phosphorus (mg/dL)	Control	6.73 ± 0.24^a	7.35 ± 0.15^b	5.97 ± 0.14^a	5.75 ± 0.15^a
	CSFA	7.40 ± 0.18^a	7.82 ± 0.10^a	6.27 ± 0.20^a	5.65 ± 0.16^a
	Sig.	NS	NS	*	NS
Ca/P ratio	Control	1.45 ± 0.03^a	1.36 ± 0.01^b	1.56 ± 0.06^a	1.48 ± 0.04^a
	CSFA	1.48 ± 0.09^a	1.25 ± 0.04^a	1.58 ± 0.05^a	1.53 ± 0.05^a
	Sig.	NS	NS	*	NS

Means with different superscripts letters in the same column are significantly different at $P < 0.05$. **: highly significant, ***: very highly significant, NS: nonsignificant. SE: standard error.
CSFA: calcium soap of fatty acid. Ca/P: calcium/phosphorus.

TABLE 3: Serum progesterone, insulin, and thyroxin concentrations of CSFA-treated and control ewes during out-of-season (mean ± SE, $N = 6$).

Parameters	Periods groups	Before treatment	Day 10 of first cycle	Day 10 of second cycle	Day 30 after with drawl
Progesterone (ng/mL)	Control	2.37 ± 0.43^a	0.96 ± 0.13^b	0.98 ± 0.26^b	0.50 ± 0.06^b
	CSFA	2.90 ± 0.27^a	3.08 ± 0.31^a	2.32 ± 0.29^a	2.10 ± 0.37^a
	Sig.	NS	***	**	**
Insulin (μU/mL)	Control	5.33 ± 0.47^a	6.32 ± 0.14^a	6.65 ± 0.15^a	6.68 ± 0.25^a
	CSFA	6.05 ± 0.11^a	5.93 ± 0.36^a	7.08 ± 0.29^a	7.23 ± 0.24^a
	Sig.	NS	NS	NS	NS
Thyroxin (μg/dL)	Control	10.70 ± 0.53^a	10.35 ± 0.72^a	8.56 ± 0.74^a	7.66 ± 0.81^a
	CSFA	9.63 ± 1.63^a	9.45 ± 1.27^a	9.5 ± 1.18^a	9.10 ± 1.06^a
	Sig.	NS	NS	NS	NS

Means with different superscripts letters in the same column are significantly different at $P < 0.05$. *: significant. NS: nonsignificant. SE: standard error. CSFA: calcium soap of fatty acid.

regulating ovarian steroidogenesis [25]. This increment in serum total cholesterol concentration in the CSFA-treated ewes may be due to action of fat supplementation which increased the lipoprotein cholesterol export by the intestine [26].

Elevation of triglycerides levels in CSFA-treated ewes was reported by Ghoreishi et al. [9] and Liel et al. [8]. This increase might be due to the depression in lipogenic enzyme activity by the liver and adipose tissues associated with feeding supplementary fat [27] or may be due to production of lipoproteins in the intestine by fat [28]. Also, Kuran et al. [29] reported a significant increase in LDL levels in CSFA supplemented ewes as reported in our results. These observations agree well with Liel et al. [8], Ghattas and Nasra [10], El-Shahat and Abo-El Maaty [30] in ewes. Funston [31] found an increase in serum cholesterol, triglycerides, and HDL-C in cows.

The effect of nutrient supply on the gonadotropic axis may result from high concentration of NADPH-dependent hepatic mixed function oxidases (MFOs) in the liver. High

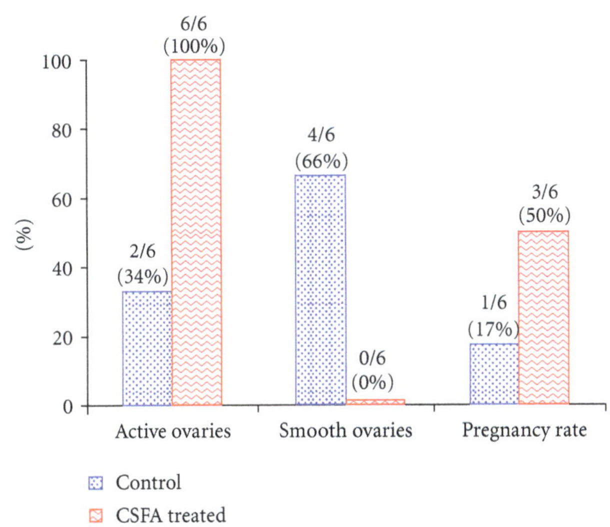

FIGURE 1: Percentage of ovarian activity, smooth ovaries, and pregnancy rate of calcium-soap-of-fatty-acid- (CSFA-) treated and control ewes during out-of-breeding season ($N = 6$).

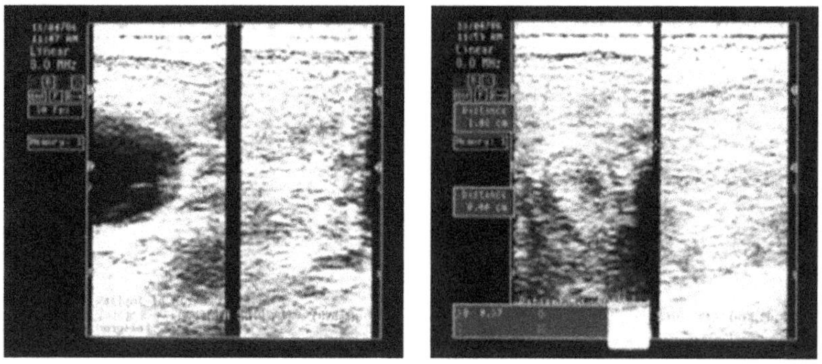

(a) (b)

Figure 2: Effect of calcium soap of fatty acid supplementation on the activity of the ovaries of ewes by using ultrasonography. (a) Control ewe nontreated had small and smooth ovary. (b) Calcium-soap-of-fatty-acid-treated ewe had normal-sized ovary with follicles.

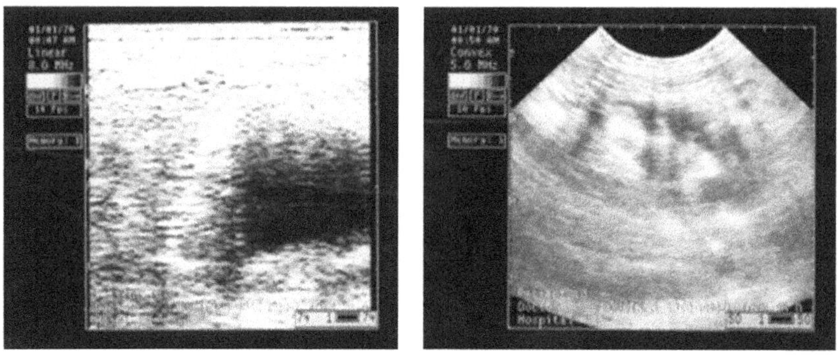

(a) (b)

Figure 3: Effect of calcium soap of fatty acid supplementation on pregnancy in ewes by using ultrasonography. (a) Control ewe nontreated was nonpregnant. (b) Calcium-soap-of-fatty-acid-treated ewe was pregnant.

MFOs result in increased steroid metabolism and in the secretion of more gonadotropins following negative feedback, which causes increased ovulation rate in ewes [32].

Regarding to serum glucose levels, there was significant ($P < 0.05$) increase in their levels in CSFA-treated ewes than control. These increases may be due to diet containing high amount of long chain fatty acids that increase hepatic gluconeogenesis due to the increase in propionate production in the rumen [33, 34]. This result agrees with Ghattas and Nasra [10] and Liel et al. [8].

There was no significant effect of CSFA on serum calcium levels during treatment and after withdrawal. These results agree with that obtained by Wilson [35], Abo-Donia et al. [36], and Ghattas and Nasra [10]. Moreover, the results of the present study revealed significant increase in serum phosphorous levels and significant decrease in the Ca/P ratio after four weeks of treatment compared with control. This increase might be due to increase in phospholipid contents in CSFA. The results disagree with that of Wilson [35] and Ghattas and Nasra [10], and these differences might be due to dose difference.

In the present study, there was significant increase in serum progesterone (P4) concentration during all times of dietary fat treatment and after withdrawal in CSFA-treated group. These results agree with El-Shahat and Abo-El Maaty [30], Ghattas and Nasra [10], and Liel et al. [8]. This increment might be due to increased availability of cholesterol which would provide increased sterol precursors for progesterone biosynthesis by the corpus lutea [37]. This reflects the beneficial effect of dietary treatment of protected fat on the ovulation and corpus lutea formation and also to early pregnancy maintenance [9]. Moreover, the increase in serum concentration of lipids was associated with an increase in the intracellular lipid droplets within the small and large steroidogenic cell types that constitute the bovine corpus luteum and provide an increased precursor for P4 biosynthesis [38]. Williams [25] reported that increased dietary lipids increase plasma cholesterol and P4 and the supply of lipoproteins which play significant role in regulating ovarian steroidogenesis.

According to results obtained by ultrasonography, the ultrasonogram of the ovaries of the CSFA-treated ewes showed presence of normal size ovaries and more than one follicle on the ovaries (100%). While the ultrasonographic examination of the ovaries of control ewes showed presence of smooth small ovaries in four ewes (66%) and presence of small follicles in two ewes (34%), the obtained results are similar with that obtained of Ghoreishi et al. [9];

El-Shahat and Abo-El Maaty [30] and Liel et al. [8]. A positive effect of CSFA on ovarian activity of Barki ewes as indicated by increasing the number of medium and large sized follicles on day zero of the second estrus cycle, and by increasing the number and size of corpora lutea 7 days later in the same cycle was recorded by Liel et al. [8]. El-Shahat and Abo-El Maaty [30] in ewes, Wehrman et al. [39] and Lammoglia et al. [40] in dairy cows reported enhanced follicular development associated with high fat supplement and increased the number of medium-sized follicles. Fat supplementation increases the growth, diameter, and mature size of preovulatory dominant follicles [41]. Higher ovulation percentage in CSFA-treated ewes was recorded also by Liel et al. [8]. The improvement in ovulation percentage may be attributed to an enhancement of LH secretion due to fat supplementation which was reported by Hightshoe et al. [42] and Funston [31]. Increased size of preovulatory follicles may be due in part to increased concentration of plasma LH which stimulates the latter stage of follicular growth. The ovulation of larger follicles may result in the formation of larger corpora lutea with increased steroidogenic capacity and result in greater progesterone production, which has been associated with higher conception rates [31].

Regarding to pregnancy rate by using ultrasonography, the percentage of pregnancy rate of CSFA treated ewes was 50% and in control was 17% when ewes were out-of-the-breeding season. This result agrees with that obtained by Thomas et al. [11] who reported that increased consumption of fats by cows resulted in increases in the number of ovarian follicles, increase in the number and size of corpora lutea, stimulation of postpartum ovarian activity, and improvement in pregnancy rate.

5. Conclusion

The dietary supplementation of CSFA in ewes during out-of-the-breeding season was effective to maintain reproductive performance as reflected by increased levels of lipid profiles, glucose, and progesterone hormone, improved the number and size of ovarian preovulatory follicles, and increased conception rate. So, CSFA may act as an important strategy to integrate nutrition, reproductive maintenance and led to improvement of animal productivity.

Conflict of Interests

Authors declare that there is no conflict of interests.

References

[1] E. S. E. Hafez, "Reproductive cycles (sheep and goats)," in *Reproduction in Farm Animals*, LEA and Febiger, Philadelephia, Pa, USA, 6th edition, 1993.

[2] H. M. Oqla, R. T. Kridli, and S. G. Haddad, "The effect of dietary fat inclusion on nutrient intake and reproductive performance in postpartum Awassi ewes," *Asian-Australasian Journal of Animal Sciences*, vol. 17, no. 10, pp. 1395–1399, 2004.

[3] K. K. Schillo, "Effects of dietary energy on control of luteinizing hormone secretion in cattle and sheep," *Journal of Animal Science*, vol. 70, no. 4, pp. 1271–1282, 1992.

[4] E. Teleni, J. B. Rowe, K. P. Croker, P. J. Murray, and W. R. King, "Lupins and energy-yielding nutrients in ewes. II. Responses in ovulation rate in ewes to increased availability of glucose, acetate and amino acids," *Reproduction, Fertility and Development*, vol. 1, no. 2, pp. 117–125, 1989.

[5] *Nutrient Requirements of Dairy Cattle*, National Academy Press, Washington DC, USA, 7th Revised edition, 2001.

[6] J. L. Espinoza, O. Lopez-Molia, J. A. Ramirez-Godinez, J. Jimenez, and A. Flores, "Milk composition, postpartum reproductive activity and growth of lambs in Pelibuey ewes fed calcium soap of long chain fatty acids," *Small Ruminant Research*, vol. 27, pp. 119–124, 1998.

[7] R. C. Rhodes, M. M. McCartor, and R. D. Randel, "Effect of feeding protein-protected lipid upon growth and reproductive development of yearling heifers," *Journal of Animal Science*, vol. 46, pp. 769–777, 1978.

[8] A. Z. A. Liel, H. M. A. Abd El-Rahman, and H. H. M. El-Nour, "Laparoscopic examination of ovarian activity and some metabolic changes in ewes supplemented with protected fat and growth hormone during estrous cycle," *Egyptian Journal of Basic and Applied Physiology*, vol. 9, pp. 307–323, 2010.

[9] S. M. Ghoreishi, M. J. Zamiri, E. Rowghani, and H. Hejazi, "Effect of a calcium soap of fatty acids on reproductive characteristics and lactation performance of fat-tailed sheep," *Pakistan Journal of Biological Sciences*, vol. 10, no. 14, pp. 2389–2395, 2007.

[10] T. A. Ghattas and A. A. Nasra, "Effects of rumen-protected polyunsaturated fatty acid on some reproductive performance in out of breeding season ewes," *Egyptian Journal of Basic and Applied Physiology*, vol. 9, pp. 291–305, 2010.

[11] M. G. Thomas, B. Bao, and G. L. Williams, "Dietary fats varying in their fatty acid composition differentially influence follicular growth in cows fed isoenergetic diets," *Journal of Animal Science*, vol. 75, no. 9, pp. 2512–2519, 1997.

[12] H. M. A. Abd El-Rahman, H. H. M. El-Nour, S. A. EL-Wakeel, and A. H. Aly, "Effect of calcium soap of fatty acids and recombinant bovine somatotropin on productive and reproductive performance of Baladi goats during early lactation," *Veterinary Medical Journal Giza*, vol. 56, pp. 367–385, 2008.

[13] J. L. Seabrook, R. K. Peel, and T. E. Engle, "The effects of replacing dietary carbohydrate with calcium salts of fatty acids on finishing lamb feedlot performance, blood metabolites, muscle fatty acid composition, and carcass characteristics," *Small Ruminant Research*, vol. 95, no. 2, pp. 97–103, 2011.

[14] C. C. Allain, L. S. Poon, C. S. G. Chan, W. Richmond, and P. C. Fu, "Enzymatic determination of total serum cholesterol," *Clinical Chemistry*, vol. 20, no. 4, pp. 470–475, 1974.

[15] P. Fossati and L. Prencipe, "Serum triglycerides determined colorimetrically with an enzyme that produces hydrogen peroxide," *Clinical Chemistry*, vol. 28, no. 10, pp. 2077–2080, 1982.

[16] M. F. Lopes-Virella, P. Stone, S. Ellis, and J. A. Coiweil, "Cholesterol determination in high density lipoproteins separated by three different methods," *Clinical Chemistry*, vol. 23, no. 5, pp. 882–884, 1977.

[17] P. Trinder, "Determination of serum glucose by enzymatic method," *Annals of Clinical Biochemistry*, vol. 6, pp. 24–28, 1969.

[18] W. T. Friedewald, R. I. Levy, and D. S. Fredrickson, "Estimation of the concentration of low-density lipoprotein cholesterol in plasma, without use of the preparative ultracentrifuge," *Clinical Chemistry*, vol. 18, no. 6, pp. 499–502, 1972.
[19] R. N. Barnett, S. B. Skodon, and M. H. Goldberg, "Performance of "kits" used for clinical chemical analysis of calcium in serum," *American Journal of Clinical Pathology*, vol. 59, no. 6, pp. 836–845, 1973.
[20] H. H. Taussky, E. Shorr, and G. Kurzmann, "A microcolorimetric method for the determination of inorganic phosphorus," *The Journal of Biological Chemistry*, vol. 202, no. 2, pp. 675–685, 1953.
[21] J. A. Katt, J. A. Duncan, L. Herbon, A. Barkan, and J. C. Marshall, "The frequency of gonadotropin releasing hormone stimulation determines the number of pituitary gonadotropin releasing hormone receptors," *Endocrinology*, vol. 116, pp. 2113–2115, 1985.
[22] R. G. Judzewitsch, M. A. Pfeifer, J. D. Best, J. C. Beard, J. B. Halter, and D. Porte Jr., "Chronic chloropropamide therapy of noninsulin-dependent diabetes augments basal and stimulated insulin secretion by increasing islet sensitivity to glucose," *The Journal of Clinical Endocrinology & Metabolism*, vol. 55, pp. 321–328, 1982.
[23] G. B. Wisdom, "Enzyme-immunoassay," *Clinical Chemistry*, vol. 22, no. 8, pp. 1243–1255, 1976.
[24] G. W. Snedecor and W. C. Cochran, *Statistical Methods*, Iowa State University Press, Ames, Iowa, USA, 8th edition, 1982.
[25] G. L. Williams, "Influence of dietary fat intake and metabolism on follicular growth in cattle," *Reproduction in Domestic Animals*, vol. 31, no. 3, pp. 539–542, 1996.
[26] R. C. Noble, "Digestion, absorption and transport of lipids in ruminant animals," in *Lipid Metabolism In Ruminant Animals*, I. W. W. Christie, Ed., pp. 57–93, Pergmon Press, Oxford, UK, 1981.
[27] J. E. Starry, "The effect of dairy fat on milk composition," in *Recent Advances in Animal Nutrition*, W. Haresign, Ed., pp. 3–33, Butter Worth, Woburn, Mass, USA, 1981.
[28] R. R. Grummer and D. J. Carroll, "Effects of dietary fat on metabolic disorders and reproductive performance of dairy cattle," *Journal of Animal Science*, vol. 69, no. 9, pp. 3838–3852, 1991.
[29] M. Kuran, A. G. Onal, J. J. Robinson, K. Mackie, B. K. Speake, and T. G. McEvoy, "A dietary supplement of calcium soaps of fatty acids enhances luteal function in sheep," *Animal Science*, vol. 69, no. 2, pp. 385–393, 1999.
[30] K. H. El-Shahat and A. M. Abo-El Maaty, "The effect of dietary supplementation with calcium salts of long chain fatty acids and/or l-carnitine on ovarian activity of Rahmani ewes," *Animal Reproduction Science*, vol. 117, no. 1-2, pp. 78–82, 2010.
[31] R. N. Funston, "Fat supplementation and reproduction in beef females," *Journal of Animal Science*, vol. 82, pp. E154–E161, 2004.
[32] S. Landau, A. Bor, H. Leibovich, Z. Zoref, Z. Nitsan, and Z. Madar, "The effect of ruminai starch degradability in the diet of Booroola crossbred ewes on induced ovulation rate and prolificacy," *Animal Reproduction Science*, vol. 38, no. 1-2, pp. 97–108, 1995.
[33] W. Chalupa, B. Vecchiarelli, A. E. Elser, D. S. Kronfeld, D. Sklan, and D. L. Palmquist, "Ruminal fermentation in vivo as influenced by long-chain fatty acids," *Journal of Dairy Science*, vol. 69, no. 5, pp. 1293–1301, 1986.
[34] J. W. Keele, R. E. Roffler, and K. Z. Beyers, "Ruminal metabolism in nonlactating cows fed whole cottonseed or extruded soybeans," *Journal of Animal Science*, vol. 67, no. 6, pp. 1612–1622, 1989.
[35] G. F. Wilson, "Stimulation of calcium absorption and reduction in susceptibility to fasting-induced hypocalcaemia in pregnant ewes fed vegetable oil," *New Zealand Veterinary Journal*, vol. 49, no. 3, pp. 115–118, 2001.
[36] F. M. Abo-Donia, F. A. Salem, and N. A. Soliman, "Incorporation of refining oil bt-products in sheep diets," *The Journal of Nutrition*, vol. 6, pp. 1279–1299, 2003.
[37] N. Savion, R. N. Laherty, D. Cohen, D. Lui, and D. Gospodarowicz, "Role of lipoproteins and 3-methylglutaryl co. enzyme A reductase in progesterone production by culture bovine granulosa cells," *Endocrinology*, vol. 11, pp. 13–22, 1982.
[38] D. E. Hawkins, K. D. Niswender, G. M. Oss et al., "An increase in serum lipids increases luteal lipid content and alters the disappearance rate of progesterone in cows," *Journal of Animal Science*, vol. 73, no. 2, pp. 541–545, 1995.
[39] M. E. Wehrman, T. H. Welsh Jr., and G. L. Williams, "Diet-induced hyperlipidemia in cattle modifies the intrafollicular cholesterol environment, modulates ovarian follicular dynamics, and hastens the onset of postpartum luteal activity," *Biology of Reproduction*, vol. 45, no. 3, pp. 514–522, 1991.
[40] M. A. Lammoglia, S. T. Willard, D. M. Hallford, and R. D. Randel, "Effects of dietary fat on follicular development and circulating concentrations of lipids, insulin, progesterone, estradiol-17β, 13,14-dihydro-15-keto-prostaglandin F2α, and growth hormone in estrous cyclic brahman cows," *Journal of Animal Science*, vol. 75, no. 6, pp. 1591–1600, 1997.
[41] R. S. Robinson, P. G. A. Pushpakumara, Z. Cheng, A. R. Peters, D. R. E. Abayasekara, and D. C. Wathes, "Effects of dietary polyunsaturated fatty acids on ovarian and uterine function in lactating dairy cows," *Reproduction*, vol. 124, no. 1, pp. 119–131, 2002.
[42] R. B. Hightshoe, R. C. Cochran, L. R. Corah, G. H. Kiracofe, D. L. Harmon, and R. C. Perry, "Effects of calcium soaps of fatty acids on postpartum reproductive function in beef cows," *Journal of Animal Science*, vol. 69, no. 10, pp. 4097–4103, 1991.

An Assessment of Whole Blood and Fractions by Nested PCR as a DNA Source for Diagnosing Canine Ehrlichiosis and Anaplasmosis

Tereza Emmanuelle de Farias Rotondano,[1] Alzira Maria Paiva de Almeida,[2] Elane Maria Camboim Lustosa,[3] Aline Antas Cordeiro,[3] Expedito Kennedy Alves Camboim,[3] Sérgio Santos de Azevedo,[3] Paulo Paes de Andrade,[4] and Marcia Almeida de Melo[3]

[1] *Departamento de Ciências Biológicas, Universidade Federal de Pernambuco, Avenue Professor Moraes Rego, s/n, Cidade Universitária, 50.670-901 Recife, PE, Brazil*
[2] *Centro de Pesquisas Aggeu Magalhães, FIOCRUZ-PE, Avenue Professor Moraes Rego, s/n, Cidade Universitária, 50.670-901 Recife, PE, Brazil*
[3] *Unidade Acadêmica de Medicina Veterinária, Universidade Federal de Campina Grande, 58.700-970 Patos, PB, Brazil*
[4] *Departamento de Genética, Universidade Federal de Pernambuco, Avenue Professor Moraes Rego, s/n, Cidade Universitária, 50.670-901 Recife, PE, Brazil*

Correspondence should be addressed to Marcia Almeida de Melo, marcia.melo@pq.cnpq.br

Academic Editors: B. Harrach and A. Reis

Ehrlichiosis and anaplasmosis are tick-borne diseases. *Ehrlichia canis* and *Anaplasma platys* infect mainly white cells and platelets, respectively. The main DNA source for PCR is peripheral blood, but the potential of blood cell fractions has not been extensively investigated. This study aims at assessment of whole blood (WB) and blood fractions potential in nested PCR (nPCR) to diagnose canine ehrlichiosis and anaplasmosis. The 16S rRNA gene was amplified in 71.4, 17.8, 31.57, and 30% of the WB, granulocyte (G), mononuclear cells (M), and buffy coat (BC) samples. Compared to the WB, the sensitivity of the PCR was 42.86% for the M, and BC fractions, 21.43% for the G, and 33.33% for the blood clot (C). There was fair agreement between the WB and M, BC and C, and slight with the G. Fair agreement occurred between the nPCR and morulae in the blood smear. One animal was coinfected with *A. platys* and *E. canis*. This study provided the first evidence of *A. platys* infection in dogs in Paraíba, Brazil, and demonstrated that WB is a better DNA source than blood fractions to detect *Ehrlichia* and *Anaplasma* by nPCR, probably because of the plasma bacterial concentration following host cell lysis.

1. Introduction

Ehrlichiosis and anaplasmosis are important, emerging zoonotic tick-borne diseases caused by gram-negative, obligate intracellular bacteria from the Anaplasmataceae family. In the host cells, the bacteria reside in inclusion bodies (morulae), which provide a hospitable environment for survival [1, 2].

Canidae can be infected by several Anaplasmataceae agents: *Ehrlichia canis*, *E. ewingii*, *E. chaffeensis*, *Anaplasma platys*, *A. phagocytophilum*, *Neorickettsia risticii*, and *N. helminthoeca*. *Ehrlichia* and *Anaplasma* infections are transmitted through the salivary secretions of attached ticks. *Ehrlichia canis* is usually transmitted by brown dog tick (*Rhipicephalus sanguineus*) bites, which can also transmit *E. ewingii* and most likely *Anaplasma platys* [1]. The occurrence of the tick *R. sanguineus* parasitizing humans in Brazil [3] serves to warn the risk of transmission of such pathogens (*A. platys* and *E. canis*) to humans [4, 5].

E. canis species mainly infect monocytes, which causes canine monocytic ehrlichiosis, and *A. platys* species infect platelets, which causes canine cyclic thrombocytopenia.

The *A. platys* platelet tropism is unique among ehrlichial-related organisms, even though all of these infections may result in thrombocytopenia [2]. *E. canis* is the main pathogen implicated in cases of canine ehrlichiosis in Brazil, but *A. platys* has recently been identified by PCR in samples from the South region with a prevalence ranging from 25.5% to 55% [1, 5].

The diagnosis of canine ehrlichiosis and anaplasmosis relies on the cultivation, serology, PCR, and direct microscopic examination of stained blood smears to identify intracytoplasmic morulae. Smear diagnosis has low sensitivity, as there are few bacteria present in the samples, morulae can be visualized only during the acute phase, and the percentage of infected cells is usually less than 1% [6]. Additionally, the presence of *A. platys* is cyclical, and the bacteria are easily mistaken as nonspecific inclusion bodies and staining artifacts [1, 7]. Serology is hampered by cross-reactions and cannot discriminate between a current infection and previous exposure to the pathogen. Moreover, antibody titers tend to persist for several months to years after treatment, making serology an unreliable tool for posttreatment diagnosis [8].

The first PCR-based diagnostic method for ehrlichiosis amplified the 16S rRNA gene and was reported by Iqbal et al. in 1994 [9]. Further improvements and the use of other target genes increased the sensitivity of the tests. The p30-based nested PCR (nPCR) assay has been shown to be more sensitive than the 16S rRNA-based nPCR assay [10], possibly because *E. canis* contains multiple copies of the p30 gene but only one copy of the 16S rRNA gene [11]. As opposed to single-step PCR, nPCR amplification of the 16S rRNA gene has been used more often to detect *E. canis* and *A. platys*. In both single step PCR and nPCR, the peripheral blood is frequently used as a DNA source [1, 5, 12]. Only a single report has described the use of mononuclear cells as a DNA source [9].

There is a high prevalence of canine ehrlichiosis, but there are few reports on the identification of the infectious agents; therefore, a practical diagnostic technique that can be routinely used in veterinary medicine must be established. The nPCR assay may fulfill this requirement, but the blood fraction that serves as the best DNA source must be determined beforehand. The aim of the present study was to compare the effectiveness of whole blood (WB) and blood fractions—buffy coat (BC), granulocytes (G), mononuclear fraction (M) and blood clot (C)—by nPCR to diagnose canine ehrlichiosis and anaplasmosis.

2. Methods

2.1. Samples and Cell Fractionation. Blood was collected from 21 dogs bearing suggestive clinical signs of either ehrlichiosis or anaplasmosis (petechia, ecchymosis, fever, and anorexia) and harboring ticks. Some animals also had intracytoplasmic morulae, as indicated by direct examination of blood smears and/or hematological parameters suggestive of ehrlichiosis and anaplasmosis. The dogs were selected from the veterinary hospital Universidade Federal de Campina Grande (UFCG), the Veterinary Medical Center Dr. Leonardo Torres at Patos, State of Paraiba, and at the Veterinary Hospital at Universidade Federal Rural de Pernambuco (UFRPE), at Recife, State of Pernambuco.

2.2. Hematology, Direct Examination of Blood Smears and Cell Fractionation. Routine platelet counts, packed cell volume, and other hematology parameters were performed at the hospitals referred to above. The reference values were those described in Jain (1993) [15]. WB smears were stained with a hematoxylin-eosin-based rapid stain (Panótico rápido, Laborclin, Brazil) and observed by microscopy (100X objective, under immersion oil). The M- and G-enriched samples were obtained from 4 mL of WB with the SepCell kit (LGC Biotecnologia, Brazil), according to the manufacturer's instructions. The BC fraction was collected from 1 mL blood that was centrifuged at 12,000 g for 10 min.

2.3. DNA Extraction. From each dog, a sample of blood was collected, and the DNA was extracted. Four milliliters of blood were extracted with sodium citrate and 1 mL without sodium citrate. The DNA samples from the WB (200 μL), BC (50 μL), M (50 μL), G (100 μL), and C (50 μL) fractions were extracted with a commercial kit (Invisorb Spin Blood Midi kit; INVITEK), following the manufacturer's instructions. The DNA from 21 WB, 19 G and 19 M, 20 BC, and 15 C samples was used in the nPCR to amplify the *E. canis* and *A. platys* 16S rRNA sequences.

2.4. Nested PCR (nPCR). The first round of PCR used 0.5 to 1.0 μg of the genomic DNA, and the primers ECC and ECB were designed to amplify a 478 base-pair (bp) fragment of the *Ehrlichia* 16S rRNA [13]. The second round of PCR used a 1.0 μL aliquot of the first reaction as a template and the EHCA sense/EHCA antisense [14] and EHPL sense/EHPL antisense (João Pessoa Araújo Jr.: pers. comm., 2010) primers, which were designed to amplify a 389 bp fragment for *E. canis* and 384 bp fragment for *A. platys*, respectively. Separate reactions were used to detect each species individually. The primers are described in Table 1. The primer design was confirmed with the software Primer 3 (http://fokker.wi.mit.edu/primer3/input.htm). The reaction mix contained 1X reaction buffer (50 mM KCl, 20 mM Tris-HCl (pH 8.4), and 0.1% Triton X-100), 1.75 mM $MgCl_2$, 0.2 mM dNTP mix, 1 μM PCR primers, 0.625 U Taq DNA polymerase, and autoclaved ultrapure water to a final volume of 25 μL. The thermocycle was as follows: 94°C for 10 minutes followed by 40 cycles at 94°C for 60 seconds, 60°C for 60 seconds, 72°C for 60 seconds, and a final step of 72°C for 4 minutes before holding at 4°C. Ultra-pure autoclaved water was used as negative control in each PCR batch. The genomic DNA from confirmed *E. canis* and *A. platys* cases was used as positive controls for the *E. canis* 16S rRNA and *A. platys* 16S rRNA genes, respectively. Ten microliters of the final products were electrophoresed at 90 volts for approximately 1 hour in 1.5% agarose gels containing ethidium bromide in Tris-Borate EDTA (TBE).

Table 1: The primer sequences for the 16S rRNA gene used to detect the *E. canis* and *A. platys* by the nPCR reactions.

Primer identification	Etiological agent	Primer sequences	Reference	Expected amplified segment length	From-to (bp)
ECC	*E.* spp.	AGAACGAACGCTGGCGGCAAGCC	Dawson et al. [13]	478 bp	13–490
ECB	*E.* spp.	CGTATTACCGCGGCTGCTGGC			
EHCA sense	*E. canis*	CAATTATTTATAGCCTCTGGCTATAGC	Wen et al. [14]	389 bp	58–446
EHCA antisense	*E. canis*	TATAGGTACCGTCATTATCTTCCCTAT			
EHPL sense	*A. platys*	TTTTTGTCGTAGCTTGCTATGATA	João Pessoa Araújo Jr., pers. comm	384 bp	49–432
EHPL antisense	*A. platys*	TGTGGGTACCGTCATTATCTTCCCCA			

The *E. canis* and *A. platys* reactions were positive when a 389 or a 384 bp fragment was detected, respectively.

2.5. Statistical Analysis. The kappa and related indices were calculated by Dag Stat software [16] to determine the agreement between the results for the WB (gold standard) and blood fractions. The McNemar test was used to evaluate the concordance among DNA sources, and the Fisher's exact test was used to determine the association between thrombocytopenia, anemia, and a positive WB nPCR. The significance level was 5% for all of the analyses.

2.6. Ethical Considerations. The animals were used according to the guidelines of Oswaldo Cruz Foundation from Brazil's Ministry of Health.

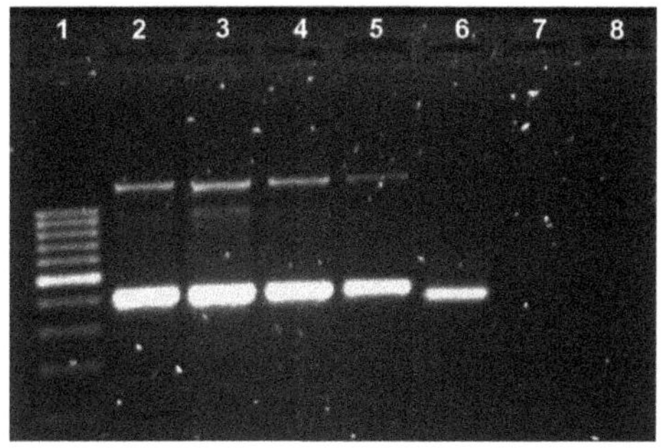

Figure 1: Detection of *Ehrlichia canis* in nPCR with EHCA sense and antisense primers for rRNA 16S gene. Lane 1: 100 base pair (bp) DNA ladder; lanes from 2 to 5: nPCR with DNA from WB; lane 6: *E. canis*-positive control and DNA from WB; lane 7: negative control; lane 8: nPCR-negative control.

3. Results

Table 2 shows the results of hematological, blood smear (direct examination), and nPCR on the WB, G, M, BC, and C samples from 21 dogs exhibiting clinical signs of ehrlichiosis. From each group, negative samples were detected. In seven animals (46.6%), identification at species level failed, as there was no amplification in the second PCR. Among them, the blood smears of five dogs were positive by direct examination and two displayed cytoplasmic inclusions.

Seven dogs (33.3%) were positive by nPCR and direct examination of blood smears (presence of morulae); inclusions within platelets were found in two blood smears. Out of the 14 blood smear-negative animals, eight (63.6%) had at least one blood fraction positive for *Ehrlichia* or *Anaplasma* by nPCR, corresponding to 57.1% false negatives by direct examination. The WB DNA samples from 66.6% (6/9) thrombocytopenic and 42.85% (3/7) anemic animals were positive by nPCR.

Among 21 WB samples, 26.6% (6/21) were negative by nPCR, and 71.4% (15/21) were positive: 46.4% (7/15) for *E. canis* (Figure 1) and 6.6% (1/15) for *A. platys. E. canis* was identified in G samples from 1.8% (3/19), in M samples from 31.6% (6/19), and in BC samples from 31.6% (6/19) animals. One BC sample was coinfected with *E. canis* and *A. platys*. Among the C samples, 7.14% (1/14) were positive for *E. canis* and 14.3% (2/14) for *A. platys*.

Among the nPCR assays carried out in all samples (WB, G, M, BC, and C) from 11 animals, at least 63.3% (7/11) were positive; WB and C samples were simultaneously positive in 9% (1/11) and WB, M, and BC in 18.1% (2/11).

The nPCR sensitivity was 42.86% when the WB was compared to the M and BC fractions (McNemar test: $X^2 = 6.13$; $P = 0.013$), 21.43% compared to the G fraction (McNemar test: $X^2 = 9.09$; $P = 0.003$), and 33.33% compared to the C fraction (McNemar test: $X^2 = 4.17$; $P = 0.041$). The kappa value showed fair agreement among WB and M (Kappa = 0.28), BC (Kappa = 0.31), and C fractions (Kappa = 0.26) and slight agreement with G fraction (Kappa = 0.13). There was also fair agreement between the presence of morulae and the nPCR results (Kappa = 0.33; McNemar test: $X^2 = 6.13$; $P = 0.0133$).

4. Discussion

The direct examination of stained blood smears to detect *Ehrlichia* in dogs has a low sensitivity rate (3 to 9%). In fact, *E. canis* morulae are difficult to detect in blood smears because this organism is usually present in very low concentrations [6]. In contrast, PCR has proven to be more sensitive for detecting *Ehrlichia*; for a 16S rRNA-based PCR assay is able to detect *E. canis* DNA from a rickettsemia, which is equivalent to one infected monocyte in 10^{36} cells [1, 5, 12]. In addition to the large sensitivity differences inherent to the techniques, genotypic variants have been reported for *E. ruminantium*, and *A. platys* infects a wide range of host cells [1, 2, 17].

Table 2: Hematological, blood smear direct examination and whole blood (WB), granulocytes (G), peripheral blood mononuclear cells (M), buffy coat (BC) and blood clot (C) PCR results of dogs with clinical signs of ehrlichiosis.

Animal ID	Packed cell volume**	Leukocytes***	Platelets****	Blood smear	PCR				
					WB	G	M	BC	C
01	37	18,100	314,000	Positive	*Ehrlichia* spp.	Negative	Negative	Negative	*
02	45	6,200	49,000	Negative	*E. canis*	*E. canis*	*E. canis*	*E. canis*	*
03	51	8,000	195,000	Negative	*Ehrlichia* spp.	Negative	Negative	Negative	Negative
04	*	*	*	Negative	*E. canis*	*E. canis*	*E. canis*	*E. canis*	*
05	27	35,300	334,000	Negative	Negative	*	*	Negative	Negative
06	46	8,200	257,000	Negative	Negative	Negative	Negative	Negative	*
07	51	6,200	199,000	Negative	*Ehrlichia* spp.	Negative	Negative	Negative	*
08	37	9,700	248,000	Negative	Negative	Negative	Negative	Negative	Negative
09	51	20,250	595,000	Positive	*Ehrlichia* spp.	Negative	Negative	Negative	*
10	*	*	*	Negative	*E. canis*	Negative	*E. canis*	*	*E. canis*
11	16	65,100	67,000	Negative	*E. canis*	*E. canis*	*E. canis*	*E. canis*	*
12	*	*	*	Positive	*E. canis*	*	*	*E. canis*/*A. platys*	*A. platys*
13	*	*	*	Positive	*E. canis*	Negative	*E. canis*	*E. canis*	Negative
14	41	*	119,000	Negative	*A. platys*	Negative	Negative	Negative	*A. platys*
15	21	12,900	116,000	Negative	Negative	Negative	Negative	Negative	Negative
16	27	14,800	148,000	Positive	*Ehrlichia* spp.	Negative	Negative	Negative	Negative
17	35	10,000	*	Negative	Negative	Negative	Negative	Negative	Negative
18	31	—	44,400	Negative	Negative	Negative	Negative	Negative	Negative
19	31	27,100	408,000	Positive	*Ehrlichia* spp.	Negative	Negative	Negative	Negative
20	41	13,100	277,920	Positive	*Ehrlichia* spp.	Negative	Negative	Negative	Negative
21	42	21,900	21,900	Negative	*E. canis*	Negative	*E. canis*	*E. canis*	Negative

ID: Identification; RV: reference value (Jain, [15]); *not performed; **Packed cell volume (RV: 37–55%); ***Leukocytes ($\times 10^3/\mu L$; RV: 6–17); ****Platelets ($\times 10^5/\mu L$; RV: 2–5).

As expected, our study demonstrates that nPCR is more sensitive for detecting *Ehrlichia* than the direct examination of stained blood smears of dogs with suggestive clinical signs. Our results show that a 50% false negative rate may occur when only direct examination is used for diagnosis. In contrast, all animals with morulae in the blood smears were positive by nPCR for at least one of the WB or fraction samples.

The nPCR was able to detect *Ehrlichia* or *Anaplasma* DNA in 71% of the samples from dogs with suggestive clinical signs. This rate is slightly higher than that registered elsewhere in Brazil [1, 5, 12]. As previously reported [1, 5], *E. canis* (46.6%) positivity in WB was higher than for *A. platys* (6.6%).

In seven (46.6%) of the samples, there was no amplification in the second PCR, and the positives were recorded as *Ehrlichia* spp. As the primers used were specific for *E. canis* and *A. platys*, the presence of other Rickettsiales, such as *A. phagocytophilum*, *E. chaffeensis*, and *E. ewingii*, should not be disregarded because they can also form cytoplasmic inclusions [18, 19]. Furthermore *E. ewingii* was already reported in dogs in Brazil [20].

Coinfection with *E. canis* and *A. platys* was observed in an animal with a positive blood smear and that was positive for *E. canis* in the WB sample by nPCR. Cytoplasmic inclusions in the platelets were not observed, possibly due to low *A. platys* load [7]. It is worth mentioning that this is the first evidence for the involvement of *A. platys* in canine anaplasmosis in the State of Paraiba, Brazil.

The blood fraction samples that were positive for *A. platys* by nPCR were WB and C (dog no. 14) and B and C (dog no. 12). Despite the small sample size, the results suggest an increased likelihood of finding *A. platys* DNA in the BC fraction, which is more enriched with platelets than the other samples.

Contrary to previous reports [21, 22], we found that there was no statistical association between thrombocytopenia ($P = 0.596$), anemia ($P = 0.299$), and the WB nPCR results. Similar to a previous report [1], anemia occurred in only 26.6% cases. These results demonstrate that thrombocytopenia is not sufficient to diagnose either canine ehrlichiosis or anaplasmosis. Santos et al. [22] also observed a high incidence of *E. canis* infection among nonthrombocytopenic dogs. In contrast, other diseases including immune-mediated thrombocytopenia, neoplasia, inflammatory diseases, or other infectious agents can provoke thrombocytopenia [23]. The differences in prevalence may reflect the diversity in strain pathogenicity or a selection bias because thrombocytopenic dogs are more likely to be tested for ehrlichiosis.

Peripheral blood has been the main source of *Ehrlichia* DNA for PCR assays because collection of this sample is less invasive than spleen and bone marrow collection. The use of serum samples for nPCR to detect *E. canis* has been suggested previously [24]. Our results support that whole blood is the best source for *Ehrlichia* DNA in PCR assays. Indeed, the Kappa value indicates a weak correlation between nPCR results from the WB samples and those obtained with the G, M, BC, or C samples; the PCR sensitivity from the M and B samples was only 42.9%. Therefore, our data and the literature support the use of WB as the best choice for DNA source for PCR *Ehrlichia* spp. detection.

This is the first assessment of the use of different blood cell fractions as DNA sources to diagnose canine ehrlichiosis and anaplasmosis by PCR. Although the pathogens only infect leukocytes and platelets, WB is a better DNA source than any of the cellular *Ehrlichia*-enriched host cell fractions. A possible explanation may be based on the assumption that WB samples contain not only intracellular *Ehrlichia* but also organisms released by host cell lysis that are not found in the fractions. In support of this hypothesis, the 16S rRNA gene was successfully amplified by Mylonakis et al. [25] by nPCR in sera samples from naturally infected dogs. Hence, these authors recommend serum-based PCR analysis for the early diagnosis of CME when WB samples are not available. Furthermore, it was demonstrated that *E. chaffeensis* reached concentrations of $\sim 10^8$ bacteria/mL in the plasma of SCID mice two weeks after infection [26]. There are no similar studies for *E. canis* or *A. platys*, but it is reasonable to assume that a similar scenario occurs in dogs infected with these pathogens, especially in the acute phase of the disease, when symptoms are severe, and platelet counts are usually reduced.

In conclusion, the present study demonstrates that canine WB is better than other cellular blood fractions as a DNA source to detect *Ehrlichia* and *Anaplasma* by PCR, most likely because of the bacterial concentration in the plasma following host cell lysis.

Conflict of Interests

The authors declare that they have no conflict of interests.

Acknowledgments

This work was supported by the Brazilian National Research Council (CNPq) and by the State of Pernambuco Research Foundation (FACEPE). It was Financially supported by the *Fundação de Amparo à Ciência e Tecnologia do Estado de Pernambuco* (FACEPE). T. E. F. Rotondano was a FACEPE fellow during the development of this study. The authors thank the Laboratório de Diagnóstico Molecular (UNESP), Botucatu, SP, Brazil for testing the samples.

References

[1] A. S. Dagnone, A. I. Souza, M. R. André, and R. Z. Machado, "Molecular diagnosis of Anaplasmataceae organisms in dogs with clinical and microscopical signs of ehrlichiosis," *Revista Brasileira de Parasitologia Veterinaria*, vol. 18, no. 4, pp. 20–25, 2009.

[2] L. A. Cohn, "Ehrlichiosis and related infections," *Veterinary Clinics of North America*, vol. 33, no. 4, pp. 863–884, 2003.

[3] F. Dantas-Torres, L. A. Figueredo, and S. P. Brandão-Filho, "*Rhipicephalus sanguineus* (Acari: Ixodidae), the brown dog tick, parasitizing humans in Brazil," *Revista da Sociedade Brasileira de Medicina Tropical*, vol. 39, no. 1, pp. 64–67, 2006.

[4] L. T. M. Figueiredo, S. J. Badra, L. E. Pereira, and M. P. J. Szabó, "Report on ticks collected in the Southeast and Mid-West regions of Brazil: analyzing the potential transmission of tick-borne pathogens to man," *Revista da Sociedade Brasileira de Medicina Tropical*, vol. 32, no. 6, pp. 613–619, 1999.

[5] C. A. N. Ramos, R. A. N. Ramos, F. R. Araújo, D. S. Guedes Jr., and I. I. F. Souza, "Ono TM. Comparação de nested-PCR com o diagnóstico direto na detecção de *Ehrlichia canis* e *Anaplasma platys* em cães," *Revista Brasileira De Parasitologia Veterinária*, vol. 18, pp. 58–62, 2009.

[6] H. F. Cadman, P. J. Kelly, L. A. Matthewman, R. Zhou, and P. R. Mason, "Comparison of the dot-blot enzyme linked immunoassay with immunofluorescence for detecting antibodies to *Ehrlichia canis*," *Veterinary Record*, vol. 135, no. 15, p. 362, 1994.

[7] C. Arraga-Alvarado, M. Palmar, O. Parra, and P. Salas, "*Ehrlichia platys* (*Anaplasma platys*) in dogs from Maracaibo, Venezuela: an ultrastructural study of experimental and natural infections," *Veterinary Pathology*, vol. 40, no. 2, pp. 149–156, 2003.

[8] T. Waner, S. Harrus, F. Jongejan, H. Bark, A. Keysary, and A. W. C. A. Cornelissen, "Significance of serological testing for ehrlichial diseases in dogs with special emphasis on the diagnosis of canine monocytic ehrlichiosis caused by *Ehrlichia canis*," *Veterinary Parasitology*, vol. 95, no. 1, pp. 1–15, 2001.

[9] Z. Iqbal, W. Chaichanasiriwithaya, and Y. Rikihisa, "Comparison of PCR with other tests for early diagnosis of canine ehrlichiosis," *Journal of Clinical Microbiology*, vol. 32, no. 7, pp. 1658–1662, 1994.

[10] R. W. Stich, Y. Rikihisa, S. A. Ewing, G. R. Needham, D. L. Grover, and S. Jittapalapong, "Detection of *Ehrlichia canis* in canine carrier blood and in individual experimentally infected ticks with a p30-based PCR assay," *Journal of Clinical Microbiology*, vol. 40, no. 2, pp. 540–546, 2002.

[11] S. Harrus and T. Waner, "Diagnosis of canine monocytotropic ehrlichiosis (*Ehrlichia canis*): an overview," *Veterinary Journal*, vol. 187, no. 3, pp. 292–296, 2011.

[12] A. C. H. Nakaghi, R. Z. Machado, M. R. André, C. D. Baldani, and M. T. Costa, "Canine ehrlichiosis: clinical, hematological, serological and molecular aspects," *Ciencia Rural*, vol. 38, no. 3, pp. 766–770, 2008.

[13] J. E. Dawson, D. E. Stallknecht, E. W. Howerth et al., "Susceptibility of white-tailed deer (*Odocoileus virginianus*) to infection with *Ehrlichia chaffeensis*, the etiologic agent of human ehrlichiosis," *Journal of Clinical Microbiology*, vol. 32, no. 11, pp. 2725–2728, 1994.

[14] B. Wen, Y. Rikihisa, J. M. Mott et al., "Comparison of nested PCR with immunofluorescent-antibody assay for detection of *Ehrlichia canis* infection in dogs treated with doxycycline," *Journal of Clinical Microbiology*, vol. 35, no. 7, pp. 1852–1855, 1997.

[15] N. C. Jain, *Essentials of Veterinary Hematology*, Lea & Febiger, Philadelphia, Pa, USA, 1993.

[16] A. Mackinnon, "A spreadsheet for the calculation of comprehensive statistics for the assessment of diagnostic tests and inter-rater agreement," *Computers in Biology and Medicine*, vol. 30, no. 3, pp. 127–134, 2000.

[17] M. T. E. P. Allsopp and B. A. Allsopp, "Novel *Ehrlichia* genotype detected in dogs in South Africa," *Journal of Clinical Microbiology*, vol. 39, no. 11, pp. 4204–4207, 2001.

[18] R. F. Ferreira, A. M. F. Cerqueira, A. M. Pereira et al., "*Anaplasma platys* diagnosis in dogs: comparison between morphological and molecular tests," *Journal of Applied Research in Veterinary Medicine*, vol. 5, pp. 113–119, 2007.

[19] Y. Rikihisa, "Diagnosis of emerging ehrlichial diseases of dogs, horses, and humans," *Journal of Veterinary Internal Medicine*, vol. 14, no. 3, pp. 250–251, 2000.

[20] L. S. Oliveira, K. A. Oliveira, L. C. Mourão et al., "First report of *Ehrlichia ewingii* detected by molecular investigation in dogs from Brazil," *Clinical Microbiology and Infection*, vol. 15, no. 2, pp. 55–56, 2009.

[21] C. Bulla, R. K. Takahira, J. P. Araújo Jr., L. A. Trinca, R. S. Lopes, and C. E. Wiedmeyer, "The relationship between the degree of thrombocytopenia and infection with *Ehrlichia canis* in an endemic area," *Veterinary Research*, vol. 35, no. 1, pp. 141–146, 2004.

[22] F. Santos, J. S. Coppede, A. L. A. Pereira et al., "Molecular evaluation of the incidence of *Ehrlichia canis, Anaplasma platys* and *Babesia* spp. in dogs from Ribeirão Preto, Brazil," *Veterinary Journal*, vol. 179, no. 1, pp. 145–148, 2009.

[23] C. B. Grindem, E. B. Breitschwerdt, W. T. Corbett, and H. E. Jans, "Epidemiologic survey of thrombocytopenia in dogs: a report on 987 cases.," *Veterinary Clinical Pathology*, vol. 20, pp. 38–43, 2002.

[24] M. E. Mylonakis, V. I. Siarkou, L. Leontides, E. Bourtzi-Hatzopoulou, V. I. Kontos, and A. F. Koutinas, "Evaluation of a serum-based PCR assay for the diagnosis of canine monocytic ehrlichiosis," *Veterinary Microbiology*, vol. 138, no. 3-4, pp. 390–393, 2009.

[25] M. E. Mylonakis, A. F. Koutinas, C. Billinis et al., "Evaluation of cytology in the diagnosis of acute canine monocytic ehrlichiosis (*Ehrlichia canis*): a comparison between five methods," *Veterinary Microbiology*, vol. 91, no. 2-3, pp. 197–204, 2003.

[26] J. S. Li and G. M. Winslow, "Survival, replication, and antibody susceptibility of *Ehrlichia chaffeensis* outside of host cells," *Infection and Immunity*, vol. 71, no. 8, pp. 4229–4237, 2003.

Shiga Toxin-Producing *Escherichia coli* Isolated from Bovine Mastitic Milk: Serogroups, Virulence Factors, and Antibiotic Resistance Properties

Hassan Momtaz,[1] Farhad Safarpoor Dehkordi,[2] Taghi Taktaz,[3] Amir Rezvani,[4] and Sajad Yarali[4]

[1] *Department of Microbiology, College of Veterinary Medicine, Islamic Azad University, Shahrekord Branch, P.O. Box 166, Shahrekord, Iran*
[2] *Young Researchers Club, Islamic Azad University, Shahrekord Branch, P.O. Box 166, Shahrekord, Iran*
[3] *Department of Clinical Sciences, College of Veterinary Medicine, Islamic Azad University, Shahrekord Branch, P.O. Box 166, Shahrekord, Iran*
[4] *College of Veterinary Medicine, Islamic Azad University, Shahrekord Branch, P.O. Box 166, Shahrekord, Iran*

Correspondence should be addressed to Hassan Momtaz, hamomtaz@yahoo.com

Academic Editors: C. DebRoy and G. Leitner

The aim of this study was to detect the virulence factors, serogroups, and antibiotic resistance properties of Shiga toxin-producing *Escherichia coli*, by using 268 bovine mastitic milk samples which were diagnosed using California Mastitis Test. After *E. coli* identification, PCR assays were developed for detection of different virulence genes, serogroups, and antibiotic resistance genes of *Escherichia coli*. The antibiotic resistance pattern was studied using disk diffusion method. Out of 268 samples, 73 (27.23%) were positive for *Escherichia coli*, and, out of 73 positive samples, 15 (20.54%) were O26 and 11 (15.06%) were O157 so they were the highest while O111 was not detected in any sample so it was the lowest serogroup. Out of 73 STEC strains, 11 (15.06%) and 36 (49.31%) were EHEC and AEEC, respectively. All of the EHEC strains had *stx1*, *eaeA*, and *ehly*, virulence genes, while in AEEC strains *stx1* had the highest prevalence (77.77%), followed by *eaeA* (55.55%). Totally, *aadA1* (65.95%) had the highest while *blaSHV* (6.38%) had the lowest prevalence of antibiotic resistance genes. The disk diffusion method showed that the STEC strains had the highest resistance to penicillin (100%), followed by tetracycline (57.44%), while resistance to cephalothin (6.38%) was the lowest.

1. Introduction

Milk is raised as a complete food especially for children and seniors. Its high value for proteins, minerals, fats, and vitamins is undeniable. It is the primary source of nutrition for young mammals before they are able to digest other types of foods. In addition, milk has been processed into various dairy products such as cheese, cream, butter, yogurt, kefir, and ice cream. Daily, millions of people use milk and dairy products. Milk production has a complex process which is done due to activity of bovine mammary glands. The hygienic quality of milking room and animals has a high importance in milk production, but in cases of low hygienic conditions several infections and illnesses occurred in udder tissue.

Mastitis is considered the most costly disease in dairy herds due to discarded milk and lowered milk production for approximately 80% of costs associated with mastitis, treatment costs, veterinary fees, labor costs early culling, and death [1]. In addition, lowered milk quality due to increased somatic cell count (SCC) in the milk decreases shelf life of milk and cheese making quality [2]. Previous study showed that bacteremia occurs in a significant proportion of cows with severe systemic disease signs [3]. Besides, the quality and hygiene of milk are changed due to mastitis and usually cannot be used for human and animal consumption. Usually in all mastitic cases the amount of milk production reduced. An increase of 25% on world milk demand between 2007 and 2020 is expected [4]. Dairy cattle with acute coliform mastitis, caused primarily by *Escherichia coli* (*E. coli*), exhibit a wide range of systemic disease severity, from mild, with only local inflammatory changes of the mammary gland, to severe, with significant systemic signs including rumen stasis, dehydration, shock, and even death [3].

E. coli strains can further be classified according to the presence of virulence factors such as enterohemorrhagic *E. coli* (EHEC), enterotoxigenic *E. coli* (ETEC), enteropathogenic *E. coli* (EPEC), attaching and effacing *E. coli* (AEEC), and Shiga toxin-producing *E. coli* (STEC or VTEC) [5–8]. Several studies showed that STEC strains are an important group for mastitis [9, 10].

Previous study showed that, from all serogroups of STEC strains, O55. O111, O124, O119, O114, O26, O157, and O44 are the most prevalent serotypes of *E. coli* isolated from mastitic milk [1]. Numerous studies to identify virulence factors of *E. coli* isolated from cows with clinical mastitis have been conducted [11]. Studies showed that Shiga toxins (*Stx1*, *Stx2*) and *eae* (intimin) are the most important virulence genes in *E. coli* strains isolated from bovine mastitic milk [10, 12, 13]. The cytotoxic necrotizing factor (*CNF*) toxins (*CNF1* and *CNF2* genes) are associated with damage to vascular endothelial cells and thrombotic microangiopathy.

Mainly, treatment of diseases caused by this bacterium often requires antimicrobial therapy; however, antibiotic-resistant strains of bacteria cause more severe diseases for longer periods of time than their antibiotic-susceptible counterparts. Several studies showed that antibiotic resistant in *E. coli* is increasing in these days [14–16]. Therefore, identification of resistance genes of bacteria seems to be so essential in reduction of treatment costs. There is no previous data about detection of virulence genes, serotypes, and antimicrobial resistance of *E. coli* strains isolated from cow in Iran so this present study was carried out for molecular characterization of STEC strains isolated from bovine mastitic milk.

2. Materials and Methods

2.1. Sampling and Detecting E. coli. Overall 268 bovine mastitic raw milk samples were collected from centers from several geographic regions of Iran, from January 2011 to March 2012. The animals selected for this study were clinically healthy, and the milk samples showed normal physical characteristics. In this study, mastitic milks were identified by the California Mastitis Test (CMT). Samples (5 mL, in sterile glass containers) were transported to the laboratory at ca. 4°C within a maximum of 6–12 h after sampling.

Samples were cultured in MacConkey (MAC) agar (Merck, Germany). Agar plates were incubated at 37°C, and bacterial growth was evaluated after 24 and 48 h. Gram-negative microorganisms were isolated from MAC agar and determined at the species level using cytochrome oxidase, triple sugar iron agar, urea, and indole tests as putatively *E. coli* [17].

2.2. DNA Isolation. Bacterial strains were overnight grown in trypticase soy agar (TSA-Merck, German) at 37°C. One colony was suspended in 100 μL of sterile distilled water. After boiling the suspension for 13 min; this was followed by freezing and subsequently centrifuged at 14,000 rpm for 15 min to pellet the cell debris [18]. The supernatant was used as a template for amplification reaction.

2.3. Polymerase Chain Reaction. Tables 1, 2, and 3 showed the list of primers which were used for detection of serogroups, virulence genes, and antibiotic resistance genes of STEC strains isolated from mastitic milk samples. Table 4 showed the PCR conditions for detection of serogroups, virulence genes, and antimicrobial resistance genes in STEC strains isolated from bovine mastitic milk samples. In all PCR reactions, a DNA thermocycler (Eppendorf Mastercycler, Eppendorf-Nethel-Hinz GmbH, Hamburg, Germany) was used. The amplified products were visualized by ethidium bromide staining after gel electrophoresis of 10 μL of the final reaction mixture in 1.5% agarose.

2.4. Antimicrobial Susceptibility Testing. Antimicrobial susceptibility tests was performed by the Kirby-Bauer disc diffusion method using Mueller-Hinton agar (HiMedia Laboratories, Mumbai, India, MV1084), according to the Clinical and Laboratory Standards Institute guidelines (CLSI) [19]. After incubating the inoculated plate aerobically at 37°C for 18–24 h in an aerobic atmosphere, the susceptibility of the *E. coli* isolates to each antimicrobial agent was measured and the results were interpreted in accordance with interpretive criteria provided by CLSI (2006). *E. coli* ATCC 25922 was used as quality control organisms in antimicrobial susceptibility determination.

2.5. Statistical Analysis. Statistical analysis was performed using *SPSS/16.0* software for significant relationship between incidences of virulence factors and antibiotics resistance genes of *E. coli* isolated from various dairy products. Statistical significance was regarded at a P value < 0.05.

3. Results

In the current study, all *E. coli* colonies were tested by applying PCR method in order to detect 16S rRNA gene of bacterium. According to data, out of 268 bovine mastitic milk samples, 73 (27.23%) were positive for presence of *E. coli* (Table 5). Therefore, it was shown that incidence of *E. coli* in bovine mastitic milk was high. From a total of 73 *E. coli* positive samples, 36 (49.31%) were AEEC and 11 (15.06%) were EHEC subtypes (Table 6). In the other hand, 26 samples (35.61%) were diagnosed as nondetected serotypes (Table 6). Results showed that all of the 11 positive EHEC serogroups had *stx1, eaeA, ehly* virulence genes, while in AEEC serogroups, 28 (77.77%), 5 (13.88%), and 20 (55.55%) samples had *stx1*, *stx2*, and *eaeA* virulence genes,

Table 1: Primers used for detection of virulence genes in Shiga toxin-producing *Escherichia coli* isolated from bovine mastitis.

Virulence factor	Primers name	Primer sequences (5′-3′)	Product size (bp)	Reference
Shiga toxin 1 (*stx1*)	Stx1f	AAATCGCCATTCGTTGACTACTTCT	366	[20]
	Stx1r	TGCCATTCTGGCAACTCGCGATGCA		
Shiga toxin 2 (*stx2*)	Stx2f	CGATCGTCACTCACTGGTTTCATCA	282	[20]
	Stx2r	GGATATTCTCCCCACTCTGACACC		
Enteropathogenic attachment and effacement (*eaeA*)	EAE1	TGCGGCACAACAGGCGGCGA	629	[21]
	EAE2	CGGTCGCCGCACCAGGATTC		
Haemolysin (*ehly*)	Hly F	CAATGCAGATGCAGATACCG	432	[22]
	Hly R	CAGAGATGTCGTTGCAGCAG		

Table 2: Primers used for detection of Shiga toxin-producing *Escherichia coli* serogroups isolated from bovine mastitis.

Primer name	Sequence	Size of product (bp)	Target gene	Reference
O26-F O26-R	CAG AAT GGT TAT GCT ACT GT CTT ACA TTT GTT TTC GGC ATC	423	*wzx*	[23]
O103-F O103-R	TTGGAGCGTTAACTGGACCT GCTCCCGAGCACGTATAAG	321	*wzx*	[23]
O111-F O111-R	TAG AGA AAT TAT CAA GTT AGT TCC ATA GTT ATG AAC ATC TTG TTT AGC	406	*wzx*	[23]
O145-F O145-R	CCATCAACAGATTTAGGAGTG TTTCTACCGCGAATCTATC	609	*wzx*	[23]
O157-F O157-R	CGG ACA TCC ATG TGA TAT GG TTG CCT ATG TAC AGC TAA TCC	259	*wzx*	[23]
O45-F O45-R	CCG GGT TTC GAT TTG TGA AGG TTG CAC AAC AGC CAC TAC TAG GCA GAA	527	*wzx1*	[24]
O91-F O91-R	GCTGACCTTCATGATCTGTTGA TAATTTAACCCGTAGAATCGCTGC	291	*gnd*	[25]
O113-F O113-R	GGGTTAGATGGAGCGCTATTGAGA AGGTCACCCTCTGAATTATGGCAG	771	*wzx*	[26]
O121-F O121-R	TGGCTAGTGGCATTCTGATG TGATACTTTAGCCGCCCTTG	322	*wzx*	[27]
O128-F O128-R	GCTTTCTGCCGATATTTGGC CCGACGGACTGATGCCGGTGATT	289	*galF*	[28]

respectively (Table 6). Significant differences ($P < 0.05$) were shown between the presences of AEEC and EHEC serogroups in mastitic milk samples.

By applying specific primers for detection of STEC serogroups in mastitic milk samples, it was indicated that, out of 73 positive samples for *E. coli*, 15 (20.54%) and 11 (15.06%) samples were positive for incidences of O26 and O157 serogroups while O111, O45, O121, and O128 serogroups had a lower incidences (0.0%, 2.73%, 2.73%, and 2.73%, resp.) (Table 7). In the other hand, 26 (35.61%) samples have been determined as nondetected serogroups. Statistical analysis of data indicated significant differences ($P < 0.05$) between total presence of O26 with O111, O45, O121, and O128 serogroups.

Distribution of antimicrobial resistance genes in Shiga toxin-producing *Escherichia coli* serogroups isolated from bovine mastitis showed that *aadA1* had the highest prevalence of antibiotic resistance genes (65.95%), followed by *SulI* (57.44%) and *dfrA1* (55.31%) while *blaSHV* (6.38%) and *CITM* (12.76%) had the lowest incidence of antibiotic resistance genes (Table 8). Besides, O26 serotype had the highest incidence of antibiotic resistance genes while O111 had the lowest incidence of antibiotic resistance genes in *E. coli* isolated from mastitic milk samples. Statistical analysis of data indicated significant differences ($P < 0.05$) between total presence of *aadA1* with *blaSHV*, *CITM* and *cmlA*, *SulI* with *blaSHV*, *CITM* and *dfrA1* with *blaSHV* gene.

The disk diffusion method indicated that the STEC serogroups had the highest resistance to penicillin (100%), followed by tetracycline (57.44%), lincomycin (55.31%), streptomycin (48.93%), ampicillin (46.80%), and sulfamethoxazole, (40.42%) but resistance to cephalothin (6.38%),

Table 3: Primers used for detection of antimicrobial resistant genes in Shiga toxin-producing *Escherichia coli* isolated from bovine mastitis.

Antibiotic	Resistant gene	Sequence	Size of product (bp)	Annealing temperature (°C)	References
Streptomycin	*aadA1*	(F) TATCCAGCTAAGCGCGAACT (R) ATTTGCCGACTACCTTGGTC	447	58	[29]
Tetracycline	*tetA*	(F) GGTTCACTCGAACGACGTCA (R) CTGTCCGACAAGTTGCATGA	577	57	[29]
Tetracycline	*tetB*	(F) CCTCAGCTTCTCAACGCGTG (R) GCACCTTGCTGATGACTCTT	634	56	[29]
Trimethoprim	*dfrA1*	(F) GGAGTGCCAAAGGTGAACAGC (R) GAGGCGAAGTCTTGGGTAAAAAC	367	45	[30]
Fluoroquinolone	*qnr*	(F) GGGTATGGATATTATTGATAAAG (R) CTAATCCGGCAGCACTATTTA	670	50	[31]
Gentamicin	*aac(3)-IV*	(F) CTTCAGGATGGCAAGTTGGT (R) TCATCTCGTTCTCCGCTCAT	286	55	[32]
Sulfonamide	*sul1*	(F) TTCGGCATTCTGAATCTCAC (R) ATGATCTAACCCTCGGTCTC	822	47	[32]
Cephalothin	*blaSHV*	(F) TCGCCTGTGTATTATCTCCC (R) CGCAGATAAATCACCACAATG	768	52	[32]
Ampicillin	*CITM*	(F) TGGCCAGAACTGACAGGCAAA (R) TTTCTCCTGAACGTGGCTGGC	462	47	[32]
Chloramphenicol	*cat1*	(F) AGTTGCTCAATGTACCTATAACC (R) TTGTAATTCATTAAGCATTCTGCC	547	55	[32]
Chloramphenicol	*cmlA*	(F) CCGCCACGGTGTTGTTGTTATC (R) CACCTTGCCTGCCCATCATTAG	698	55	[32]

ciprofloxacin (10.63%), and nitrofurantoin (10.63%) was the lowest (Table 9). Significant differences were seen between level of resistance to penicillin with cephalothin, ciprofloxacin, and nitrofurantoin ($P < 0.05$) and tetracycline and lincomycin only with cephalothin.

4. Discussion

Our results showed that the STEC strains can cause mastitis in bovine and reduce milk quality for human consumption because some of mastitic cases are subclinical and its diagnosis only is based on the accurate diagnostic tests. Therefore, application of accurate and sensitive assays for detection of subclinical mastitic milks is essential. The rules of milk inspection and control are more important in cases where raw milk is consumed. Several outbreaks of diseases due to *E. coli* [33, 34] showed that inspection and control of food and especially foods with animal origin is a golden key to reducing the risk of contamination.

There are many studies which showed that the STEC strains are the most prevalent resources for milk-poisoning [7, 35, 36]. Our results showed that the milk of animals with mastitis and especially subclinical mastitis is the main resource for STEC strains. In addition to unsanitary conditions in milk collection and processing, methods of milking, unsanitary conditions of milking machine, and preventing contamination of raw milk with extrinsic factors like staff, insects, and dust, the primary hygiene of milk can be important in presences of STEC strains in milk. Unfortunately, the mechanism of mastitis in bovine herds is not clear. *E. coli* is one of the most frequent bacteria in the environments and, following parturition and the onset of lactation, the immune system is less able to react appropriately to bacterial challenges. Therefore, mastitis occurred due to *E. coli*. A combination of metabolic and hormonal influences may temporarily suppress the immune system in the periparturient period. Additionally, the altered nutritional and energy demands that occur in the periparturient cow during the last trimester and early lactation increase fat metabolism, leading to a buildup of ketone metabolites (ketosis), which also negatively impact the microbicidal properties of circulating neutrophils and increase the cow's susceptibility to mastitis [37]. This temporary and transient immunosuppression increases the cow's susceptibility to opportunistic organisms and increases the likelihood for environmental bacteria to invade the udder and cause mastitis [37, 38].

Our results showed that 27.23% of all milk samples were positive for presence of *E. coli* and from these positive samples, O26 serogroup, *stx1* gene, *aadA1* antibiotic resistance

TABLE 4: PCR conditions for detection of serogroups, virulence genes and antimicrobial resistance genes in Shiga toxin-producing *Escherichia coli* in bovine mastitis.

Gene	PCR program	PCR volume (50 μL)
O157, O145, O103, O26, O111	1 cycle: 95°C—3 min 30 cycle: 95°C—20 s 58°C—40 s 72°C—30 s 1 cycle: 72°C—8 min	5 μL PCR buffer 10X 1.5 mM $MgCl_2$ 200 μM dNTP (Fermentas) 0.5 μM of each primers F and R 1.25 U Taq DNA polymerase (Fermentas) 2.5 μL DNA template
O91, O128, O121, O113, O45	1 cycle: 94°C—6 min 34 cycle: 95°C—50 s 58°C—70 s 72°C—55 s 1 cycle: 72°C—10 min	5 μL PCR buffer 10X 2 mM $MgCl_2$ 150 μM dNTP (Fermentas) 0.75 μM of each primers F and R 1.5 U Taq DNA polymerase (Fermentas) 3 μL DNA template
stx1, stx2, eaeA, ehly	1 cycle: 95°C—3 min 34 cycle: 94°C—60 s 56°C—45 s 72°C—60 s 1 cycle: 72°C—10 min	5 μL PCR buffer 10X 2 mM $MgCl_2$ 200 μM dNTP (Fermentas) 0.5 μM of each primers F and R 1.5 U Taq DNA polymerase (Fermentas) 5 μL DNA template
aadA1, tetA, tetB, dfrA1, qnr, aac(3)-IV, sul1, blaSHV, CITM, cat1, cmlA	1 cycle: 94°C—8 min 32 cycle: 95°C—60 s 55°C—70 s 72°C—2 min 1 cycle: 72°C—8 min	5 μL PCR buffer 10X 2.5 mM $MgCl_2$ 200 μM dNTP (Fermentas) 0.5 μM of each primers F and R 2 U Taq DNA polymerase (Fermentas) 3 μL DNA template

TABLE 5: Prevalence of *Escherichia coli* isolated from bovine mastitis.

Number of samples	Number of positive samples
268	73 (27.23%)

gene, and resistance to penicillin antibiotic have the highest frequencies in bovine mastitic milk samples. Previous study [1] showed that, from a total of 181 mastitic milk samples, 57 were positive for *E. coli* and, from these numbers, 19.2%, 15.8%, 12.3%, 12.3%, 10.5%, 7%, 7%, and 3.5% were O55, O111, O124, O119, O114, O26, O157, and O44 serogroups which was inconsistent with our results. Another study [39] showed that, from 40 mastitic milk samples, 77.4% of the isolates belonged to four different O serogroups (O26, O86, O111, and O127) which was in agreement with our results.

TABLE 6: Distribution of virulence factors in *Escherichia coli* subtypes isolated from bovine mastitis.

Subtypes	Number of positive samples	Virulence gene
Nondetected	26 (35.61%)	—
EHEC	11 (15.06%)	*stx1, eaeA, ehly: 11* (100%)
AEEC	36 (49.31%)	*stx1: 28* (77.77%) *stx2: 5* (13.88%) *eaeA: 20* (55.55%) *stx1, eaeA: 23* (63.88%) *stx2, eaeA: 8* (22.22%) *stx1, stx2, eaeA: 5* (13.88%)
Total	73 (27.23%)	

Bean et al. [40] evaluated the "health status" of cows from which isolates were obtained to study virulence genes. In addition to it, in the majority of cases, presence of STEC strains is related to attendance of various virulence genes. Previous study in Egypt [39] revealed that all *E. coli* strains which were isolated from mastitic milk samples had *stx1*, *stx2*, *hylA*, *Flic(h7)*, *stb*, *F41*, *K99*, *sta*, *F17*, *LT-I*, *LT-II*, and *eaeA* virulence genes. Another study confirmed that the *stx2* and *eaeA* genes were the most prevalent virulence factors in cow's environment that is contaminated by feces, and it is also a frequent cause of bovine mastitis [41]. Study in Turkey indicated that genes encoding Shiga toxins 1 and 2 (*stx1* and *stx2*), intimin (*eaeA*), heat-stable enterotoxin a (*Sta*), and F5 (K99), F41, and F17 fimbriae were the most prevalent virulence factors which were isolated from clinical bovine mastitis cases [9].

Previous study from Iran showed that out of 400 samples, 42 specimens were found to be *E. coli* positive and 14 out of 42 isolates carried the *eaeA* gene, 4 isolates were positive for the gene of F41fimbriae and 10 for *stxI* and *stxII* genes [42]. Another investigation on mastitic milk samples during 17 months showed that the most common virulence gene detected was *stx1*, with a prevalence of 31%, followed by *cnf2* (7.5%), *vt2e* (6.25%), and *eaeA* (4%) which was in agreement with our study [40].

Some studies indicated that, in addition to virulence genes like *stx1*, *stx2*, *eae*, and *ehly*, the presence of STEC strains is mainly accompanied by attendance of antibiotic resistance genes [11, 43]. Unfortunately studying of the antibiotic resistance genes in *E. coli* strains isolated from mastic milk samples has been done very rare. In one study, of the 123 *E. coli* strains isolated from milk, 15 (10.7%) had a single virulence gene detected by PCR and *CNF2* is the most common virulence gene which was identified [11], but our study showed that the *aadA1* was the most common virulence gene in mastitic milk samples (65.95%). Another study showed that S and P fimbriae, *CNF1*, and *CNF2* are the most common virulence genes in *E. coli* isolated from mastitic milk samples [44]. Despite the presence of these numerous antibiotic resistance genes in *E. coli* strains isolated from mastitic milk samples,

Table 7: Prevalence of Shiga toxin-producing *Escherichia coli* serogroups isolated from bovine mastitis.

Serogroup	O157	O26	O103	O111	O145	O45	O91	O113	O121	O128	Nondetected
Total (73)	11 (15.06%)	15 (20.54%)	3 (4.10%)	— —	3 (4.10%)	2 (2.73%)	6 (8.21%)	3 (4.10%)	2 (2.73%)	2 (2.73%)	26 (35.61%)

Table 8: Distribution of antimicrobial resistance genes in Shiga toxin-producing *Escherichia coli* serogroups isolated from bovine mastitis.

	aadA1	*tetA*	*tetB*	*dfrA1*	*qnr*	*aac(3)-IV*	*sul1*	*blaSHV*	*CITM*	*cat1*	*cmlA*
O157 (11)	7	6	4	5	6	2	9	1	1	3	2
O26 (15)	12	8	3	7	5	3	6	—	1	5	2
O103 (3)	2	1	2	3	—	2	3	—	—	2	—
O111 (-)	—	—	—	—	—	—	—	—	—	—	—
O145 (3)	2	2	1	2	1	—	1	—	—	1	1
O45 (2)	1	1	1	—	1	—	—	—	1	2	—
O91 (6)	4	3	2	4	2	4	4	2	—	2	—
O113 (3)	2	2	—	3	—	2	2	—	1	1	1
O121 (2)	1	—	1	1	1	—	2	—	2	—	1
O128 (2)	—	—	2	1	1	—	—	—	—	—	—
Total (47)	31 (65.95%)	23 (48.93%)	16 (34.04%)	26 (55.31%)	17 (36.17%)	13 (27.65%)	27 (57.44%)	3 (6.38%)	6 (12.76%)	16 (34.04%)	7 (14.89%)

developing resistance against common antibiotic drugs is not unexpected. Our results showed that resistance to penicillin, tetracycline, and lincomycin was the highest, while previous study showed that the predominantly observed resistance was to tetracycline (92.2%), streptomycin (90.4%), nalidixic acid (88.3%), amikacin (86.5%), and cephalothin (84.8%). Multidrug resistance was found among 152 isolates (65.8%) [36]. Langoni et al. [45] reported a discrete level of resistance to tetracycline (13.0%) and ampicillin (12.0%) among *E. coli* isolates from bovine mastitis which was lower than our results. Studies performed in the United States indicate that there is no correlation among increased resistance and antimicrobials that are commonly used in dairy cattle for treatment of mastitis [46, 47]. In Switzerland [48], there was no increased antibiotic resistance of mastitis pathogens during the last 20 years, indicating different points of view about this theme. Our results are in contrast with previous study in Switzerland and, in addition to common used antibiotics, the *E. coli* strains which were isolated from mastitic milk samples in our study even had resistance to chloramphenicol and nitrofurantoin. Chloramphenicol and nitrofurantoin are forbidden antibiotics, and the high antibiotic resistance to them in our study indicated the irregular and unauthorized uses of these antibiotics in veterinary treatment in Iran. Unfortunately, veterinarians in many fields of veterinary such as large animal internal medicine, poultry, and even aquaculture use these antibiotics as a basic one. Therefore, in a very short period of time, antibiotic resistance will appear. Therefore, prescription of antibiotics and prescribed antibiotics has the highest effects on providing of antibiotic resistance. In addition to our study, the multiple antibiotic resistance has been reported by Spînu et al. [49], Rangel and Marin [50], Maidhof et al. [51], Mora et al. [52], and Lira et al. [53]. In total the finding which is common between our study and previous researches [54–56] is the high resistance of STEC strains isolated from milk

Table 9: Antibiotic resistance properties in STEC serogroups isolated from bovine mastitis (disk diffusion method).

STES Serogroups	P10*	TE30	S10	C30	SXT	GM10	NFX5	L2	CF30	CIP5	TMP5	F/M300	AM10
O157 (11)	11	9	6	4	8	2	4	5	1	2	3	1	6
O26 (15)	15	11	10	6	4	2	3	10	—	1	5	1	8
O103 (3)	3	3	1	1	2	1	—	2	—	—	2	1	2
O111 (-)	—	—	—	—	—	—	—	—	—	—	—	—	—
O145 (3)	3	—	1	1	1	—	—	1	—	—	1	—	—
O45 (2)	2	1	1	2	—	—	1	—	1	—	—	—	1
O91 (6)	6	—	3	1	2	1	2	4	—	1	1	1	3
O113 (3)	3	1	—	1	—	2	—	2	—	—	2	—	1
O121 (2)	2	1	—	1	1	—	—	1	1	—	—	1	1
O128 (2)	2	1	1	1	1	—	1	1	—	1	1	—	—
Total (47)	47 (100)	27 (57.44)	23 (48.93)	18 (38.29)	19 (40.42)	8 (17.02)	11 (23.40)	26 (55.31)	3 (6.38)	5 (10.63)	15 (31.91)	5 (10.63)	22 (46.80)

*In this table, P10: penicillin (10 u/disk); TE30: tetracycline (30 μg/disk); S10: streptomycin (10 μg/disk); C30: chloramphenicol (30 μg/disk); SXT: sulfamethoxazole (25 μg/disk); GM10: gentamycin (10 μg/disk); NFX5: enrofloxacin (5 μg/disk); L2: lincomycin (2 μg/disk); CF30: cephalothin (30 μg/disk); CIP5: ciprofloxacin (5 μg/disk); TMP5: trimethoprim (5 μg/disk); F/M300: nitrofurantoin (300 μg/disk); AM10: ampicillin (10 u/disk).

to tetracycline. Therefore, in these situation not only in our country (Iran), nut also all around the world, prescription of tetracycline and penicillin is not effective for the cases of coliforms bovine mastitis.

On the other hand, in the current situation in Iran, the use of cephalothin, ciprofloxacin, and nitrofurantoin, due to low antibiotic resistance, can be more effective for treatment of diseases caused by *E. coli*. This survey indicated the highest antimicrobial resistance in O26 and O157 serogroups. Totally *E. coli* antibiotic resistance against common antibiotics which are used in veterinary in Iran was so high.

We recommended (i) vaccination of dairy animals (if necessary), observe hygiene in animal's platform, improving methods of milking, checking milking halls in order to detect *E. coli* especially in the animal feces monthly, fumigating milking halls frequently, observing hygiene during milking for prevent *E.coli* mastitis; (ii) using PCR method as an accurate, safe, and fast diagnostic one for accurate detection of pathogens in mastitic milks; (iii) using simple disk diffusion method in order to evaluate the antibiotic resistance of pathogens in mastitis cases; (iv) due to antibiotic resistance especially in *E. coli*, the veterinarians should pay more attention to prescribing the antibiotics; (v) in order to prevent antibiotic resistance in bacteria, we should apply antibiotics more cautiously in animals, detect resistance genes, and finally use different antibiotics periodically. Our results recommended the use of PCR for detection of antibiotic resistance genes of bacteria as a safe, rapid, and accurate method in laboratories.

Acknowledgments

The authors would like to thank Dr. E. Tajbakhsh, Mr. M. Momeni, and Dr. M. H. Fazeli at the Biotechnology Research Center and Large Animal Clinic of the Islamic Azad University of Shahrekord for their important technical and clinical support.

References

[1] M. H. Salwa, M. A. Ammar, R. A. Aisha et al., "Molecular and virulence characterization of *Escherichia coli*strains isolated from persistent bovine mastitis," *Journal of American Science*, vol. 7, pp. 614–624, 2011.

[2] Y. Ma, C. Ryan, D. M. Barbano, D. M. Galton, M. A. Rudan, and K. J. Boor, "Effects of somatic cell count on quality and shelf-life of pasteurized fluid milk," *Journal of Dairy Science*, vol. 83, no. 2, pp. 264–274, 2000.

[3] J. R. Wenz, G. M. Barrington, F. B. Garry, R. P. Dinsmore, and R. J. Callan, "Use of systemic disease signs to assess disease severity in dairy cows with acute coliform mastitis," *Journal of the American Veterinary Medical Association*, vol. 218, no. 4, pp. 567–572, 2001.

[4] Food and Agriculture Organization Statistics (FAO Statistics), Annual Agricultural Data, 2007.

[5] I. Holko, T. Bisova, Z. Holkova, and V. Kmet, "Virulence markers of *Escherichia coli* strains isolated from traditional cheeses made from unpasteurised sheep milk in Slovakia," *Food Control*, vol. 17, no. 5, pp. 393–396, 2006.

[6] H. Karch, P. I. Tarr, and M. Bielaszewska, "Enterohaemorrhagic *Escherichia coli* in human medicine," *International Journal of Medical Microbiology*, vol. 295, no. 6-7, pp. 405–418, 2005.

[7] N. Solomakos, A. Govaris, A. S. Angelidis et al., "Occurrence, virulence genes and antibiotic resistance of *Escherichia coli* O157 isolated from raw bovine, caprine and ovine milk in Greece," *Food Microbiology*, vol. 26, no. 8, pp. 865–871, 2009.

[8] Q. Wang, X. Ruan, D. Wei et al., "Development of a serogroup-specific multiplex PCR assay to detect a set of *Escherichia coli* serogroups based on the identification of their O-antigen gene clusters," *Molecular and Cellular Probes*, vol. 24, no. 5, pp. 286–290, 2010.

[9] L. Güler and K. Gündüz, "Virulence properties of *Escherichia coli* isolated from clinical bovine mastitis," *Turkish Journal of Veterinary and Animal Sciences*, vol. 31, no. 5, pp. 361–365, 2007.

[10] D. Kobori, E. C. Rigobelo, C. Macedo, J. M. Marin, and F. A. Avila, "Virulence properties of Shiga toxin-producing *Escherichia coli* isolated from cases of bovine mastitis in Brazil," *Revue d'Elevage et de Medecine Veterinaire des pays Tropicaux*, vol. 57, pp. 15–20, 2004.

[11] J. R. Wenz, G. M. Barrington, F. B. Garry, R. P. Ellis, and R. J. Magnuson, "Escherichia coli isolates' serotypes, genotypes, and virulence genes and clinical coliform mastitis severity," *Journal of Dairy Science*, vol. 89, no. 9, pp. 3408–3412, 2006.

[12] J. C. Paton and A. W. Paton, "Pathogenesis and diagnosis of Shiga toxin-producing *Escherichia coli* infections," *Clinical Microbiology Reviews*, vol. 11, no. 3, pp. 450–479, 1998.

[13] L. H. Wieler, E. Vieler, C. Erpenstein et al., "Shiga toxin-producing *Escherichia coli* strains from bovines: association of adhesion with carriage of *eae* and other genes," *Journal of Clinical Microbiology*, vol. 34, no. 12, pp. 2980–2984, 1996.

[14] T. Lehtolainen, T. Pohjanvirta, S. Pyörälä, and S. Pelkonen, "Association between virulence factors and clinical course of *Escherichia coli* mastitis," *Acta Veterinaria Scandinavica*, vol. 44, no. 3-4, pp. 203–205, 2003.

[15] V. Srinivasan, B. E. Gillespie, M. J. Lewis et al., "Phenotypic and genotypic antimicrobial resistance patterns of *Escherichia coli* isolated from dairy cows with mastitis," *Veterinary Microbiology*, vol. 124, no. 3-4, pp. 319–328, 2007.

[16] L. Suojala, T. Pohjanvirta, H. Simojoki et al., "Phylogeny, virulence factors and antimicrobial susceptibility of *Escherichia coli* isolated in clinical bovine mastitis," *Veterinary Microbiology*, vol. 147, no. 3-4, pp. 383–388, 2011.

[17] S. M. Franck, B. T. Bosworth, and H. W. Moon, "Multiplex PCR for enterotoxigenic, attaching and effacing, and shiga toxin-producing *Escherichia coli* strains from calves," *Journal of Clinical Microbiology*, vol. 36, no. 6, pp. 1795–1797, 1998.

[18] U. Reischl, M. T. Youssef, J. Kilwinski et al., "Real-time fluorescence PCR assays for detection and characterization of Shiga toxin, intimin, and enterohemolysin genes from Shiga toxin-producing *Escherichia coli*," *Journal of Clinical Microbiology*, vol. 40, no. 7, pp. 2555–2565, 2002.

[19] Clinical and Laboratory Standards Institute (CLSI), *Performance Standards for Antimicrobial Disk Susceptibility Tests, Approved Standard-Ninth Edition (M2-A9)*, Clinical and Laboratory Standards Institute, Wayne, Pa, USA, 2006.

[20] M. J. Brian, M. Frosolono, B. E. Murray et al., "Polymerase chain reaction for diagnosis of enterohemorrhagic *Escherichia coli* infection and hemolytic-uremic syndrome," *Journal of Clinical Microbiology*, vol. 30, no. 7, pp. 1801–1806, 1992.

[21] A. E. Heuvelink, N. C. A. J. van de Kar, J. F. G. M. Meis, L. A. H. Monnens, and W. J. G. Melchers, "Characterization of verocytotoxin-producing *Escherichia coli* O157 isolates from patients with haemolytic uraemic syndrome in Western Europe," *Epidemiology and Infection*, vol. 115, no. 1, pp. 1–14, 1995.

[22] M. Idress, U. Mussarat, Y. Badshah, R. Qamar, and H. Bokhari, "Virulence factors profile of drug-resistant *Escherichia coli* isolates from urinary tract infections in Punjab, Pakistan," *European Journal of Clinical Microbiology and Infectious Diseases*, vol. 29, no. 12, pp. 1533–1537, 2010.

[23] B. Possé, L. de Zutter, M. Heyndrickx, and L. Herman, "Metabolic and genetic profiling of clinical O157 and non-O157 Shiga-toxin-producing *Escherichia coli*," *Research in Microbiology*, vol. 158, no. 7, pp. 591–599, 2007.

[24] C. DebRoy, P. M. Fratamico, E. Roberts, M. A. Davis, and Y. Liu, "Development of PCR assays targeting genes in O-antigen gene clusters for detection and identification of *Escherichia coli* O45 and O55 serogroups," *Applied and Environmental Microbiology*, vol. 71, no. 8, pp. 4919–4924, 2005.

[25] S. Perelle, F. Dilasser, J. Grout, and P. Fach, "Identification of the O-antigen biosynthesis genes of *Escherichia coli* O91 and development of a O91 PCR serotyping test," *Journal of Applied Microbiology*, vol. 93, no. 5, pp. 758–764, 2002.

[26] C. DebRoy, E. Roberts, J. Kundrat, M. A. Davis, C. E. Briggs, and P. M. Fratamico, "Detection of *Escherichia coli* serogroups O26 and O113 by PCR amplification of the wzx and wzy genes," *Applied and Environmental Microbiology*, vol. 70, no. 3, pp. 1830–1832, 2004.

[27] P. M. Fratamico, C. E. Briggs, D. Needle, C. Y. Chen, and C. DebRoy, "Sequence of the *Escherichia coli* O121 O-antigen gene cluster and detection of enterohemorrhagic *E. coli* O121 by PCR amplification of the wzx and wzy genes," *Journal of Clinical Microbiology*, vol. 41, no. 7, pp. 3379–3383, 2003.

[28] J. Shao, M. Li, Q. Jia, Y. Lu, and P. G. Wang, "Sequence of *Escherichia coli* O128 antigen biosynthesis cluster and functional identification of an α-1,2-fucosyltransferase," *FEBS Letters*, vol. 553, no. 1-2, pp. 99–103, 2003.

[29] L. P. Randall, S. W. Cooles, M. K. Osborn, L. J. V. Piddock, and M. J. Woodward, "Antibiotic resistance genes, integrons and multiple antibiotic resistance in thirty-five serotypes of *Salmonella enterica* isolated from humans and animals in the UK," *Journal of Antimicrobial Chemotherapy*, vol. 53, no. 2, pp. 208–216, 2004.

[30] C. S. Toro, M. Farfán, I. Contreras et al., "Genetic analysis of antibiotic-resistance determinants in multidrug-resistant Shigella strains isolated from Chilean children," *Epidemiology and Infection*, vol. 133, no. 1, pp. 81–86, 2005.

[31] H. Mammeri, M. van de Loo, L. Poirel, L. Martinez-Martinez, and P. Nordmann, "Emergence of plasmid-mediated quinolone resistance in *Escherichia coli* in Europe," *Antimicrobial Agents and Chemotherapy*, vol. 49, no. 1, pp. 71–76, 2005.

[32] T. T. H. Van, J. Chin, T. Chapman, L. T. Tran, and P. J. Coloe, "Safety of raw meat and shellfish in Vietnam: an analysis of *Escherichia coli* isolations for antibiotic resistance and virulence genes," *International Journal of Food Microbiology*, vol. 124, no. 3, pp. 217–223, 2008.

[33] European Food Safety Authority (EFSA), "The community summary report on trends and sources of zoonoses, zoonotic agents, antimicrobial resistance and foodborne outbreaks in the European Union in 2006," *EFSA Journal*, vol. 130, pp. 1–352, 2007.

[34] I. A. Gillespie, S. J. O'Brien, G. K. Adak, T. Cheasty, and G. Willshaw, "Foodborne general outbreaks of Shiga toxin-producing *Escherichia coli* O157 in England and Wales 1992–2002: where are the risks?" *Epidemiology and Infection*, vol. 133, no. 5, pp. 803–808, 2005.

[35] H. S. Hussein and T. Sakuma, "Invited review: prevalence of Shiga toxin-producing *Escherichia coli* in dairy cattle and their products," *Journal of Dairy Science*, vol. 88, no. 2, pp. 450–465, 2005.

[36] R. Stephan, S. Schumacher, S. Corti, G. Krause, J. Danuser, and L. Beutin, "Prevalence and characteristics of Shiga toxin-producing *Escherichia coli* in Swiss raw milk cheeses collected at producer level," *Journal of Dairy Science*, vol. 91, no. 7, pp. 2561–2565, 2008.

[37] W. Suriyasathaporn, C. Heuer, E. N. Noordhuizen-Stassen, and Y. H. Schukken, "Hyperketonemia and the impairment of udder defense: a review," *Veterinary Research*, vol. 31, no. 4, pp. 397–412, 2000.

[38] A. Diez-Fraile, E. Meyer, and C. Burvenich, "Sympathoadrenal and immune system activation during the periparturient period and their association with bovine coliform mastitis. A review," *Veterinary Quarterly*, vol. 25, no. 1, pp. 31–44, 2003.

[39] K. M. Osman, A. M. Mustafa, M. A. K. Aly, and G. S. AbdEl-hamed, "Serotypes, virulence genes, and intimin types of Shiga toxin-producing *Escherichia coli* and enteropathogenic *Escherichia coli* isolated from mastitic milk relevant to human health in Egypt," *Vector-Borne and Zoonotic Diseases*, vol. 12, no. 4, pp. 297–305, 2012.

[40] A. Bean, J. Williamson, and R. T. Cursons, "Virulence genes of *Escherichia coli* strains isolated from mastitic milk," *Journal of Veterinary Medicine Series B*, vol. 51, no. 6, pp. 285–287, 2004.

[41] I. M. Moussa, M. H. Ashgan, H. A. Alwathnani, K. F. Mohamed, and A. A. Al-Doss, "Multiplex polymerase chain reaction for detection and characterization of shiga toxigenic *Escherichia coli* (STEC)," *African Journal of Biotechnology*, vol. 9, no. 28, pp. 4356–4363, 2010.

[42] H. Momtaz, "Investigation of virulence factors in *Escherichia coli*isolated from clinical and subclinical bovine mastitis," *Bulgarian Journal of Veterinary Medicine*, vol. 13, pp. 122–126, 2010.

[43] K. de Verdier, A. Nyman, C. Greko, and B. Bengtsson, "Antimicrobial resistance and virulence factors in *Escherichia coli* from swedish dairy calves," *Acta Veterinaria Scandinavica*, vol. 54, no. 1, article 2, 2012.

[44] T. Lehtolainen, A. Shwimmer, N. Y. Shpigel, T. Honkanen-Buzalski, and S. Pyörälä, "In vitro antimicrobial susceptibility of *Escherichia coli* isolates from clinical bovine mastitis in Finland and Israel," *Journal of Dairy Science*, vol. 86, no. 12, pp. 3927–3932, 2003.

[45] H. Langoni, W. N. de Araújo, A. V. da Silva, and L. C. de Souza, "Tratamento da mastite bovina com amoxicilina e enrofloxacina bem como com a sua associação," *Área de Zoonoses e Saúde Pública*, vol. 67, pp. 177–180, 2000.

[46] R. J. Erskine, R. D. Walker, C. A. Bolin, P. C. Bartlett, and D. G. White, "Trends in antibacterial susceptibility of mastitis pathogens during a seven-year period," *Journal of Dairy Science*, vol. 85, no. 5, pp. 1111–1118, 2002.

[47] J. A. Makovec and P. L. Ruegg, "Antimicrobial resistance of bacteria isolated from dairy cow milk samples submitted for bacterial culture: 8,905 samples (1994–2001)," *Journal of the American Veterinary Medical Association*, vol. 222, no. 11, pp. 1582–1589, 2003.

[48] M. Roesch, V. Perreten, M. G. Doherr, W. Schaeren, M. Schällibaum, and J. W. Blum, "Comparison of antibiotic resistance of udder pathogens in dairy cows kept on organic and on conventional farms," *Journal of Dairy Science*, vol. 89, no. 3, pp. 989–997, 2006.

[49] M. Spînu, L. Köbölkúti, D. Cadar et al., "Changes in antibiotic resistance indices of animal *Escherichia coli*strains with number of isolate," *Annals of the Romanian Society for Cell Biology*, vol. 17, pp. 361–366, 2012.

[50] P. Rangel and J. M. Marin, "Analysis of *Escherichia coli* isolated from bovine mastitic milk," *Pesquisa Veterinaria Brasileira*, vol. 29, no. 5, pp. 363–368, 2009.

[51] H. Maidhof, B. Guerra, S. Abbas, H. M. Elsheikha, T. S. Whittam, and L. Beutin, "A multiresistant clone of Shiga toxin-producing *Escherichia coli* O118:[H16] is spread in cattle and humans over different European countries," *Applied and Environmental Microbiology*, vol. 68, no. 12, pp. 5834–5842, 2002.

[52] A. Mora, J. E. Blanco, M. Blanco et al., "Antimicrobial resistance of Shiga toxin (verotoxin)-producing *Escherichia coli* O157:H7 and non-O157 strains isolated from humans, cattle, sheep and food in Spain," *Research in Microbiology*, vol. 156, no. 7, pp. 793–806, 2005.

[53] W. M. Lira, C. Macedo, and J. M. Marin, "The incidence of Shiga toxin-producing *Escherichia coli* in cattle with mastitis in Brazil," *Journal of Applied Microbiology*, vol. 97, no. 4, pp. 861–866, 2004.

[54] E. Rahimi, S. S. Chaleshtori, and P. Parsaei, "Prevalence and antimicrobial resistance of *Escherichia coli* o157 isolated from traditional cheese, ice cream and yoghurt in Iran," *African Journal of Microbiology Research*, vol. 5, no. 22, pp. 3706–3710, 2011.

[55] C. M. Schroeder, C. Zhao, C. DebRoy et al., "Antimicrobial resistance of *Escherichia coli* O157 isolated from humans, cattle, swine, and food," *Applied and Environmental Microbiology*, vol. 68, no. 2, pp. 576–581, 2002.

[56] A. Skočková, S. Cupáková, R. Karpíšková, and B. Janštová, "Detection of tetracycline resistance genes in *Escherichia coli* from raw cow's milk," *Journal of Microbiology, Biotechnology and Food Sciences*, vol. 1, pp. 777–784, 2012.

Permissions

The contributors of this book come from diverse backgrounds, making this book a truly international effort. This book will bring forth new frontiers with its revolutionizing research information and detailed analysis of the nascent developments around the world.

We would like to thank all the contributing authors for lending their expertise to make the book truly unique. They have played a crucial role in the development of this book. Without their invaluable contributions this book wouldn't have been possible. They have made vital efforts to compile up to date information on the varied aspects of this subject to make this book a valuable addition to the collection of many professionals and students.

This book was conceptualized with the vision of imparting up-to-date information and advanced data in this field. To ensure the same, a matchless editorial board was set up. Every individual on the board went through rigorous rounds of assessment to prove their worth. After which they invested a large part of their time researching and compiling the most relevant data for our readers. Conferences and sessions were held from time to time between the editorial board and the contributing authors to present the data in the most comprehensible form. The editorial team has worked tirelessly to provide valuable and valid information to help people across the globe.

Every chapter published in this book has been scrutinized by our experts. Their significance has been extensively debated. The topics covered herein carry significant findings which will fuel the growth of the discipline. They may even be implemented as practical applications or may be referred to as a beginning point for another development. Chapters in this book were first published by Hindawi Publishing Corporation; hereby published with permission under the Creative Commons Attribution License or equivalent.

The editorial board has been involved in producing this book since its inception. They have spent rigorous hours researching and exploring the diverse topics which have resulted in the successful publishing of this book. They have passed on their knowledge of decades through this book. To expedite this challenging task, the publisher supported the team at every step. A small team of assistant editors was also appointed to further simplify the editing procedure and attain best results for the readers.

Our editorial team has been hand-picked from every corner of the world. Their multi-ethnicity adds dynamic inputs to the discussions which result in innovative outcomes. These outcomes are then further discussed with the researchers and contributors who give their valuable feedback and opinion regarding the same. The feedback is then collaborated with the researches and they are edited in a comprehensive manner to aid the understanding of the subject.

Apart from the editorial board, the designing team has also invested a significant amount of their time in understanding the subject and creating the most relevant covers. They scrutinized every image to scout for the most suitable representation of the subject and create an appropriate cover for the book.

The publishing team has been involved in this book since its early stages. They were actively engaged in every process, be it collecting the data, connecting with the contributors or procuring relevant information. The team has been an ardent support to the editorial, designing and production team. Their endless efforts to recruit the best for this project, has resulted in the accomplishment of this book. They are a veteran in the field of academics and their pool of knowledge is as vast as their experience in printing. Their expertise and guidance has proved useful at every step. Their uncompromising quality standards have made this book an exceptional effort. Their encouragement from time to time has been an inspiration for everyone.

The publisher and the editorial board hope that this book will prove to be a valuable piece of knowledge for researchers, students, practitioners and scholars across the globe.

List of Contributors

Adriano Savoia Morales, Juliana Fragoso de Araujo, Vasco Tulio de Moura Gomes, Thais Sebastiana Porfida Ferreira, Pedro Henrique Nogueira de Lima Filsner, Maria Roberta Felizardo and Andrea Micke Moreno
Laboratorio de Sanidade Suına e Virologia, Faculdade de Medicina Veterinaria e Zootecnia (FMVZ), Universidade de Sao Paulo (USP), 05508 270 Sao Paulo, SP, Brazil

Adrienny Trindade Reis Costa
Instituto de Pesquisas Veterinarias Especializadas-IPEVE, Rua Esmeralda, 786, 304111-191 Belo Horizonte, MG, Brazil

Dalia dos Prazeres Rodrigues
Laboratorio de Enterobacterias, FIOCRUZ, Avenida Brasil, 4365, Pavilhao Rocha Lima, 3 andar, Manguinhos, 21040-360 Rio de Janeiro, RJ, Brazil

Expedito K. A. Camboim, Arthur P. Almeida, Felıcio G. Junior, Marcia A. Melo and Franklin Riet-Correa
Unidade Academica de Medicina Veterinaria, Universidade Federal de Campina Grande, 58708 Patos, PB, Brazil

Michelle Z. Tadra-Sfeir
Laboratorio de Fixacao Biologica de Nitrogenio, Departamento de Bioquımica e Biologia Molecular, Universidade Federal do Parana, 80060 Curitiba, PR, Brazil

Paulo P. Andrade
Departamento de Genetica, Universidade Federal de Pernambuco, 50670 Recife, PE, Brazil

Chris S. McSweeney
CSIRO Livestock Industries, Queensland Bioscience Precinct, St Lucia, QLD 4067, Australia

Mari Vainionpaa, Marja Raekallio, Marjatta Snellman and Outi Vainio
Department of Equine and Small Animal Medicine, Pharmacology and Toxicology, Faculty of Veterinary Medicine, University of Helsinki, Koetilantie 7, 00014 Helsinki, Finland

Esa-Pekka Tienhaara
Kosonkuja 3, 04370 Rusutjarvi, Finland

Jouni Junnila
4Pharma Ltd, 02130 Espoo, Finland

Bozena Dworecka-Kaszak, Alicja Krutkiewicz and Malgorzata Bieganska
Mycology Division, Preclinical Science Department, Faculty of Veterinary Medicine, Warsaw University of Life Sciences, Ciszewskiego 8, 02-789 Warsaw, Poland

Daniel Szopa
Molecular Genetic Division, Mother and Child institute, Kasprzaka 17a, 01-211 Warsaw, Poland

Miroslaw Kleczkowski
Division of Laboratory Diagnostics, Department of Pathology and Veterinary Diagnostics, Faculty of Veterinary Medicine, Warsaw University of Life Sciences, Nowoursynowska 159, 02-776 Warsaw, Poland

Andrea Zatelli, Marco Pierantozzi and Paola D'Ippolito
Clinica Veterinaria Pirani, Nephrology and Urology Division, Via Majakowski 2/L, M, N, 42124 Reggio Emilia, Italy

Mauro Bigliati
Istituto Farmaceutico Candioli, Via Manzoni 2, 10192 Beinasco, Italy

Eric Zini
Istituto Veterinario di Novara, S.P. 9, 28060 Granozzo con Monticello, Italy
Department of Veterinary Clinical Sciences, University of Padua, 35020 Agripolis, Legnaro, Italy

Rahil Farzan
Young Researchers Club, Islamic Azad University, Shahrekord Branch, Shahrekord 166, Iran

Ebrahim Rahimi
Department of Food Hygiene, College of Veterinary Medicine, Islamic Azad University, Shahrekord Branch, Shahrekord 166, Iran

Negar Souod
Young Researchers Club, Islamic Azad University, Jahrom Branch, Jahrom 74135-355, Iran

Bruna Rocha Passos Barbosa, Nara Thiers Cacciatori Galleti Bernardes, Laila Andreia Rodrigues Beserra and Fábio Gregori
Department of Preventive Veterinary Medicine and Animal Health, Faculty of Veterinary Medicine, University of Sao Paulo, Avenida Prof. Dr. Orlando Marques de Paiva 87, Cidade Universitaria, 05508-270 Sao Paulo, SD, Brazil

A. Nikkhah, F. Amiri and H. Amanloo
Department of Animal Sciences, Faculty of Agricultural Sciences, University of Zanjan, Zanjan 313-45195, Iran

Germana Beha, Giuseppe Sarli, Barbara Brunetti, Domenico Ferrara and Cinzia Benazzi
Department of Veterinary Medical Science, University of Bologna, 40064 Ozzano Emilia, Italy

Francesco Sassi
Institute for Cancer Research and Treatment (IRCC), Fourth Floor, 10060 Candiolo, Italy

Robert Klopfleisch and Achim D. Gruber
Institut fur Tierpathologie, Universitat Berlin, Robert-von-Ostertag-Strasse 15, 14163 Berlin, Germany

M. Mahouachi
Ecole Superieure d'Agriculture du Kef, Le Kef 7119, Tunisia

N. Atti
INRA-Tunisie, Laboratoire des Productions Animales et Fourrageres, Rue Hedi Karray, Ariana 2080, Tunisia

H. Hajji
INRA-Tunisie, Laboratoire des Productions Animales et Fourrageres, Rue Hedi Karray, Ariana 2080, Tunisia
Institut National Agronomique de Tunis, Tunis 2019, Tunisia

Nurcan Donmez and I. Kısadere
Department of Physiology, Faculty of Veterinary Medicine, University of Kyrgyzstan-Turkey Manas, Bishkek 720044, Kyrgyzstan

H. H. Donmez
Department of Histology and Embryology, Faculty of Veterinary Medicine, University of Kyrgyzstan-Turkey Manas, Bishkek 720044, Kyrgyzstan

E. Keskin
Department of Physiology, Faculty of Veterinary Medicine, Selcuk University, 42075 Konya, Turkey

Huda Yahia Hamid
Department of Anatomy, Faculty of Veterinary Medicine, University of Khartoum, Khartoum 13314, Sudan
Department of Veterinary Preclinical Sciences, Faculty of Veterinary Medicine, Universiti Putra Malaysia, Selangor, 43400 Serdang, Malaysia

Md Zuki Abu Bakar Zakaria and Goh Yong Meng
Department of Veterinary Preclinical Sciences, Faculty of Veterinary Medicine, Universiti Putra Malaysia, Selangor, 43400 Serdang, Malaysia

Abd. Wahid Haron
Department of Veterinary Clinical Studies, Faculty of Veterinary Medicine, Universiti Putra Malaysia, Selangor, 43400 Serdang, Malaysia

Noordin Mohamed Mustapha
Department of Veterinary Pathology & Microbiology, Faculty of Veterinary Medicine, Universiti Putra Malaysia, Selangor, 43400 Serdang, Malaysia

Keijiro Mizukami, Akira Yabuki, Hye-Sook Chang and Osamu Yamato
Laboratory of Clinical Pathology, Department of Veterinary Medicine, Kagoshima University, 1-21-24 Korimoto, Kagoshima, Kagoshima 890-0065, Japan

Takuji Kawamichi
Japan Border Collie Health Network, 1-14-8 Manabigaoka, Tarumi-ku, Hyogo, Kobe 655-0004, Japan

Hiroshi Koie
Department of Veterinary Medicine, College of Bioresource Sciences, Nihon University, 1866 Kameino, Kanagawa, Fujisawa 252-0880, Japan

Shinji Tamura
Tamura Animal Clinic, 7-16 Yoshimien, Saeki-ku, Hiroshima, Hiroshima 731-5132, Japan

Satoru Matsunaga
Japan Animal Referral Medical Center, 2-5-8 Kuji, Takatsu-ku, Kanagawa, Kawasaki 213-0032, Japan

Shigeki Imamoto
Shinjo Animal Hospital, 104-1 Katsuragi, Nara, Katsuragi 639-2144, Japan

Miyoko Saito
Laboratory of Veterinary Surgery II, School of Veterinary Medicine, Azabu University, 1-17-71 Fuchinobe, Kanagawa, Sagamihara 229-8501, Japan

Daisuke Hasegawa
Department of Veterinary Science, Nippon Veterinary and Life Science University, 1-7-1 Kyounan-chou, Tokyo, Musashino 180-8602, Japan

Naoaki Matsuki and Satoshi Tamahara
Department of Veterinary Clinical Pathobiology, Graduate School of Agricultural and Life Sciences, The University of Tokyo, 1-1-1 Yayoi, Tokyo, Bunkyo-ku 113-8657, Japan

Shigenobu Sato
Sato Animal Hospital, 6-38-20 Goinishi, Chiba, Ichihara 290-0038, Japan

Byung-suk Jeon and Byung-IL Yoon
Laboratory of Histology and Molecular Pathogenesis, College of Veterinary Medicine and Institute of Veterinary Science, Kangwon National University, Chuncheon, 200-701, Republic of Korea

Zahra Boroomand and Keramat Asasi
Poultry Research Center, School of Veterinary Medicine, Shiraz University, Shiraz, Iran

Ali Mohammadi
Department of Pathobiology, School of Veterinary Medicine, Shiraz University, Shiraz, Iran

Fatma Colakoglu and Hasan Huseyin Donmez
Department of Histology and Embryology, Faculty of Veterinary Medicine, Selcuk University, 42075 Konya, Turkey

A. Kavaguchi De Grandis, C. Boulocher, E. Viguier, T. Roger and S. Sawaya
Universite de Lyon et Vet Agro Sup, Campus Veterinaire de Lyon, UPSP ICE, 69280 Marcy l'Etoile, France

Guilherme Augusto Marietto-Goncalves and Raphael Lucio Andreatti Filho
Laboratory of Avian Pathology, School of Veterinary Medicine and Animal Science, Universidade Estadual Paulista (UNESP), 18618-970 Botucatu, SP, Brazil

Fabrizio Grandi
Department of Pathology, Botucatu Medical School, Universidade Estadual Paulista (UNESP), 18618-970 Botucatu, SP, Brazil
Laboratory of Investigative and Comparative Pathology, School of Veterinary Medicine and Animal Science, Universidade Estadual Paulista (UNESP), 18618-970 Botucatu, SP, Brazil

K. Rypula and M. Porowski
Division of Infectious Diseases and Veterinary Administration, Department of Epizootiology with Clinic of Birds and Exotic Animals, Faculty of Veterinary Medicine, Wrocław University of Environmental and Life Sciences, Grunwaldzki Square 45, 50-366 Wrocław, Poland

J. Kaba
Division of Infectious Diseases and Epidemiology, Department of Large Animal Diseases, Faculty of Veterinary Medicine, Warsaw University of Life Sciences—SGGW, Nowoursynowska 159c, 02-776 Warsaw, Poland

M. Gorczykowski
Divison of Parasitology, Department of Internal Diseases with Clinic of Horses, Dogs and Cats, Faculty of Veterinary Medicine, Agricultural University of Wrocław, Poland

A. Deniz
Bayer HealthCare Animal Health, Leverkusen, Germany

Afshin Raoofi
Department of Clinical Sciences, Faculty of Veterinary Medicine, University of Tehran, P.O. Box 14155-6453, Tehran, Iran

Alireza Rahmani Shahraki
Club of Young Researchers, Islamic Azad University, Shahrekord Branch, P.O. Box 166, Shahrekord, Iran

Abdolrasool Namjoo
Department of Clinical Sciences, Faculty of Veterinary Medicine, Islamic Azad University, Shahrekord Branch, P.O. Box 166, Shahrekord, Iran

Hasan Momtaz
Department of Microbiology, Faculty of Veterinary Medicine, Islamic Azad University, Shahrekord Branch, P.O. Box 166, Shahrekord, Iran

Paula Fajardo, Lorenzo Pastrana, Isabel Rodrıguez, Clara Fucinos and Nelson P. Guerra
Departamento de Quımica Analıtica y Alimentaria, Facultade de Ciencias de Ourense, Universidade de Vigo, As Lagoas s/n, 32004 Ourense, Spain

Jesus Mendez
Cooperativas Orensanas Sociedad Cooperativa Ltda (COREN), Polıgono San Ciprian de Vinas, 32901 Ourense, Spain

Salisu Buhari
Department of Veterinary Clinical Studies, Faculty of Veterinary Medicine, Universiti Putra Malaysia, 43400 Serdang, Selangor, Malaysia
Department of Veterinary Surgery & Radiology, Faculty of Veterinary Medicine, Usmanu Danfodiyo University Sokoto, PMB Sokoto, Nigeria

Kalthum Hashim
Department of Veterinary Clinical Studies, Faculty of Veterinary Medicine, Universiti Putra Malaysia, 43400 Serdang, Selangor, Malaysia

Goh Yong Meng
Department of Veterinary Preclinical Studies, Faculty of Veterinary Medicine, Universiti Putra Malaysia, 43400 Serdang, Selangor, Malaysia

Noordin Mohamed Mustapha
Department of Veterinary Pathology and Microbiology, Faculty of Veterinary Medicine, Universiti Putra Malaysia, 43400 Serdang, Selangor, Malaysia

Siew Hua Gan
Human Genome Centre, School of Medical Sciences, Universiti Sains Malaysia, Kelantan, 16150 Kubang Kerian, Malaysia

Y. C. Wang and J. L. Deng
College of Veterinary Medicine, Sichuan Agricultural University, Yaan, Sichuan 625014, China

S. W. Xu
Department of Veterinary Medicine, Northeast Agricultural University, Harbin 150030, China

X. Peng and H. M. Cui
Sichuan Key Laboratory of Animal Disease and Human Health, Yaan, Sichuan 625014, China

Z. C. Zuo, Y. Wang and Z. H. Ren
Sichuan Key Laboratory of Environmental Hazards Disease, Yaan, Sichuan 625014, China

Aline S. Hora, Karen M. Asano, Leonardo J. Richtzenhain and Paulo E. Brandão
Department of Preventive Veterinary Medicine and Animal Health, College of Veterinary Medicine, University of Sao Paulo, Avenida Professor Dr. Orlando Marques de Paiva 87, Cidade Universitaria, 05508-270 Sao Paulo, SP, Brazil
Coronavirus Research Group, College of Veterinary Medicine, University of Sao Paulo, Avenida Professor Dr. Orlando Marques de Paiva 87, Cidade Universitaria, 05508-270 Sao Paulo, SP, Brazil

Juliana M. Guerra, Ramon G. Mesquita and Paulo Maiorka
Department of Pathology, College of Veterinary Medicine, University of Sao Paulo, Avenida Professor Dr. Orlando Marques de Paiva 87, Cidade Universitaria, 05508-270 Sao Paulo, SP, Brazil

Cristina Roman Amigo, Debora Dirani Sena de Gobbi, Vasco Tulio de Moura Gomes, Pedro Henrique Nogueira de Lima Filsner, Barbara Letıcia Pereira Costa, Maria Garcia Spindola, Thais Sebastiana Porfida Ferreira, Paulo Eduardo Brandao and Andrea Micke Moreno
Departamento de Medicina Veterinaria Preventiva e Saude Animal, Faculdade de Medicina Veterinaria e Zootecnia (FMVZ), Universidade de Sao Paulo (USP), Avenida Professor Dr. Orlando Marques de Paiva 87 Cidade Universitaria, 05508 270 Sao Paulo, SP, Brazil

Danilo do Prado Perina
Departamento de Zootecnia, Escola Superior de Agricultura "Luiz de Queiroz" (ESALQ), Universidade de Sao Paulo (USP), Avenida Padua Dias 11, Agronomia, 13418-900 Piracicaba, SP, Brazil

Omer Cetin, Hilal Colak and Enver Baris Bingol
Department of Food Hygiene and Technology, Faculty of Veterinary Medicine, Istanbul University, Avcilar, 34320 Istanbul, Turkey

Hamparsun Hampikyan
The School of Vocational Studies, Beykent University, Buyukcekmece, 34500 Istanbul, Turkey

Hayat H. M. El-Nour
Department of Biology, Animal Reproduction Research Institute, El-Ahram, Giza, Egypt

Soad M. Nasr
Department of Parasitology and Animal Diseases, National Research Center, El-Behouse Street, P.O. Box 12622, Dokki, Giza, Egypt

Walid R. Hassan
Ultrasonography Unit, Animal Reproduction Research Institute, El-Ahram, Giza, Egypt

Tereza Emmanuelle de Farias Rotondano
Departamento de Ciencias Biologicas, Universidade Federal de Pernambuco, Avenue Professor Moraes Rego, s/n, Cidade Universitaria, 50.670-901 Recife, PE, Brazil

Alzira Maria Paiva de Almeida
Centro de Pesquisas Aggeu Magalhaes, FIOCRUZ-PE, Avenue Professor Moraes Rego, s/n, Cidade Universitaria, 50.670-901 Recife, PE, Brazil

Elane Maria Camboim Lustosa, Aline Antas Cordeiro, Expedito Kennedy Alves Camboim, Sergio Santos de Azevedo and Marcia Almeida de Melo
Unidade Academica de Medicina Veterinaria, Universidade Federal de Campina Grande, 58.700-970 Patos, PB, Brazil

Paulo Paes de Andrade
Departamento de Genetica, Universidade Federal de Pernambuco, Avenue Professor Moraes Rego, s/n, Cidade Universitaria, 50.670-901 Recife, PE, Brazil

Hassan Momtaz
Department of Microbiology, College of Veterinary Medicine, Islamic Azad University, Shahrekord Branch, P.O. Box 166, Shahrekord, Iran

Farhad Safarpoor Dehkordi
Young Researchers Club, Islamic Azad University, Shahrekord Branch, P.O. Box 166, Shahrekord, Iran

Taghi Taktaz
Department of Clinical Sciences, College of Veterinary Medicine, Islamic Azad University, Shahrekord Branch, P.O. Box 166, Shahrekord, Iran

Amir Rezvani and Sajad Yarali
College of Veterinary Medicine, Islamic Azad University, Shahrekord Branch, P.O. Box 166, Shahrekord, Iran

www.ingramcontent.com/pod-product-compliance
Ingram Content Group UK Ltd.
Pitfield, Milton Keynes, MK11 3LW, UK
UKHW052007051026
15624UKWH00003B/611

9 781632 412102